T0228993

Complications, Considerations, and Consequences of Colorectal Surgery

Editor

SCOTT R. STEELE

SURGICAL CLINICS
OF NORTH AMERICA

www.surgical.theclinics.com

Consulting Editor
RONALD F. MARTIN

February 2013 • Volume 93 • Number 1

ELSEVIER

1600 John F. Kennedy Blvd., Suite 1800, Philadelphia, PA 19103-2899

http://www.surgical.theclinics.com

SURGICAL CLINICS OF NORTH AMERICA Volume 93, Number 1
February 2013 ISSN 0039–6109, ISBN-13: 978-1-4557-7333-6

Editor: John Vassallo, j.vassallo@elsevier.com
Developmental Editor: Teia Stone

Surgical Clinics of North America (ISSN 0039–6109) is published bimonthly by Elsevier Inc., 360 Park Avenue South, New York, NY 10010-1710. Months of publication are February, April, June, August, October, and December. Business and Editorial Offices: 1600 John F. Kennedy Blvd., Suite 1800, Philadelphia, PA 19103-2899. Periodicals postage paid at New York, NY and additional mailing offices. Subscription prices are $339.00 per year for US individuals, $575.00 per year for US institutions, $166.00 per year for US students and residents, $415.00 per year for Canadian individuals, $714.00 per year for Canadian institutions, $468.00 for international individuals, $714.00 per year for international institutions and $229.00 per year for Canadian and foreign students/residents. To receive student/resident rate, orders must be accompanied by name of affiliated institution, date of term, and the *signature* of program/residency coordinator on institution letterhead. Orders will be billed at individual rate until proof of status is received. Foreign air speed delivery is included in all *Clinics* subscription prices. All prices are subject to change without notice. POSTMASTER: Send address changes to *Surgical Clinics*, Elsevier Health Sciences Division, Subscription Customer Service, 3251 Riverport Lane, Maryland Heights, MO 63043. **Customer Service (orders, claims, online, change of address): Telephone: 1-800-654-2452 (U.S. and Canada); 314-447-8871 (outside U.S. and Canada). Fax: 314-447-8029. E-mail: journalscustomerservice-usa@elsevier.com (for print support); journalsonline support-usa@elsevier.com (for online support).**

Reprints. For copies of 100 or more, of articles in this publication, please contact the Commercial Reprints Department, Elsevier Inc., 360 Park Avenue South, New York, New York 10010-1710. Tel. (212) 633-3812, Fax: (212) 462-1935, e-mail: reprints@elsevier.com.

The Surgical Clinics of North America is also published in Spanish by McGraw-Hill Interamericana Editores S.A., P.O. Box 5-237 06500 Mexico D.F. Mexico; and in Portuguese by Interlivros Edicoes Ltda., Rua Comandante Coelho 1085, CEP 21250, Rio de Janeiro, Brazil; and in Greek by Paschalidis Medical Publications, Athens Greece.

The Surgical Clinics of North America is covered in *MEDLINE/PubMed (Index Medicus)*, *EMBASE/Excerpta Medica*, *Current Contents/Clinical Medicine*, *Current Contents/Life Sciences*, *Science Citation Index*, and *ISI/BIOMED*.

Printed and bound by CPI Group (UK) Ltd, Croydon, CR0 4YY

Transferred to digital print 2012

Contributors

CONSULTING EDITOR

RONALD F. MARTIN, MD, FACS
Staff Surgeon, Department of Surgery, Marshfield Clinic, Marshfield, Wisconsin; Clinical Associate Professor, University of Wisconsin School of Medicine and Public Health, Madison, Wisconsin; Colonel, Medical Corps, United States Army Reserve

GUEST EDITOR

SCOTT R. STEELE, MD, FACS, FASCRS
Chief, Colon and Rectal Surgery, Madigan Army Medical Center, Fort Lewis; Clinical Associate Professor, Department of Surgery, University of Washington, Seattle, Washington

AUTHORS

ANDREA C. BAFFORD, MD, FACS
Assistant Professor of Surgery, Section of Colon and Rectal Surgery, Division of General and Oncologic Surgery, Department of Surgery, University of Maryland Medical Center, University of Maryland School of Medicine, Baltimore, Maryland

JOSHUA I.S. BLEIER, MD, FACS, FASCRS
Assistant Professor of Surgery, Division of Colon and Rectal Surgery, Department of Surgery, Hospital of the University of Pennsylvania, Philadelphia, Pennsylvania

SARAH Y. BOOSTROM, MD
Consultant; Assistant Professor of Surgery, Division of Colon and Rectal Surgery, Mayo Clinic, Rochester, Minnesota

BRAD CHAMPAGNE, MD, FACS, FASCRS
Associate Professor of Surgery, Department of Colon and Rectal Surgery, Case Western Reserve University Medical Center, Cleveland, Ohio

PAUL J. CHESTOVICH, MD
Resident in General Surgery, Department of Surgery, David Geffen School of Medicine, University of California Los Angeles, Los Angeles, California

BRADLEY DAVIS, MD, FACS, FASCRS
Associate Professor, Department of Surgery, University of Cincinnati, Cincinnati, Ohio

KURT G. DAVIS, MD, FACS, FASCRS
Associate Professor of Surgery, Uniformed Services University of the Health Sciences, Bethesda, Maryland; Chief, General Surgery; General Surgery Residency Program Director, Section of Colon and Rectal Surgery, Department of Surgery, William Beaumont Army Medical Center, Fort Bliss, Texas

ERIC J. DOZOIS, MD, FACS, FASCRS
Consultant; Professor of Surgery, Division of Colon and Rectal Surgery, Mayo Clinic, Rochester, Minnesota

DAVID A. ETZIONI, MD, MSHS, FACS
Senior Associate Consultant, Department of Surgery, Mayo Clinic Arizona; Associate Professor, Mayo Clinic College of Medicine, Phoenix, Arizona

TODD D. FRANCONE, MD, FACS, FASCRS
Assistant Professor of Surgery and Oncology, Department of Colon and Rectal Surgery, University of Rochester Medical Center, Rochester, New York

DAVID M. GOURLAY, MD, FACS
Associate Professor of Surgery, Division of Pediatric Surgery, Department of Surgery, Medical College of Wisconsin, Milwaukee, Wisconsin

JASON F. HALL, MD, MPH, FACS
Senior Surgeon, Department of Colon and Rectal Surgery, Lahey Clinic, Burlington; Assistant Professor of Surgery, Tufts University School of Medicine, Boston, Massachusetts

SAMANTHA K. HENDREN, MD, MPH, FACS
Assistant Professor, Department of Surgery, University of Michigan, Ann Arbor, Michigan

STEVEN R. HUNT, MD
Associate Professor, Section of Colon and Rectal Surgery, Department of Surgery, Washington University School of Medicine, St Louis, Missouri

JENNIFER L. IRANI, MD
Instructor in Surgery, Department of Surgery, Harvard Medical School; Associate Surgeon, Brigham and Women's Hospital, Boston, Massachusetts

ERIC K. JOHNSON, MD, FACS, FASCRS
Assistant Professor of Surgery, Uniformed Services University of the Health Sciences, Bethesda, Maryland; Section of Colon and Rectal Surgery, Department of Surgery, Madigan Army Medical Center, Joint Base Lewis-McChord, Tacoma, Washington

ANJALI S. KUMAR, MD, MPH, FACS
Assistant Professor of Surgery, Section of Colon and Rectal Surgery, MedStar Washington Hospital Center, Georgetown University School of Medicine, Washington, DC

MARY R. KWAAN, MD, MPH
Assistant Professor of Surgery, Division of Colon and Rectal Surgery, University of Minnesota, Minneapolis, Minnesota

SANG W. LEE, MD, FACS, FASCRS
Associate Professor of Surgery, Division of Colon and Rectal Surgery, NY Presbyterian Hospital, Weill-Cornell Medical College, New York, New York

ANNE Y. LIN, MD
Assistant Professor, Department of Surgery, David Geffen School of Medicine, University of California Los Angeles, Los Angeles, California

KIM C. LU, MD, FACS, FASCRS
Associate Professor, Division of Gastrointestinal and General Surgery, Department of Surgery, Oregon Health & Science University, Portland, Oregon

JUSTIN A. MAYKEL, MD, FACS, FASCRS
Chief, Division of Colon and Rectal Surgery, Department of Surgery, UMass Memorial Medical Center; Assistant Professor of Surgery, University of Massachusetts Medical School, Worcester, Massachusetts

GENEVIEVE B. MELTON, MD, MA, FACS, FASCRS
Associate Professor of Surgery, Division of Colon and Rectal Surgery, University of Minnesota, Minneapolis, Minnesota

HUSEIN MOLOO, MD, MSc, FRSCS
Surgical Oncologist, Division of General Surgery, The Ottawa Hospital, Clinical Investigator, Ottawa Hospital Research Institute; Assistant Professor of Surgery, University of Ottawa, Ottawa, Ontario, Canada

ARDEN M. MORRIS, MD, MPH
Associate Professor, Department of Surgery, University of Michigan, Ann Arbor, Michigan

VINCENT OBIAS, MD, FACS
Assistant Professor of Surgery, Chief, Division of Colon and Rectal Surgery, George Washington University, Washington, DC

SONIA RAMAMOORTHY, MD, FACS, FASCRS
Associate Professor of Surgery; Chief, Colon and Rectal Surgery, University of California, San Diego, La Jolla, California

DAVID E. RIVADENEIRA, MD, FACS, FASCRS
Chief, Colon and Rectal Surgery, Saint Catherine of Siena Medical Center, Smithtown, New York

SHARON L. STEIN, MD, FACS
Director, Case Acute Intestinal Failure Unit; Surgical Director, Inflammatory Bowel Disease Center of Excellence, Digestive Health Institute; Assistant Professor of Surgery, Division of Colon and Rectal Surgery, University Hospital/Case Medical Center, Cleveland, Ohio

JAMES YOO, MD
Chief, Section of Colon and Rectal Surgery; Assistant Professor, Department of Surgery, David Geffen School of Medicine, University of California Los Angeles, Los Angeles, California

Contents

This review discusses the preoperative evaluation of patients preparing for elective colorectal resection, touching on several specific categories of morbidity, including cardiac, pulmonary, hepatic, renal, and surgical site complications. For each of these, the evidence for practices that optimize patient function and minimize risk is reviewed. Finally, authors discuss how to counsel high-risk surgical patients, including those for whom elective surgery is not recommended.

Enhanced recovery after surgery or "fast-track" pathways are a multimodal approach to the perioperative management of patients undergoing colorectal surgery designed to improve the overall quality of care. These pathways use existing evidence to streamline and standardize the perioperative management of patients to improve pain management, speed intestinal recovery, and ultimately facilitate a more rapid hospital discharge, thus minimizing complications, decreasing the use of hospital resources and health care costs, and improving overall patient care and satisfaction. Fast-track protocols are safe for patients and offer improvement in intestinal recovery and hospital discharge.

This article reviews the evidence regarding intraoperative techniques used by surgeons to prevent postoperative complications. The specific prophylactic measures examined include proximal diversion and use of drains after colorectal anastomoses, omentoplasty, adhesion prevention, and optimal wound closure.

Abdominal surgeons are often asked to manage challenging pathologic conditions with limited preoperative information. As such, unexpected intraoperative findings are commonly encountered. Often, there is little peer-reviewed evidence on which to base management decisions. This article reviews common unexpected surgical challenges and provides recommendations based on the latest available literature.

Intestinal anastomosis is an essential part of surgical practice, and with it comes the inherent risk of complications including leaks, strictures, and bleeding, which result in significant morbidity and occasional mortality. Understanding the myriad of risk factors and the strength of the data helps guide a surgeon as to the safety of undertaking an operation in which a primary anastomosis is to be considered. This article reviews the risk factors, management, and outcomes associated with anastomotic complications.

Rectal resection is the most common treatment of rectal cancer and inflammatory bowel disease. The surgical techniques for removing and reconstructing the rectum have evolved significantly over the past 50 years. Technological advances including retractors, stapling devices, energy delivery systems, and minimally invasive approaches, as well as the nerve-sparing total mesorectal excision, have revolutionized the surgical treatment. Surgical exposure and precise technique affect the ability to preserve the pelvic autonomic nerves, directly influencing postoperative urinary and sexual function. The complex interplay between all these factors demands attention because of the associated short-term and long-term impact on patient quality of life.

Total proctocolectomy with ileal pouch anal anastomosis (IPAA) preserves fecal continence as an alternative to permanent end ileostomy in select patients with ulcerative colitis and familial adenomatous polyposis. The procedure is technically demanding, and surgical complications may arise. This article outlines both the early and late complications that can occur after IPAA, as well as the workup and management of these potentially morbid conditions.

Stomas are created for a wide range of indications such as temporary protection of a high-risk anastomosis, diversion of sepsis, or permanent relief of obstructed defecation or incontinence. Yet this seemingly benign procedure is associated with an overall complication rate of up to 70%. Therefore, surgeons caring for patients with gastrointestinal diseases must be proficient not only with stoma creation but also with managing postopera-tive stoma-related complications. This article reviews the common compli-cations associated with ostomy creation and strategies for their management.

Although medical management can control symptoms in a recurring incur-able disease, such as Crohn's disease, surgical management is reserved for disease complications or those problems refractory to medical man-agement. In this article, we cover general principles for the surgical man-agement of Crohn's disease, ranging from skin tags, abscesses, fistulae, and stenoses to small bowel and extraintestinal disease.

Optimal management of rectal prolapse requires multiple clinical consider-ations with respect to treatment options, particularly for surgeons who must counsel and give realistic expectations to rectal prolapse patients. Rectal prolapse outcomes are good with respect to recurrence. Although posterior rectopexy remains most popular in the United States, increas-ingly surgeons perform ventral rectopexy to repair rectal prolapse. Func-tional outcomes vary and are fair after rectal prolapse repair. Although incarceration with rectal prolapse is rare, it is potentially life threatening and requires immediate and effective measures to adequately address in the acute setting.

Recurrent pelvic surgery is technically challenging. This article discusses this complex topic in patients with both benign and malignant disease. Perspectives regarding a safe approach to patients who may require reo-perative pelvic surgery are discussed with a focus on work-up, technical approach, and the importance of an experienced multidisciplinary team.

Laparoscopic colorectal surgery may be comparable with open tech-niques when considering oncological and long-term follow-up outcomes; however, there are a few operative complications specific to laparoscopic colorectal surgery. This article reviews the array of complications and dis-cusses them in detail.

Enterocutaneous fistula and its variations are some of the most difficult problems encountered in the practice of general surgery. Reliable

evidence that can be used to direct the care of patients afflicted with this
malady is limited. There are controversies in several areas of care. This
article addresses some of the gray areas of care for the patient with enterocutaneous fistula. There is particular attention directed toward the phe-
nomenon of enteroatmospheric fistula, as well as prevention and
abdominal wall reconstruction, which is often required in these individuals.

Colorectal disease in pediatric patients includes a spectrum of diseases,
many of which have a significant impact on quality of life and warrant
long-term follow-up and treatment into adulthood. Although many diseases, such as inflammatory bowel disease and colon cancer, are managed similar to adults, other disease processes are more common to
pediatric patients and are the focus of this article.

Robotic approaches in all surgical realms have seen tremendous growth
over the previous few years. Taking advantage of 3-dimensional visualization, improved articulation, and the opportunity for an enhanced ability to
suture/operate in the deep pelvis all provide theoretical and real advantages in colorectal surgery. This article reviews the potential advantages
and disadvantages, current indications, future directions, and lessons
learned for robotic approaches in colorectal surgery.

SURGICAL CLINICS
OF NORTH AMERICA

FORTHCOMING ISSUES

April 2013
Multidisciplinary Breast Management
George M. Fuhrman, MD, and
Tari A. King, MD, *Guest Editors*

June 2013
Pancreatic Surgery
Stephen W. Behrman, MD, FACS, and
Ronald F. Martin, MD, FACS, *Guest Editors*

August 2013
Vascular Surgery
Girma Tefera, MD, *Guest Editor*

RECENT ISSUES

December 2012
Surgical Critical Care
John A. Weigelt, MD, *Guest Editor*

October 2012
Contemporary Management of Esophageal Malignancy
Chadrick E. Denlinger, MD, and
Carolyn E. Reed, MD, *Guest Editors*

August 2012
Recent Advances and Future Directions in Trauma Care
Jeremy W. Cannon, MD, SM, *Guest Editor*

June 2012
Pediatric Surgery
Kenneth S. Azarow, MD, and
Robert A. Cusick, MD, *Guest Editors*

ISSUE OF RELATED INTEREST

Critical Care Clinics October 2012 (Vol. 28, Issue 4)
Cardiopulmonary Resuscitation
Wanchun Tang, MD, *Guest Editor*

DOWNLOAD Free App!

Review Articles THE CLINICS

NOW AVAILABLE FOR YOUR iPhone and iPad

Foreword

Complications, Considerations, and Consequences of Colorectal Surgery

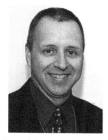

Ronald F. Martin, MD
Consulting Editor

We are more interconnected than we may think. "It's a small world" is an axiomatic cliché that gets tossed about from time to time but it kind of is. The world of surgery is even smaller. As we enter into the interview season for the applicants for surgical residency for 2013, I get to read and reacquaint with many friends and acquaintances through their letters of recommendation. I recently participated in a conference co-sponsored by the American College of Surgeons and the Accreditation Council for Graduate Medical Education on Transitions to Practice; there I saw many of our colleagues from around the country and realized that we all share the same concerns and largely the same problems no matter where we work. Even more proof, as I type this today, I am delayed in travel because of Hurricane Sandy, which by the time one reads this may be a distant memory for many. Yet, while stuck in New England (a great place to be stuck, in my opinion), so many of the contributors to this issue and other surgical colleagues have reached out to help me. We surgeons are not the only collegial group by any stretch of the imagination, but we are tightly connected.

This issue, and many other issues, of the *Surgical Clinics of North America* is an important byproduct of our collegiality. Dr Steele and I both serve the country in a uniformed capacity; he, full time, and I, when called. We have never been downrange together but every time I need his help or advice, he is right there in a moment. As anybody who has ever met him will tell you, his energy is infectious and his diligence is boundless. Most, if not all, the contributors to this series are cut from similar cloth. They have a passion for their craft and their profession and sense of duty to improve our knowledge base.

Surg Clin N Am 93 (2013) xiii–xiv
http://dx.doi.org/10.1016/j.suc.2012.11.001
0039-6109/13/$ – see front matter © 2013 Elsevier Inc. All rights reserved.

I am occasionally propositioned via email to write for e-journals for pay. The argument usually alleges that publishers use us contributors for slave labor and get rich off of our efforts. Without going into a serious debate on the economics of publishing, I would suggest it isn't that simplistic an analysis. I don't know the people who are blast e-mailing me and it is unclear as to what product they have a passion for. They may be inventing the better mousetrap—or not.

I can say without fear of equivocation that through the *Clinics* series I have been allowed and encouraged by our publishers to find the best content put in the best context possible with the best authors we can gather. Every guest editor and I review all materials and we reach out to contributors who we feel can really put matters into useful perspective. The best part of this process is the enthusiasm with which requests are almost universally greeted. These excellent people with very busy schedules readily grab at the chance to be part of this project with very, very few exceptions. We have made numerous friendships and have learned a great deal from one another along the way.

We surgeons are scattered all over geographically and we all have very different practices in very different environments, but time and time again we come together to solve problems. Whether it is helping with disasters like Hurricane Katrina or the Haitian earthquake, serving the country at home or abroad, or just taking a phone call from a colleague who needs an ear or help at 0230, we routinely answer the call.

This series is written mostly by surgeons and for surgeons. We extend our community to include those who have an interest in the problems we address for both our contributor base and our readership. There is a pretty fair chance that there are still hard times ahead for those in our line of work. If we can maintain the same level of collaboration and selfless contribution that this series has seen, we will all be better off for it. I am most grateful to Dr Steele and his colleagues for this excellent effort. As always, we value and appreciate the input of our readership and will continue to strive to improve this series to meet the needs of our fellow surgeons and their patients. Thank you to all who offer us feedback and suggestions to improve this effort.

Ronald F. Martin, MD
Department of Surgery
Marshfield Clinic
1000 North Oak Avenue
Marshfield, WI 54449, USA

E-mail address:
martin.ronald@marshfieldclinic.org

Preface

Complications, Considerations, and Consequences of Colorectal Surgery

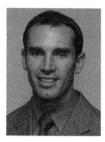

Scott R. Steele, MD
Guest Editor

Complications, no matter how "trivial," have long-standing implications for both surgeons and patients alike. For patients, the manifestations are often all too obvious. As a mentor once told me, "It is the wise surgeon who remembers the patient takes all the risks." For surgeons, even in this era of evidence-based medicine, many of us may still harken back to the last time we did something and base decisions, at least in part, from the results. We are also not infrequently called on to manage difficult clinical situations, whether as a result of the underlying disease process or from therapeutic endeavors, that leave us pondering as to how to proceed. In this issue of *Surgical Clinics of North America*, our objective was to fully explore the complex nature of complications following colorectal surgery in order to help optimize patient outcomes in what is likely an already problematical state of affairs.

Drs Morris and Hendren set the stage for the issue by providing an overview of the evaluation of colorectal surgery patients and how risk stratification and intervention can help to optimize outcomes. Drs Chestovich, Lin, and Yoo discuss the role of "fast-track" pathways, including superb guidance on how enhanced recovery protocols can lead to a return of gastrointestinal function and hospital discharge safely, even in this era of minimally invasive surgery. Regarding intraoperative considerations, Drs Etzioni and Moloo present an in-depth review of the adjuncts available in the operating room. The authors highlight data concerning which ones have more solid evidence behind their use versus those that are more anecdotal. As a crucial component of decision-making in the operating room, Drs Hall and Stein outline the principles of how to approach several unique, but not too uncommon, scenarios of encountering unexpected findings. Rounding out this section, Drs Rivadeneira and Davis present

Surg Clin N Am 93 (2013) xv–xvi
http://dx.doi.org/10.1016/j.suc.2012.10.001
0039-6109/13/$ – see front matter Published by Elsevier Inc.

surgical.theclinics.com

what I feel is the most up-to-date and thorough review of predicting and dealing with one of the most feared complications in colorectal surgery—the anastomotic leak. Additionally, they present a step-wise strategy for the evaluation and treatment of other anastomotic complications including stricture and bleeding.

As assorted clinical settings can have a major impact on both diagnostic and therapeutic considerations in colorectal surgery, the authors have compiled a comprehensive review with respect to the patient's underlying condition and specific procedure. Drs Bleier and Maykel begin with a thorough summary detailing the patient undergoing a proctectomy, including some technical aspects and management strategies for dealing with those who are struggling with poor postoperative function following an otherwise successful surgery. Drs Francone and Champagne tackle the difficult scenario of what to do when the pouch patient has problems, while Drs Irani and Bafford explore how to avoid problems with patients requiring an ostomy, and the management of several complications ranging from stricture to hernia and prolapse. Drs Kim and Hunt provide insight into the principles of operative and medical management for Crohn patients, highlighting technical aspects as they pertain to the various sites and processes that Crohn can manifest as. Drs Melton-Meaux and Kwaan provide a detailed analysis of the data surrounding rectal prolapse patients, including an overview of outcomes for both the abdominal and the perineal approaches. Drs Boostrom and Dozois deliver an extensive review of one of the most difficult situations—the reoperative pelvis. In addition to providing technical tips, they delineate the importance of a multidisciplinary team, and the surgeon's role within that team. Drs Kumar and Lee discuss the unique complications that can occur with minimally invasive procedures, as well as strategies as to how to both prevent and manage them. Rounding out this issue, Drs Johnson and Davis present an extensive evaluation of the described techniques of dealing with patients with enterocutaneous fistulas as well as the technical aspects and expected outcomes with abdominal wall reconstruction in enterocutaneous fistula (ECF) patients. Dr Gourlay highlights a thorough approach to many of the more commonly encountered pediatric colorectal conditions, stratifying these into the newborn, toddler, and adolescent phases. Finally, Drs Ramamoorthy and Obias review the unique aspects involved with the emergence of robotics in colorectal surgery, and how to safely and effectively embark in this endeavor.

The authors of each of these articles are experts in their respective fields, and it has been my privilege and pleasure to work with them in developing this issue. I would like to personally thank each one of them for taking time out of their busy schedules to provide the most up-to-date management on these topics. It is my wish that this issue serve as a guide for surgeons who unfortunately find themselves faced with these taxing and unfortunate situations. In closing, I would like to extend my gratitude to Dr Ronald Martin for allowing me to serve as a guest editor on this important topic.

Scott R. Steele, MD
Colon & Rectal Surgery
Madigan Army Medical Center
9040A Fitzsimmons Drive
Fort Lewis, WA 98431, USA
Department of Surgery
University of Washington
Seattle, WA, USA

E-mail address:
scott.steele1@us.army.mil

Evaluating Patients Undergoing Colorectal Surgery to Estimate and Minimize Morbidity and Mortality

Samantha K. Hendren, MD, MPH*, Arden M. Morris, MD, MPH

KEYWORDS

- Preoperative evaluation • Complications • Morbidity • Risk stratification

KEY POINTS

- Compared with other common surgical procedures, colorectal operations carry a high risk for morbidity and mortality.
- Risk assessment, and intervention when possible, may decrease patient morbidity and mortality for elective operations.
- Several strategies and evidence-based guidelines are available to assess organ system and surgical site risk.

INTRODUCTION

Compared with other common surgical procedures, colorectal surgery carries a high risk for morbidity and mortality. The American College of Surgeons' National Surgical Quality Improvement Program reports a 30-day complication rate of 27% for colorectal resection, compared with a rate of 11% for other general and vascular surgery procedures.[1,2] The same study reports a mortality rate of 4% after colorectal resection. Clearly, not all patients are at equal risk for morbidity and mortality; adverse outcomes vary by patient characteristics outside of the surgeon's control including demographic factors, diagnosis, disease severity, and comorbid conditions.[1] However, observed variations in risk-adjusted morbidity rates suggest that at least some complications may be preventable.[3,4]

Although reduction of patient risk is inherently limited in emergency cases, it may be possible to predict and even decrease patient risk for elective operations. This review discusses the preoperative evaluation of patients preparing for elective colorectal resection, touching on several specific categories of morbidity, including cardiac,

Department of Surgery, University of Michigan, 1500 East Medical Center Drive, TC-5343, Ann Arbor, MI 48109, USA
* Corresponding author.
E-mail address: Hendren@med.umich.edu

Surg Clin N Am 93 (2013) 1–20
http://dx.doi.org/10.1016/j.suc.2012.09.005
0039-6109/13/$ – see front matter © 2013 Elsevier Inc. All rights reserved.

pulmonary, hepatic, renal, and surgical site complications. For each of these, the evidence for practices that optimize patient function and minimize risk is discussed. Finally, the authors discuss how to counsel high-risk surgical patients, including those for whom elective surgery is not recommended.

OVERALL PREOPERATIVE EVALUATION: BEST PRACTICES

Operative risk is the probability of an adverse outcome or death associated with surgery or anesthesia. A thorough and meticulous assessment of operative risk should include evaluation of 4 components: the patient, the procedure, the provider, and the anesthetic.[5,6] This review focuses on risk associated with the patient. Risk associated with the procedure—that is, colon or rectal resection—is high by definition.

At the patient level, a general preoperative evaluation to assess risk is performed for 2 purposes. First, for individual patients, the potential benefit of an operation must be weighed against the risk of an adverse postoperative medical or surgical event. The benefits of colon and rectal resection are obvious in the urgent setting (obstruction or perforation) but less clear in the elective setting. For example, a small malignant growth in an elderly patient with heart failure may take years to affect health, whereas a major operation poses a clear risk of 1-year mortality. Several long-standing principles of surgical treatment have become less clear with time and rigorous scrutiny, such as the timing and optimal treatment of diverticulitis.[7,8] Nonetheless, as surgeons we are bound to consider (1) the potential *benefit of an operation* and the duration of benefit, (2) the immediate and long-term *risk of an operation*, and (3) the *risk of avoiding an operation* and the time span of risk.

The second purpose of preoperative risk assessment is to identify comorbid disease that may be mitigated by medical or procedural intervention. In the presence of any comorbid disease, the following considerations must be weighed:

- What is the patient's health status?
- What are the types and severity of the comorbid disease?
- How urgent is the operation?
- If the operation is delayed, can the burden of comorbid disease be reduced with treatment?
- If the operation cannot be delayed, how should medical management be optimized in the short-term?

To this end, the initial assessment consists of a comprehensive history especially focused on cardiac and pulmonary disease, physical examination to confirm diagnoses, record review, and review of radiologic and laboratory data. Medications must be reviewed to assess both preoperative medication-associated risk and whether protective medications are optimized.

CARDIAC EVALUATION AND OPTIMIZATION

After a comprehensive history-taking and physical examination, the next step to assess cardiac risk is performing electrocardiogram for patients older than 50 years or who have a history or physical examination suspicious for cardiac risk factors. The American College of Cardiologists (ACC) and the American Heart Association (AHA)[9,10] recommend a preoperative cardiology consult for patients at highest risk for an adverse perioperative cardiac event—that is, patients with the following:

- Unstable angina
- Myocardial infarction between 7 and 30 days before the surgery

- Decompensated heart failure
- Significant arrhythmias
- Severe valvular disease

A cardiology consultation can help to assess the relative risks of anesthesia and benefits of operation and to optimize cardiac function before noncardiac surgery. Noting that patients with stable cardiac disease undergoing vascular surgery have not derived benefit from preoperative cardiac revascularization,[11] the most recent ACC/AHA perioperative guidelines[9,10] strongly discourage cardiac testing that will not change management. Patients with low-to-intermediate cardiac risk factors, such as diabetes, mild stable angina, previous myocardial infarction, and compensated heart failure, can undergo intermediate-risk procedures without interventional testing. For patients whose risk is less clear, there are several well-supported and widely used risk assessment instruments.[12]

American Society of Anesthesiologists' Physical Status Classification

The American Society of Anesthesiologists' (ASA) classification is one of the oldest and most widely used means of assessing patients' global physical status before an operation.[5,13] The system was not initially designed for risk prediction per se, although there is a correlation between the ASA score and the postoperative adverse cardiac and other outcomes. Rather, the ASA score is a means of assessing any individual patient's baseline health, and therefore the system does not include a measure of the risk of the procedure. The initial classification system included the first 5 items in the following list, with a subsequent sixth item added to describe brain-dead potential organ donors:

Class 1: A normal healthy patient
Class 2: A patient with mild systemic disease
Class 3: A patient with severe systemic disease
Class 4: A patient with severe systemic disease that is a constant threat to life
Class 5: A moribund patient who is not expected to survive without the operation
Class 6: A declared brain-dead patient whose organs are being removed for donation

Revised Cardiac Risk Index

The simplest and most current method of risk assessment is the revised cardiac risk index (RCRI),[14] which includes the following 6 independent predictors of a major postoperative cardiac event:

- High-risk surgery (present by definition in the current population)
- Insulin-dependent diabetes
- Renal failure (defined as serum creatinine level >2 mg/dL)
- History of ischemic heart disease
- History of congestive heart failure
- History of cerebrovascular disease

Each predictor is equally weighted. An RCRI score 0/6 is associated with less than 1% perioperative cardiac risk; RCRI score 1/6, with 1.3% or less risk (low risk); RCRI score 2/6, with 4% to 7% risk (intermediate risk); and RCRI score 3/6 or more, with 9% to 11% risk (high risk). Beyond a statistical calculation of risk, the implications of RCRI are not entirely clear but may have promise for risk reduction. For example, recent studies report a benefit of aggressive beta-blockade (target heart rate <65) for those with RCRI score 2/6 or more and possible harm (stroke, death) of using beta-blockade in those with RCRI score less than 2.[14–16]

PULMONARY EVALUATION AND OPTIMIZATION

Pulmonary complications are relatively common events after colorectal resection. Bilimoria and colleagues[2] studied patients who underwent 28,692 colorectal resection from the American College of Surgeons National Surgical Quality Improvement Program (ACS-NSQIP) and found that several of the most common postoperative complications were pulmonary (prolonged ventilation [4.9% of patients], pneumonia [4.2%], and unplanned reintubation [3.6%]).

Risk factors for postoperative pulmonary complications include the patient's comorbid conditions, the type of operation planned, and the perioperative course. A systematic review of risk factors for postoperative pulmonary complications revealed the following comorbid conditions to be independent risk factors (pooled, adjusted odds ratios): older age (3.9), ASA Class (3.1), abnormalities in chest radiograph (4.8), congestive heart failure (CHF) (2.9), arrhythmia (2.9), functional dependence (1.7), chronic obstructive pulmonary disease (COPD) (2.4), weight loss (1.6), medical comorbid condition (1.5), cigarette use (1.4), impaired sensorium (1.4), corticosteroid use (1.3), and alcohol use (1.2).[17] Abnormal findings of a pulmonary physical examination may also be a strong predictor of postoperative pulmonary complications (odds ratio 5.8), although only a few high-quality studies have included this factor.[17] The elderly are at particular risk for pulmonary complications after colorectal resection. Bentram and colleagues[1] found that pulmonary complications were significantly more common in elderly patients, with a pneumonia rate of 6.3%.

Obstructive sleep apnea (OSA) is estimated to affect approximately 5% of people in Western countries, and the possible perioperative significance of diagnosed or undiagnosed sleep apnea is an area of current research interest.[18] It is not entirely clear whether OSA increases postoperative pulmonary complications; however, physiologic studies have suggested that sleep apnea may be associated with post-operative hemodynamic instability, myocardial ischemia, stroke, mental confusion, and wound breakdown, via the mechanism of "rapid eye movement (REM) sleep rebound."[18] There are limited empirical data on sleep apnea in patients who undergo colorectal resection.[18] Nevertheless, this history is important to elicit from patients preoperatively so that a plan for perioperative management can be made; this usually includes the patient bringing continuous positive airway pressure (CPAP) or other devices used at home to the hospital. Sleep apnea may also be associated with a difficult airway or with pulmonary hypertension, of which the anesthesiologist will need to be aware.[17,19]

The type of operation is also associated with the risk of pulmonary complications, with upper abdominal, lower abdominal, and any abdominal operation having risks of 19.7%, 7.7% and 14.2%, respectively.[17] It is likely that these risks are lower with minimally invasive operations. General anesthesia and longer duration of surgery are also associated with increased risk.[17] Arozullah and colleagues[20,21] used the Veterans Affairs' National Surgical Quality Improvement Program (VA-NSQIP) database to create and validate a risk scoring index for postoperative pneumonia and postoperative respiratory failure (**Table 1**). They found that many of the factors were not modifiable, but at least these indices give the provider and the patient a risk estimate for discussion.

In contrast to pulmonary surgery, preoperative pulmonary testing, such as chest radiograph, arterial blood gas (ABG), and spirometry, does not clearly predict

Table 1
Risk indices for predicting pulmonary complications after major, noncardiothoracic surgery

Postoperative Pneumonia Risk Index		Postoperative Respiratory Failure Risk Index	
Score 0–15 risk 0.2%		Score ≤10 risk 0.5%	
Score 16–25 risk 1.2%		Score 11–19 risk 2.2%	
Score 26–40 risk 4.6%		Score 20–27 risk 5.0%	
Score 41–55 risk 10.8%		Score 28–40 risk 11.6%	
Score >55 risk 15.9%		Score >40 risk 30.5%	
Preoperative Risk Factor	**Score**	**Preoperative Risk Factor**	**Score**
Type of surgery		Type of surgery	
Abdominal aortic aneurysm repair	15	Abdominal aortic aneurysm	27
Thoracic	14	Thoracic	21
Upper abdominal	10	Neurosurgery, upper abdominal, or peripheral vascular	14
Neck	8	Neck	11
Neurosurgery	8	Emergency surgery	11
Vascular	3	Albumin (<30 g/L)	9
Age		Blood urea nitrogen (>30 mg/dL)	8
≥80 y	17	Partially or fully dependent functional status	7
70–79 y	13	History of COPD	6
60–69 y	9	Age (y)	
50–59 y	4	≥70	6
Functional status		60–69	4
Totally dependent	10		
Partially dependent	6		
Weight loss >10% in past 6 mo	7		
History of chronic obstructive pulmonary disease	5		
General anesthesia	4		
Impaired sensorium	4		
History of cerebrovascular accident	4		
Blood urea nitrogen level			
<2.86 mmol/L (<8 mg/dL)	4		
7.85–10.7 mmol/L (22–30 mg/dL)	2		
≥10.7 mmol/L (≥30 mg/dL)	3		
Transfusion >4 units	3		
Emergency surgery	3		
Steroid use for chronic condition	3		
Current smoker within 1 y	3		
Alcohol (>2 drinks/d in past 2 wk)	2		

Definition of respiratory failure was mechanical ventilator greater than 48 hours or unplanned intubation.

Data from Arozullah AM, Khuri SF, Henderson WG, et al. Development and validation of a multifactorial risk index for predicting postoperative pneumonia after major noncardiac surgery. Ann Intern Med 2001;135(10):847–57; and Arozullah AM, Daley J, Henderson WG, et al. Multifactorial risk index for predicting postoperative respiratory failure in men after major noncardiac surgery. The National Veterans Administration Surgical Quality Improvement Program. Ann Surg 2000;232(2):242–53.

postoperative pulmonary complications for abdominal surgery.[17,19] For general surgery, these tests only occasionally change management and are not routinely recommended.[22] History and physical examination that evaluate for the risk factors noted above (and including the assessment of whether the patient can climb 2 flights of stairs) probably identify the same patients as "high risk." However, *selective* use of these tests may help the provider to differentiate a pulmonary versus cardiac cause of dyspnea or may help the pulmonologist to optimize chronic pulmonary disease in the patient before surgery.[23,24]

What can be done preoperatively and perioperatively to modify the risk for patients preparing for elective abdominal operations? In 2007, Bapoje and colleagues[19] summarized the evidence for perioperative interventions in *Chest* (**Box 1**). For patients with chronic pulmonary disease, consultation with the pulmonologist may be warranted.[19] The goal is to ensure that the patient's pulmonary condition is optimized, whether it is COPD, asthma, or any other chronic pulmonary disease. Suboptimal medical management or an episode of pulmonary infection should be treated before elective surgery is performed.

Smoking cessation is an important preoperative intervention before elective operation, and it should take place as early as possible before elective surgery.[23,24] Evidence is mixed about the effect of preoperative smoking cessation on risk of pulmonary complications, but systematic reviews of studies support a beneficial effect.[25,26] Controversy about the timing of smoking cessation before surgery followed studies by Warner and colleagues[27,28] that suggested a higher risk of pulmonary complications among coronary artery bypass grafting (CABG) patients who quit fewer than 8 weeks before surgery. These data resulted in hesitation among surgeons to recommend cessation immediately before surgery. However, a recent meta-analysis of studies comparing cessation within 8 weeks with continuing smoking did not show any adverse effect of smoking cessation on postoperative outcomes.[26] As such, smoking cessation at any time before elective surgery should be encouraged.[26] Preoperative smoking cessation interventions have been found to have promising results.[29] Systematic reviews of preoperative smoking cessation intervention trials (generally including nicotine replacement and counseling) showed overall success in cessation (40%–89%), decreased short-term morbidity, and for intensive interventions, a positive effect on long-term cessation.[29,30]

Box 1
Evidence-based perioperative care to minimize pulmonary complications

Preoperative

  Smoking cessation

  Inspiratory muscle training

Intraoperative

  Avoidance of pancuronium (long-acting neuromuscular blockade)

Postoperative

  Lung expansion maneuvers

  CPAP

  Selective (rather than routine) NG decompression

Data from Refs.[19,22,31]

On the day of surgery, a careful reassessment of the patient with chronic pulmonary disease should be performed, and the surgery should be canceled if symptoms are worse than usual. Anesthetic techniques can be tailored to decrease risk in patients at high risk for postoperative pulmonary complications. A full review of anesthetic management is beyond the scope of this review but may include bronchodilators, neuroaxial blockade (eg, epidural) in selected circumstances (controversy exists about its benefit), avoidance of long-acting neuromuscular blockade, and use of lung recruitment maneuvers and positive end-expiratory pressure (PEEP) in intubated patients.[23,31] Use of intraoperative PEEP in particular has been the subject of a Cochrane meta-analysis; a lower risk of postoperative atelectasis was found, but there was no difference in pulmonary complications or mortality based on available trials.[32]

From the surgeon's perspective, minimally invasive surgery may be associated with a decreased risk for postoperative pulmonary complications; however, data from randomized trials seldom report pulmonary complications and data are insufficient to conclude that pulmonary complications are definitively less after laparoscopic approach.[31] Also, some patients with severe pulmonary disease may tolerate pneumoperitoneum poorly.[19] Routine nasogastric tube (NGT) placement should be avoided because it is associated with increased risk of postoperative pulmonary complications.[31,33] Some investigators have advocated transverse rather than midline abdominal incisions as a way to decrease pulmonary complications, but meta-analysis reveals that pulmonary complication rates are similar between groups.[34,35]

Postoperatively, there are several issues particular to patients with chronic pulmonary disease. Optimal pain control can help in avoiding atelectasis; however, pulmonary patients may be at increased risk for respiratory depressant effects of narcotics and benzodiazepines.[23] As such, local, regional, and nonnarcotic pain control methods should be considered. These methods may include epidural analgesia, which may decrease risk for postoperative pulmonary complications, although the evidence is mixed. In a meta-analysis, there was a 7.5% versus 12.8% ($P = .04$) risk of postoperative pneumonia among patients who received thoracic epidural analgesia.[36] In addition, more intensive monitoring in a step-down unit or with continuous pulse oximetry should be considered for both patients with COPD and those with sleep apnea.[23]

Although there is a lack of data regarding methods to optimize outcomes in patients with diagnosed or undiagnosed OSA, some authors have raised the concern that outpatient surgery may be contraindicated in patients with OSA because of a possible risk for increased apnea due to effects of surgery and pain medications (REM sleep rebound).[19] These risks may last for more than 3 days after surgery.

Lung expansion maneuvers including incentive spirometry, deep breathing exercises, and CPAP seem to decrease pulmonary complications and are recommended as preoperative and postoperative interventions.[19,31] However, results of trials vary. Incentive spirometry has not been specifically shown to be superior to other deep breathing exercises or to chest physiotherapy. In fact, a meta-analysis of randomized controlled trials performed by the Cochrane collaboration showed no effect of incentive spirometry compared with no respiratory intervention or with other respiratory interventions.[37] This result highlights the poor methodological quality of many studies that have suggested decreased pulmonary complications with lung expansion therapies. Nevertheless, a systematic review of trials of these treatments suggests that lung expansion techniques in general are beneficial.[31] Although incentive spirometry is not superior to other techniques, it has the advantages of being inexpensive, easy to teach, and able to give feedback to the patient and provider about the patient's performance.[24,31] CPAP may be useful specifically for patients who cannot perform other lung expansion techniques effectively.[19]

In summary, pulmonary complications are common after major abdominal surgery, including colorectal resection. Predictive models have been developed to identify patients at high risk for postoperative pulmonary complications. These patients may benefit from preoperative optimization under the care of a pulmonologist. There are several evidence-based practices to minimize patients' risk of pulmonary complications, including smoking cessation, avoidance of long-acting neuromuscular blockade, effective pain management, postoperative lung expansion maneuvers, and selective rather than routine nasogastric tube use. The role of minimally invasive surgery on postoperative pulmonary complications and the risks associated with OSA are topics for further research.

HEPATIC EVALUATION AND OPTIMIZATION

Cirrhosis and portal hypertension incur major risk for perioperative mortality and a host of perioperative complications. The surgeon must check the platelet count, INR, serum aspartate aminotransferase, alanine aminotransferase, alkaline phosphatase, and bilirubin levels in the following patients:

- Those with *a history of* heavy alcohol use, intravenous drug use, high-risk sexual history
- Those with *physical findings of* palmar erythema, gynecomastia, testicular atrophy, splenomegaly, hepatomegaly, ascites, caput medusa, varices, or jaundice

Any patient with a positive finding in history and abnormal laboratory values should undergo a careful preoperative evaluation by a hepatologist. The Child-Turcotte-Pugh (CTP) classification of cirrhosis[38] was developed to predict the risk of adverse outcomes after portosystemic shunt procedures, and over time, it has proved to be a reliable predictor of perioperative mortality for extrahepatic surgery (**Table 2**).[39]

The Model for End-stage Liver disease (MELD) score[40] was developed to predict the perioperative morbidity and mortality before transplant, without the inclusion of more subjective physical findings. The MELD score is hard to calculate without electronic means; MELD = $3.78 \times \ln(\text{bilirubin [mg/dL]}) + 11.2 \times \ln(\text{INR}) + 9.57 \times \ln(\text{creatinine [mg/dL]}) + 6.43$. Similar to the CTP system, the MELD score has been used more recently as a predictor of extrahepatic operative risk.

Patients with CTP class A or MELD score less than 10 can undergo surgery without excessive risk after a consultation with a hepatologist and optimization. For CTP class

Table 2						
Child-Turcotte-Pugh classification of cirrhosis						
	Albumin	INR	Bilirubin	Ascites	Encephalopathy	**Perioperative Mortality Rate**
Class A	>3.5	<1.7	<2	Absent	None	10%
Class B	2.8–3.5	1.7–2.3	2–3	Moderate	Mild-	30%
Class C	<2.8	>2.3	>3	Tense	Moderate to severe	75%

Data from Mansour A, Watson W, Shayani V, et al. Abdominal operations in patients with cirrhosis: still a major surgical challenge. Surgery 1997;122(4):730–5 [discussion: 735–6].

B or MELD score 10 to 15, a transplant should be considered if possible. If the operation cannot be delayed, patient risk can be reduced through the following:

- Correction of coagulopathy with vitamin K or fresh frozen plasma
- Minimization of ascites with potassium-sparing diuretics and paracentesis
- Reduction of hepatic encephalopathy with lactulose
- Improvement of nutrition with total parented nutrition (TPN)
- Antibiotic prophylaxis
- Use of transjugular intrahepatic portosystemic shunts to reduce portal hypertension and intraoperative bleeding.[41]

Elective surgery among patients with a CTP class C or MELD score greater than 15 is strongly discouraged.

RENAL EVALUATION AND OPTIMIZATION

It has long been recognized that patients with renal failure are at increased risk for postoperative morbidity and mortality.[42,43] A large population-based study of hospital discharges from 1993 to 2007 documented that patients on dialysis undergoing colorectal resection operations had an increased risk of in-hospital death (22% vs 3%, $P<.0001$). Mortality for elective procedures in patients undergoing dialysis was 10%. These patients also had an increased risk for postoperative complications (52% vs 34%) and increased length of stay (median 13 days vs 7 days). These results partly reflect that patients undergoing dialysis had higher rates for vascular and infectious indications for colorectal resection; however, patients undergoing dialysis still had a significantly increased risk of death and complications even in adjusted analyses. Patients undergoing dialysis were especially predisposed to infectious and pulmonary complications, and investigators cite the immunosuppressive effect of uremia, dialysis-induced hypoxemia, and hypoproteinemia as the possible mechanisms. Patients with chronic kidney disease not requiring dialysis also seem to be at increased risk for postoperative complications, especially acute renal failure.[44]

Acute kidney injury (AKI) is a common complication of colorectal resection surgery. This is sometimes defined as an increase in serum creatinine level greater than 50% over the baseline value.[45] A single-institution study of 339 patients who underwent colectomy documented a rate of AKI (as defined above) of 12% (increased to 23% among patients who had a major surgical complication).[46] A larger study based on data from the ACS-NSQIP documented a 2.1% risk of postoperative renal failure among elderly patients undergoing colorectal resection.[1] These varying results not only reflect differences in measurement of outcomes but also raise the question of whether some of these events are predictable and/or preventable.

Risk factors for AKI after various types of surgery have been examined in observational studies. It seems that patients' baseline health status, the type of operation, and intraoperative/perioperative events are all associated with the risk for AKI. Particularly at risk are older patients who undergo cardiovascular surgery with baseline renal disease; blood loss and/or sepsis perioperatively increase the risk further.[45] There are limited data about risk factors, specifically among patients who undergo colorectal resection; however, several large observational studies have examined the risk among cohorts of major surgical patients. Kheterpal and colleagues studied 15,102 patients from a single institution who had normal renal function preoperatively and underwent major noncardiac surgery.[47] They found that 0.8% developed acute renal failure and that the following factors were independently associated with this result: age, emergency (v. elective) surgery, liver disease, body mass index (BMI), calculated as the weight in kilograms divided by the height in meters squared, high-risk surgery, peripheral vascular occlusive disease, COPD, intraoperative vasopressor use, and intraoperative diuretic use.[47] A large retrospective study of patients who underwent orthopedic surgery found that among 17,938 patients from 1 institution, the rate of renal injury was 0.55% (defined as doubling of baseline serum creatinine level).[48] Using case-control methodology, independent risk factors included higher BMI, higher preoperative serum creatinine levels, operative duration, COPD, liver disease, congestive heart failure, hypertension, and other heart problems.[48] Unfortunately, fluid administration and drug exposures were not included as potential risk factors in this study.

There is not yet a robust base of evidence for preventing postoperative AKI or for optimizing perioperative management of the patient with chronic kidney disease. Much of the work in this area has focused on patients who undergo cardiac surgery.[44] However, the basic principles apply to general surgery and are reviewed here (**Box 2**).

There is essentially no proven intervention to prevent AKI postoperatively; however, certain principles of perioperative management may be helpful. The most obvious and feasible practices to prevent AKI are the systematic avoidance of drugs that are toxic to the kidney, including aminoglycoside antibiotics, nonsteroidal antiinflammatory drugs, and intravenous contrast dye. For patients with renal

---

Box 2
Principles for perioperative management of the patient with chronic kidney disease

Possibly helpful strategies

Recognize chronic kidney disease (glomerular filtration rate <60 mL/min/1.73m^2) or decreased renal function (serum creatinine level $\geq$1.5 mg/dL)

Optimize medical management of hypertension preoperatively and perioperatively

Optimize glycemic control preoperatively and perioperatively

Avoid hypovolemia and hypotension

Avoid contrast dye

Avoid nephrotoxic drugs (aminoglycoside antibiotics, nonsteroidal antiinflammatory drugs)

Use Statins

Perform hydration (with or without sodium bicarbonate) for contrast-dye procedures, if required

Administer *N*-acetylcysteine for contrast-dye procedures, if required

Strategies with insufficient data to support use in perioperative patients

Calcium channel blockers

Fenoldopam

Mannitol

Possibly harmful

Renal-dose dopamine

Loop diuretics (eg, furosemide)

angiotensin converting enzyme inhibitor (ACE-I) and angiotensin receptor blocker (ARB)

Data from Eilers H, Liu KD, Gruber A, et al. Chronic kidney disease: implications for the perioperative period. Minerva Anestesiol 2010;76(9):725–36.

insufficiency, hydration and perhaps *N*-acetylcysteine administration for these procedures is recommended.[45]

Avoidance of hypertension, hypotension, and hypovolemia are recommended. To achieve this, it is suggested to optimize the volume status and judiciously use vasodilator and vasopressor agents perioperatively. As with sepsis management, goal-directed resuscitation, with invasive hemodynamic monitoring as needed, may be useful in preventing end-organ dysfunction, including AKI. In general, diuretics should be avoided because they have not been shown to decrease the risk for AKI and may exacerbate the risk due to hypovolemia.[45] From the surgeon's perspective, avoiding bleeding that requires transfusion and using minimally invasive surgical techniques are associated with decreased risk.

Most cardio-protective and renal-protective medications have not been proven helpful in preventing postoperative AKI. ACE-I and ARB therapies do not seem to prevent AKI and may even be harmful in certain perioperative circumstances, especially when hypotension is anticipated.[45] However, statins may decrease the risk for AKI. A large population-based study from Ontario, Canada, showed that statin use was associated with a 16% decreased risk of AKI as well as decreased mortality after major elective surgery, after adjusting for associated comorbidities.[49] Effective glycemic control, beginning with preoperative optimization, is probably a worthwhile effort in patients at risk for AKI. Patients in surgical intensive care unit randomly assigned to aggressive glycemic control had decreased risks of serious renal injury.[50]

Optimizing the perioperative management of patients on dialysis undergoing elective surgery requires collaboration between the surgeon, anesthesiologist, and nephrologist. The recommended features of optimization include ensuring that metabolic status is adequately corrected with dialysis; the blood filtration requirement may actually increase perioperatively because of catabolic state.[51] Also, correction of chronic anemia, control of hypertension and blood glucose level, optimization of fluid status and mineral metabolism disorders, and management of congestive heart failure should be optimized preoperatively under the guidance of the medical specialists caring for the patient.[51] It is also important for surgeons and anesthesiologists to be aware that pulmonary hypertension is relatively common among patients on dialysis with arteriovenous fistulas for dialysis access, and this complicates hemodynamic management, if present.[51] Finally, the choices and dosing of anesthetic drugs and medications and fluid used perioperatively must be adjusted to account for dialysis and/or decreased renal functioning, as appropriate.

Several technical considerations apply to patients with chronic renal insufficiency or renal failure. First, the surgeon and anesthesiologist should stop and consult with the nephrologist before placing central venous catheters, including peripherally inserted central catheter lines. Complications of these lines—even if temporary—may create difficulties for future dialysis access, and they should be avoided if possible (especially subclavian vein access). Intravenous access and blood pressure cuffs should be avoided on the arm used for dialysis access. Also, if blood transfusion is required and the patient is a possible candidate for renal transplantation, human-leukocyte-antigen-matched blood may be preferred.[51]

Also, patients with end-stage renal disease (ESRD) may be at increased risk of infectious complications because of immunosuppressive effects of ESRD and may be infected with drug-resistant organisms because of dialysis access infection treatment and frequent exposure to health care institutions. As such, patients may need to be isolated and/or receive tailored extended-spectrum antibiotic prophylaxis.[51] In general, dialysis should be performed the day before elective surgery, and if a dialysis-access catheter is present, it should not be used for purposes other than dialysis perioperatively, except in an emergency.

In summary, patients on dialysis and with chronic kidney disease are at increased risk for surgical complications. Recognizing these patients and tailoring their management to minimize renal insult is recommended. Perioperative management strategies include optimizing the management of hypertension, optimizing glycemic control, avoiding hypovolemia and hypotension, avoiding contrast dye (or using hydration and possibly N-acetylcysteine for contrast studies if absolutely required), avoiding nephrotoxic drugs, and possibly using statins perioperatively. Consultation with a pharmacist or nephrologist may be helpful in managing complex medication dosing issues after surgery.

SURGICAL SITE COMPLICATIONS: PREDICTING AND REDUCING RISK

In addition to the "medical" complications discussed above, colorectal resection surgery is associated with a variety of postoperative complications, most notably surgical site infections (SSIs) including anastomotic leak (**Table 3**).[2]

Thus far we have concentrated on identifying and optimizing those patients at risk for cardiac, pulmonary, and other "medical" complications. However, there is less evidence on how to optimize patients' condition preoperatively to prevent SSIs.

Table 3
Complications of 28,692 patients undergoing colorectal resection

Complication	n	%
Superficial SSI	2540	8.9
Ventilator >48 h	1400	4.9
Sepsis	1251	4.4
Pneumonia	1216	4.2
Urinary tract infection	1206	4.2
Organ space SSI	1140	4.0
Unplanned reintubation	1029	3.6
Septic shock	667	2.3
Deep venous thrombosis	532	1.9
Wound disruption	531	1.9
Deep SSI	509	1.8
Bleeding requiring transfusion	310	1.1
Acute renal failure	294	1.0
Progressive renal insufficiency	261	0.9
Cardiac arrest	253	0.9
Pulmonary embolism	211	0.7
Stroke	116	0.4
Myocardial infarction	111	0.4
Mortality	1142	4.0

Data from national ACS-NSQIP database; patients could experience more than one of the listed complications.
Abbreviation: CVA, cerebrovascular accident.
Adapted from Bilimoria KY, Cohen ME, Ingraham AM, et al. Effect of postdischarge morbidity and mortality on comparisons of hospital surgical quality. Ann Surg 2010;252(1):183–90.

SSIs are extremely common and costly after colorectal resection.[52] Risk factors for SSI may include ASA score, obesity, tobacco use, COPD, surgical wound class, age, blood loss, longer operative duration, and intraoperative contamination.[52] SSIs were prospectively studied among 534 patients undergoing colorectal resection in a 24-hospital prospective study in Switzerland (2008–2010).[53] Based on multivariable analysis, 4 significant risk factors were identified: (1) contamination class III to IV, (2) obesity, (3) open (vs laparoscopic) surgery, and (4) ASA grade III to IV.[53] Based on these results, a simple scoring system was created that predicted both all SSIs and organ–space SSIs (**Fig. 1**). Patients with multiple risk factors had very high rates of SSIs. It is notable that these factors are modifiable only to a limited extent in the preoperative setting, other than encouraging weight loss before operations that are elective.

Anastomotic leak is a surgeon's most dreaded complication after colorectal resection. Risk factors for anastomotic leak have been reported in a variety of mainly retrospective studies and may include sex, ASA class, obesity, alcohol abuse, smoking, steroid use, operative duration, low rectal anastomosis, blood loss, transfusion, and fecal contamination.[54] Risk factors for anastomotic leak were studied *prospectively* in 51 US hospitals participating in a trial of perioperative antibiotic prophylaxis.[55] Of the 672 patients evaluated, 3.6% had anastomotic leak, and the risk factors in univariate analysis included low albumin level (<3.5 g/dL), longer operation, steroid use, and male sex. However, in multivariable analysis, only low albumin level and male sex were independent risk factors, whereas steroid use was of borderline significance ($P = .06$).[55] Not significant in this study were BMI, COPD, smoking, diabetes, age, and rectal (vs colon) resection.[55] However, another research has demonstrated that low pelvic anastomosis is associated with higher anastomotic leak rates, compared with high colorectal anastomosis.[56]

In another publication that prospectively studied anastomotic leak after colectomy using a detailed multihospital clinical registry, only fecal contamination and higher blood loss were independently associated with anastomotic leak.[54] Factors in operative care that may reduce leak rates include routine leak testing[57] and diverting ileostomy for low rectal anastomosis,[58–60] which decreases symptomatic leak rates and

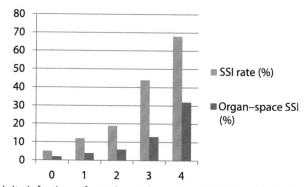

Fig. 1. Surgical site infections after colorectal resection. COLA (contamination, obesity, laparoscopic, and ASA class) score = 1 point each for contamination class III to IV, obesity, open (vs laparoscopic) surgery, and ASA grade III to IV. (*Data from* Gervaz P, Bandiera-Clerc C, Buchs NC, et al. Scoring system to predict the risk of surgical-site infection after colorectal resection. Br J Surg 2012;99(4):589–95; and Suding P, Jensen E, Abramson MA, et al. Definitive risk factors for anastomotic leaks in elective open colorectal resection. Arch Surg 2008;143(9):907–11; [discussion: 911–2].)

the need for reoperation in randomized trials. Again, these risk factors are in general not modifiable in the preoperative setting.

One risk factor for anastomotic leak and mortality that might be modifiable is malnutrition. Malnourished patients are at increased risk for morbidity and mortality; for example, a prospective study of 608 patients who underwent gastrointestinal surgery showed that malnourished patients had a postoperative complication rate of 40% (vs 15% for other patients).[61] However, evidence is mixed for the ability of preoperative nutrition interventions to change this risk.[62] Selected meta-analyses by Klein (1997) and colleagues[63] and Heyland (2001)[64] suggested that severely malnourished patients given preoperative nutrition support had a modest reduction in postoperative complications of about 10%. However, other studies and meta-analyses have not shown a beneficial effect.[62]

Helpful reviews by Salvino and colleagues[62] and Hebbar and colleagues[65] summarize the issue of preoperative nutrition support. Patients should be considered for preoperative nutrition support before colorectal resection *only* if *severely* malnourished and if operation can be safely postponed for 7 to 14 days, which is the duration of nutrition support that may improve outcomes.[62,66] The European Society for Clinical Nutrition and Metabolism has published guidelines for the use of enteral and parenteral nutrition in the preoperative setting.[66,67] It recommends 7 to 10 days of preoperative TPN for severely malnourished patients who cannot tolerate enteral nutrition.[67] Severe malnutrition is defined as weight loss greater than 10% to 15% within 6 months; BMI less than 18 kg/m^2; subjective global assessment, Grade C; or serum albumin level less than 30 g/L (without evidence of hepatic or renal dysfunction).[67] Oral or other enteral feedings are considered preferable where possible, and immunonutrition should be considered.[62,67,68]

Other potentially modifiable risk factors include alcohol and tobacco abuse. Smoking and "hazardous drinking" (3 or more drinks per day) are commonplace factors that have both been shown to be associated with increased complications after surgery.[30] The mechanism for this association is physiologic effect that smoking has on pulmonary, cardiovascular, immune, and healing function.[30] Heavy alcohol use has short-term effects on cardiac, immune, stress response, and muscular functioning, in addition to well-known effects on the liver, pancreas, and nervous system.[30] Physiologic effects of these drugs take up to 6 months to return to normal, but short-term abstinence programs have been studied in an effort to decrease surgical complications.

Tonnesen and colleagues[30] have reviewed the evidence for interventions to decrease the surgical risks of smoking and alcohol. There have been at least 6 trials of smoking cessation programs, with a subset studying the effect on rates of postoperative complications. Trials in general and orthopedic surgery showed dramatically decreased complication rates with smoking cessation of 3 to 8 weeks duration, but no effect from cessation for 1 to 3 weeks.[30] The 2002 randomized trial by Moller and colleagues[69] showed a reduction in overall complication rate from 52% in controls to 18% in the smoking intervention group ($P = .0003$), with dramatic reductions in wound-related complications (5% vs 31%, $P = .001$), cardiovascular complications (0% vs 10%, $P = .08$), and reoperation (4% vs 15%, $P = .07$).

For alcohol interventions, the evidence is mixed. The most promising randomized trial reported on an intensive intervention with a high rate of alcohol abstinence for 4 weeks before colorectal resection surgery. This study showed a dramatic decrease in complication rates after surgery (reduced from 74% to 31% ($P = .02$).[70] However, other studies have not replicated these success rates in abstinence or in complication rates, possibly due to weaker intervention designs with low rates of alcohol abstinence.[30] The investigators stress that intensive interventions with a goal of cessation (not cutting down) of smoking and drinking will likely result in decreased complication rates, whereas low-intensity interventions with poor compliance may have little effect.[30]

RISK REDUCTION THROUGH "PREHABILITATION"

An exciting development in perioperative care is the concept of *prehabilitation*: an intervention (physical training) to enhance functional capacity in anticipation of a forthcoming physiologic stressor (surgery).[71] Prehabilitation might target frail and/or elderly patients before elective operations, with a goal of decreasing complications and/or the functional decline that may follow surgery and its recovery.

In the setting of orthopedic surgery, several small studies have shown promising results of prehabilitation before knee and spine surgery.[72–74] Patients who underwent total knee arthroplasty randomized to prehabilitation had improved postoperative function and strength and decreased pain.[73] In spine surgery, a small randomized trial of a multimodal prehabilitation program showed that intervention patients had faster functional recovery, shorter length of stay, and higher satisfaction.[74] In colorectal surgery, Carli and colleagues[71] randomized 112 patients to a prehabilitation program of strengthening and stationary bicycle, versus a control regimen of walking and breathing exercises; however, they found no improvement in exercise capacity. The trial was limited by poor patient compliance, a relatively young patient population that may have limited benefit from the intervention, and the fact that both groups received an exercise intervention. Several clinical trials are in progress to study this promising method for optimizing patients' physical status before surgery.

SURGICAL RISK AND PATIENT EXPECTATIONS: COUNSELING THE HIGH-RISK SURGICAL PATIENT

Fortunately, most surgical consultations are made for clear operative indications and the most difficult doctor–patient communication task is to convey the rationale, process, and risks of the procedure. However, in some cases, the relative risks and benefits of operating are less clear and may require a leap of faith or impart a sense of foreboding. In these situations, surgical judgment must be exercised and may be challenged. Reaching out to colleagues, either in a multidisciplinary setting or by requesting a second opinion, can help to alleviate this burden. Although it may be true that "good judgment comes from experience; experience comes from bad judgment," not every lesson must be learned through first-hand experience.

A separate challenge arises when a patient or family does not yet understand that operative risks clearly outweigh the benefits.[75] Although there is little empirical support, several techniques to reduce long-term patient and family stress have been identified that have face value, especially if there is only a limited previous doctor–patient relationship.[76,77] First, the setting should be private, and the patient should have an advocate available; the patient or family should be able to sit; the surgeon should sit rather than stand, make good eye contact, and have ample time for the discussion. Second, to begin the discussion, the surgeon should initiate introductions and clarify the family relationships. The surgeon should judge the mood by eliciting what the patient and family know about the disease and expect in terms of next steps.[75] The importance of first hearing the patient's perspective cannot be overstated. If bad news is to be delivered, a "warning shot" such as "I have bad news" is warranted. The surgeon should then briefly review the results of previous tests and interventions. Next, the surgeon should communicate the recommendation not to operate and reasons why. The final step may be the most difficult: listen, permit the patient and family to react, and elicit their questions. It is strongly recommended not to leave the room or end the conversation if the patient and family are angry—rather, to keep listening and talking if possible. Third, the surgeon should follow-up at a later time to clarify any misperceptions and answer any further questions. After all, the stress of communicating bad news peaks for the surgeon just before speaking, but peaks for the patient and family at the end of the conversation and may persist for years.

SUMMARY

Risk assessment, and intervention when possible, may decrease patient morbidity and mortality for elective operations. Several strategies and evidence-based guidelines are available to assess organ system and surgical site risk. It is imperative for surgeons to not only be familiar with them but also use them routinely to optimize patient outcomes.

REFERENCES

1. Bentrem DJ, Cohen ME, Hynes DM, et al. Identification of specific quality improvement opportunities for the elderly undergoing gastrointestinal surgery. Arch Surg 2009;144(11):1013–20.
2. Bilimoria KY, Cohen ME, Ingraham AM, et al. Effect of postdischarge morbidity and mortality on comparisons of hospital surgical quality. Ann Surg 2010; 252(1):183–90.
3. Cohen ME, Bilimoria KY, Ko CY, et al. Effect of subjective preoperative variables on risk-adjusted assessment of hospital morbidity and mortality. Ann Surg 2009; 249(4):682–9.
4. Campbell DA Jr, Henderson WG, Englesbe MJ, et al. Surgical site infection prevention: the importance of operative duration and blood transfusion–results of the first American College of Surgeons-National Surgical Quality Improvement Program Best Practices Initiative. J Am Coll Surg 2008;207(6):810–20.
5. Saklad M. Grading of patients for surgical procedures. Anesthesiology 1941;2(3): 281–4.
6. Cohn SL. Cardiac risk stratification before noncardiac surgery. Cleve Clin J Med 2006;73(Suppl 1):S18–24.
7. Chapman J, Davies M, Wolff B, et al. Complicated diverticulitis: is it time to rethink the rules? Ann Surg 2005;242(4):576–81 [discussion: 581–73].
8. Rafferty J, Shellito P, Hyman NH, et al. Practice parameters for sigmoid diverticulitis. Dis Colon Rectum 2006;49(7):939–44.
9. Fleisher LA, Beckman JA, Brown KA, et al. 2009 ACCF/AHA focused update on perioperative beta blockade incorporated into the ACC/AHA 2007 guidelines on perioperative cardiovascular evaluation and care for noncardiac surgery. J Am Coll Cardiol 2009;54(22):e13–118.
10. Feisher LA, Beckman JA, Brown KA, et al. ACC/AHA 2007 guidelines on perioperative cardiovascular evaluation and care for noncardiac surgery: executive summary: a report of the American College of Cardiology/American Heart Association Task Force on Practice Guidelines (Writing Committee to Revise the 2002 Guidelines on Perioperative Cardiovascular Evaluation for Noncardiac Surgery) Developed in Collaboration With the American Society of Echocardiography, American Society of Nuclear Cardiology, Heart Rhythm Society, Society of Cardiovascular Anesthesiologists, Society for Cardiovascular Angiography and Interventions, Society for Vascular Medicine and Biology, and Society for Vascular Surgery. J Am Coll Cardiol 2007;50(17):1707–32.

11. McFalls EO, Ward HB, Moritz TE, et al. Coronary-artery revascularization before elective major vascular surgery. N Engl J Med 2004;351(27):2795–804.
12. Barnett S, Moonesinghe SR. Clinical risk scores to guide perioperative management. Postgrad Med J 2011;87(1030):535–41.
13. Dripps RD. New classification of physical status. Anesthesiol 1963;24(1):111.
14. Lee TH, Marcantonio ER, Mangione CM, et al. Derivation and prospective validation of a simple index for prediction of cardiac risk of major noncardiac surgery. Circulation 1999;100(10):1043–9.
15. Auerbach AD, Goldman L. Beta-blockers and reduction of cardiac events in noncardiac surgery: scientific review. JAMA 2002;287(11):1435–44.
16. Devereaux PJ, Yang H, Yusuf S, et al. Effects of extended-release metoprolol succinate in patients undergoing non-cardiac surgery (POISE trial): a randomised controlled trial. Lancet 2008;371(9627):1839–47.
17. Smetana GW, Cohn SL, Mercado DL, et al. Update in perioperative medicine. J Gen Intern Med 2006;21(12):1329–37.
18. Kaw R, Michota F, Jaffer A, et al. Unrecognized sleep apnea in the surgical patient: implications for the perioperative setting. Chest 2006;129(1):198–205.
19. Bapoje SR, Whitaker JF, Schulz T, et al. Preoperative evaluation of the patient with pulmonary disease. Chest 2007;132(5):1637–45.
20. Arozullah AM, Khuri SF, Henderson WG, et al. Development and validation of a multifactorial risk index for predicting postoperative pneumonia after major noncardiac surgery. Ann Intern Med 2001;135(10):847–57.
21. Arozullah AM, Daley J, Henderson WG, et al. Multifactorial risk index for predicting postoperative respiratory failure in men after major noncardiac surgery. The National Veterans Administration Surgical Quality Improvement Program. Ann Surg 2000;232(2):242–53.
22. Qaseem A, Snow V, Fitterman N, et al. Risk assessment for and strategies to reduce perioperative pulmonary complications for patients undergoing noncardiothoracic surgery: a guideline from the American College of Physicians. Ann Intern Med 2006;144(8):575–80.
23. Cook MW, Lisco SJ. Prevention of postoperative pulmonary complications. Int Anesthesiol Clin 2009;47(4):65–88.
24. Behr J. Optimizing preoperative lung function. Curr Opin Anaesthesiol 2001; 14(1):65–9.
25. Theadom A, Cropley M. Effects of preoperative smoking cessation on the incidence and risk of intraoperative and postoperative complications in adult smokers: a systematic review. Tob Control 2006;15(5):352–8.
26. Myers K, Hajek P, Hinds C, et al. Stopping smoking shortly before surgery and postoperative complications: a systematic review and meta-analysis. Arch Intern Med 2011;171(11):983–9.
27. Warner MA, Divertie MB, Tinker JH. Preoperative cessation of smoking and pulmonary complications in coronary artery bypass patients. Anesthesiology 1984;60(4):380–3.
28. Warner MA, Offord KP, Warner ME, et al. Role of preoperative cessation of smoking and other factors in postoperative pulmonary complications: a blinded prospective study of coronary artery bypass patients. Mayo Clin Proc 1989; 64(6):609–16.
29. Thomsen T, Villebro N, Moller AM. Interventions for preoperative smoking cessation. Cochrane Database Syst Rev 2010;(7):CD002294.
30. Tonnesen H, Nielsen PR, Lauritzen JB, et al. Smoking and alcohol intervention before surgery: evidence for best practice. Br J Anaesth 2009;102(3):297–306.

31. Lawrence VA, Cornell JE, Smetana GW. Strategies to reduce postoperative pulmonary complications after noncardiothoracic surgery: systematic review for the American College of Physicians. Ann Intern Med 2006;144(8):596–608.
32. Imberger G, McIlroy D, Pace NL, et al. Positive end-expiratory pressure (PEEP) during anaesthesia for the prevention of mortality and postoperative pulmonary complications. Cochrane Database Syst Rev 2010;(9):CD007922.
33. Nelson R, Edwards S, Tse B. Prophylactic nasogastric decompression after abdominal surgery. Cochrane Database Syst Rev 2007;(3):CD004929.
34. Brown SR, Goodfellow PB. Transverse verses midline incisions for abdominal surgery. Cochrane Database Syst Rev 2005;(4):CD005199.
35. Seiler CM, Deckert A, Diener MK, et al. Midline versus transverse incision in major abdominal surgery: a randomized, double-blind equivalence trial (POVATI: ISRCTN60734227). Ann Surg 2009;249(6):913–20.
36. Popping DM, Elia N, Marret E, et al. Protective effects of epidural analgesia on pulmonary complications after abdominal and thoracic surgery: a meta-analysis. Arch Surg 2008;143(10):990–9 [discussion: 1000].
37. Guimaraes MM, El Dib R, Smith AF, et al. Incentive spirometry for prevention of postoperative pulmonary complications in upper abdominal surgery. Cochrane Database Syst Rev 2009;(3):CD006058.
38. Pugh RN, Murray-Lyon IM, Dawson JL, et al. Transection of the oesophagus for bleeding oesophageal varices. Br J Surg 1973;60(8):646–9.
39. Mansour A, Watson W, Shayani V, et al. Abdominal operations in patients with cirrhosis: still a major surgical challenge. Surgery 1997;122(4):730–5 [discussion: 735–6].
40. Kamath PS, Wiesner RH, Malinchoc M, et al. A model to predict survival in patients with end-stage liver disease. Hepatology 2001;33(2):464–70.
41. Kim JJ, Dasika NL, Yu E, et al. Cirrhotic patients with a transjugular intrahepatic portosystemic shunt undergoing major extrahepatic surgery. J Clin Gastroenterol 2009;43(6):574–9.
42. Schneider CR, Cobb W, Patel S, et al. Elective surgery in patients with end stage renal disease: what's the risk? Am Surg 2009;75(9):790–3 [discussion: 793].
43. Drolet S, Maclean AR, Myers RP, et al. Morbidity and mortality following colorectal surgery in patients with end-stage renal failure: a population-based study. Dis Colon Rectum 2010;53(11):1508–16.
44. Eilers H, Liu KD, Gruber A, et al. Chronic kidney disease: implications for the perioperative period. Minerva Anestesiol 2010;76(9):725–36.
45. Josephs SA, Thakar CV. Perioperative risk assessment, prevention, and treatment of acute kidney injury. Int Anesthesiol Clin 2009;47(4):89–105.
46. Causey MW, Maykel JA, Hatch Q, et al. Identifying risk factors for renal failure and myocardial infarction following colorectal surgery. J Surg Res 2011;170(1): 32–7.
47. Chen M, Cook KD, Kheterpal I, et al. A triaxial probe for on-line proteolysis coupled with hydrogen/deuterium exchange-electrospray mass spectrometry. J Am Soc Mass Spectrom 2007;18(2):208–17.
48. Davis K, Kielar A, Jafari K. Effectiveness of ultrasound-guided radiofrequency ablation in the treatment of 36 renal cell carcinoma tumours compared with published results of using computed tomography guidance. Can Assoc Radiol J 2012;63(Suppl 3):S23–32.
49. Molnar AO, Coca SG, Devereaux PJ, et al. Statin use associates with a lower incidence of acute kidney injury after major elective surgery. J Am Soc Nephrol 2011; 22(5):939–46.

50. van den Berghe G, Wouters P, Weekers F, et al. Intensive insulin therapy in critically ill patients. N Engl J Med 2001;345(19):1359–67.
51. Trainor D, Borthwick E, Ferguson A. Perioperative management of the hemodialysis patient. Semin Dial 2011;24(3):314–26.
52. Murray BW, Huerta S, Dineen S, et al. Surgical site infection in colorectal surgery: a review of the nonpharmacologic tools of prevention. J Am Coll Surg 2010; 211(6):812–22.
53. Gervaz P, Bandiera-Clerc C, Buchs NC, et al. Scoring system to predict the risk of surgical-site infection after colorectal resection. Br J Surg 2012;99(4):589–95.
54. Leichtle SW, Mouawad NJ, Welch KB, et al. Risk factors for anastomotic leakage after colectomy. Dis Colon Rectum 2012;55(5):569–75.
55. Suding P, Jensen E, Abramson MA, et al. Definitive risk factors for anastomotic leaks in elective open colorectal resection. Arch Surg 2008;143(9):907–11 [discussion 911–2].
56. Vignali A, Fazio VW, Lavery IC, et al. Factors associated with the occurrence of leaks in stapled rectal anastomoses: a review of 1,014 patients. J Am Coll Surg 1997;185(2):105–13.
57. Kwon S, Morris A, Billingham R, et al. Routine leak testing in colorectal surgery in the surgical care and outcomes assessment program. Arch Surg 2012;147(4):345–51.
58. Chude GG, Rayate NV, Patris V, et al. Defunctioning loop ileostomy with low anterior resection for distal rectal cancer: should we make an ileostomy as a routine procedure? A prospective randomized study. Hepatogastroenterology 2008; 55(86–87):1562–7.
59. Matthiessen P, Hallbook O, Rutegard J, et al. Defunctioning stoma reduces symptomatic anastomotic leakage after low anterior resection of the rectum for cancer: a randomized multicenter trial. Ann Surg 2007;246(2):207–14.
60. Montedori A, Cirocchi R, Farinella E, et al. Covering ileo-or colostomy in anterior resection for rectal carcinoma. Cochrane Database Syst Rev 2010;(5):CD006878.
61. Schiesser M, Muller S, Kirchhoff P, et al. Assessment of a novel screening score for nutritional risk in predicting complications in gastro-intestinal surgery. Clin Nutr 2008;27(4):565–70.
62. Salvino RM, Dechicco RS, Seidner DL. Perioperative nutrition support: who and how. Cleve Clin J Med 2004;71(4):345–51.
63. Klein S, Kinney J, Jeejeebhoy K, et al. Nutrition support in clinical practice: review of published data and recommendations for future research directions. National Institutes of Health, American Society for Parenteral and Enteral Nutrition, and American Society for Clinical Nutrition. JPEN J Parenter Enteral Nutr 1997;21(3):133–56.
64. Heyland DK, Montalvo M, Mac Donald S, et al. Total parenteral nutrition in the surgical patient: a meta-analysis. Can J Surg 2001;44(2):102–11.
65. Hebbar R, Harte B. Do preoperative nutritional interventions improve outcomes in malnourished patients undergoing elective surgery? Cleve Clin J Med 2007; 74(Suppl 1):S8–10.
66. Weimann A, Braga M, Harsanyi L, et al. ESPEN guidelines on enteral nutrition: surgery including organ transplantation. Clin Nutr 2006;25(2):224–44.
67. Braga M, Ljungqvist O, Soeters P, et al. ESPEN guidelines on parenteral nutrition: surgery. Clin Nutr 2009;28(4):378–86.
68. Gustafsson UO, Ljungqvist O. Perioperative nutritional management in digestive tract surgery. Curr Opin Clin Nutr Metab Care 2011;14(5):504–9.
69. Moller AM, Villebro N, Pedersen T, et al. Effect of preoperative smoking intervention on postoperative complications: a randomised clinical trial. Lancet 2002; 359(9301):114–7.

70. Tonnesen H, Rosenberg J, Nielsen HJ, et al. Effect of preoperative abstinence on poor postoperative outcome in alcohol misusers: randomised controlled trial. BMJ 1999;318(7194):1311–6.

71. Carli F, Charlebois P, Stein B, et al. Randomized clinical trial of prehabilitation in colorectal surgery. Br J Surg 2010;97(8):1187–97.

72. Jaggers JR, Simpson CD, Frost KL, et al. Prehabilitation before knee arthroplasty increases postsurgical function: a case study. J Strength Cond Res 2007;21(2): 632–4.

73. Topp R, Swank AM, Quesada PM, et al. The effect of prehabilitation exercise on strength and functioning after total knee arthroplasty. PM R 2009;1(8):729–35.

74. Nielsen PR, Jorgensen LD, Dahl B, et al. Prehabilitation and early rehabilitation after spinal surgery: randomized clinical trial. Clin Rehabil 2010;24(2):137–48.

75. Loewy EH. Talking with patients. Textbook of healthcare ethics. New York: Plenium Press; 1996. p. 192–5.

76. Miller SJ, Hope T, Talbot DC. The development of a structured rating schedule (the BAS) to assess skills in breaking bad news. Br J Cancer 1999;80(5–6): 792–800.

77. Ptacek JT, Eberhardt TL. Breaking bad news. A review of the literature. JAMA 1996;276(6):496–502.

Fast-Track Pathways in Colorectal Surgery

Paul J. Chestovich, MD[a], Anne Y. Lin, MD[b], James Yoo, MD[c],*

KEYWORDS

- Fast-track • Enhanced recovery after surgery • ERAS • Colorectal surgery

KEY POINTS

- Enhanced recovery after surgery (ERAS) or "fast-track" pathways are a multimodal approach to the perioperative management of patients undergoing colorectal surgery designed to improve the overall quality of care.
- Typical fast-track management includes proper patient selection, avoidance of bowel preparation unless indicated, multimodal pain management including epidural catheters, use of a laparoscopic approach when possible, avoidance of excessive fluid administration, early diet advancement and ambulation, and adherence to Surgical Care Improvement Project (SCIP) measures.
- Fast-track protocols are safe for patients and offer improvement in intestinal recovery and hospital discharge.
- A higher rate of hospital readmissions should be expected, although the overall hospital days will be lower than in standard perioperative management.

INTRODUCTION

Fast-track pathways, also known as ERAS pathways, were first introduced in the mid-1990's and are a more recent addition to the care of patients undergoing colorectal procedures.[1] The purpose of these pathways is to use current evidence in a streamlined multidisciplinary manner with the aim of minimizing surgical pain and enhancing recovery, leading to fewer complications, more rapid hospital discharge, and improved overall outcomes. These pathways encompass all facets of perioperative care, including preoperative planning, intraoperative management, and postoperative

[a] Department of Surgery, David Geffen School of Medicine, University of California Los Angeles, 757 Westwood Plaza, B711, Los Angeles, CA 90095, USA; [b] Department of Surgery, David Geffen School of Medicine, University of California Los Angeles, 10833 Le Conte, 72-247 CHS, Los Angeles, CA 90095, USA; [c] Department of Surgery, David Geffen School of Medicine, University of California, Los Angeles, 10833 Le Conte Avenue, 72-253 CHS, Los Angeles, CA 90095, USA
* Corresponding author.
E-mail address: jayoo@mednet.ucla.edu

Surg Clin N Am 93 (2013) 21–32
http://dx.doi.org/10.1016/j.suc.2012.09.003
0039-6109/13/$ – see front matter © 2013 Elsevier Inc. All rights reserved.

care. Success is achieved by making evidence-based management decisions aimed to expedite recovery and minimize complications after surgery, which ultimately decreases the use of hospital resources and health care costs.

Several small trials have been performed in the past several years comparing traditional perioperative management with a fast-track approach in colorectal surgery.[2–8] These studies demonstrated more rapid return of bowel function, shorter inpatient hospital stays, and fewer complications, although 2 studies[3,8] noted an increased rate of readmissions after fast-track surgery. Systematic review and meta-analysis has supported these findings with decreased hospital stay and no change in mortality, complications, or readmissions.[9] From this information, fast-track protocols are a safe useful tool for any surgeon performing colorectal procedures.

PREOPERATIVE EVALUATION AND PATIENT SELECTION

Proper patient selection is the first and perhaps most important component of a fast-track pathway. Not all patients should be considered for this type of management. The best candidates for fast-track protocol are primarily healthy individuals requiring straightforward procedures for diverticulitis, polyps, or nonobstructive malignancy (**Box 1**). Generally, any patient with American Society of Anesthesiologists (ASA) score 1 or 2 and select ASA 3 patients may be included. Finally, the patient should be well informed and amenable to fast-track management because active patient participation will directly affect the success of the program. In ideal circumstances, the protocol should be discussed with the patient in a preoperative clinic visit, and the goals, advantages, and risks discussed in detail.

Box 1
Indications and contraindications to fast-track management in colorectal surgery

Ideal patients for fast-track management

Straightforward elective procedures

ASA 1, 2, possibly 3

Ambulatory preoperatively

Good nutritional status

No prior abdominal surgery

Compliant, reliable, and amenable to fast-track management

Relative contraindications—use fast-track management with caution

Contraindication to epidural analgesia

Psychiatric issues

Poor social support

Difficult or unconventional procedure

Absolute contraindications to fast-track management

Emergent procedures (obstruction, perforation, ischemia)

ASA 4 or higher

Patients who are nonmobile or have limited mobility

Severe malnutrition

Noncompliant or reluctant to participate in the fast-track program

There are also several patient groups in which fast-track management is inadvisable. These include patients who are malnourished, immobile, or minimally mobile. Patients requiring emergent procedures should also be avoided, such as for ischemia, obstruction, or perforation. Medical comorbidities should be considered, and all patients with ASA 4 or higher and some ASA 3 patients would not be well suited for fast-track management. The specific procedure should be considered in the decision, and difficult procedures, such as those requiring extensive dissection or lysis of adhesions, would be best managed via standard postoperative protocols. Owing to the higher readmission rates after discharge from fast-track protocols, a patient's social support and psychiatric history should be considered, and patients who may be unreliable, or may have difficulty returning for complications or follow-up, should be fast-tracked with caution.

BOWEL PREPARATION

Mechanical bowel preparation before elective colorectal surgery was previously considered the standard of care for decades. It was thought to decrease infectious complications and anastomotic dehiscence by decreasing intraluminal fecal mass and bacterial load. Although tolerated by most patients, cathartic bowel preparation may cause dehydration and potentially severe electrolyte toxicities, especially in elderly patients with renal insufficiency,[10] and should not be treated lightly.

Recently, use of bowel preparation has been extensively studied. Meta-analyses of multiple trials have concluded that bowel preparation is unnecessary and fails to decrease infectious complications or improve outcomes after colorectal surgery.[11–13] Many surgeons continue using bowel preparation for patients requiring a low rectal anastomosis because of concern that the column of stool may cause anastomotic disruption. Detailed subgroup analysis comparing patients with and without bowel preparation has failed to find a difference in anastomotic leakage, infectious complications, mortality, peritonitis, or reoperation in both colon and rectal procedures. Furthermore, no difference was found between oral bowel preparation and enemas.[11] However, in patients receiving cathartic bowel preparation, the addition of oral antibiotics may reduce infectious complications compared with prep alone.[14]

Current clinical practice guidelines from the Canadian Society of Colon and Rectal surgeons endorses omitting bowel preparation for open left-sided and right-sided colon surgery but has found insufficient evidence for patients undergoing laparoscopic or low anterior resection procedures. Some surgeons may prefer a bowel preparation in certain scenarios, such as resection of a small nontattooed lesion (<2 cm), or if there may be a need to perform an intraoperative colonoscopy. This preference is particularly relevant to laparoscopic procedures when the location of a lesion is uncertain and manual palpation is not possible. Some surgeons may also prefer to use a bowel preparation in all laparoscopic procedures to make colon manipulation easier, and guidelines published by the Society of Alimentary Gastrointestinal Endoscopic Surgeons (SAGES) have endorsed the use of bowel preparations in laparoscopic colorectal surgery.[15]

At present there is no study specifically investigating the use of cathartic bowel preparation in a fast-track pathway, although some studies investigating fast-track protocols omitted bowel preparation,[6,16] whereas others included a standard bowel preparation.[4,8] It is up to the specific surgeon as to the inclusion of a bowel preparation, but the general recommendation is to avoid routine use unless specifically indicated.[2]

LAPAROSCOPIC VERSUS OPEN PROCEDURES

Laparoscopy has revolutionized the modern practice of surgery and has become a standard method for performing colon resection. Properly performed laparoscopic colon surgery achieves appropriate surgical margins, accurate staging, and equivalent survival when compared with open surgery.[17] A meta-analysis of long-term outcomes comparing laparoscopic to open colorectal surgery for cancer resection found no difference in tumor recurrence, cancer-related mortality, as well as reoperations for hernia or adhesions.[18]

When considering inclusion in a fast-track protocol, the laparoscopic approach to colon resection offers several advantages. In trials comparing laparoscopic and open colon surgery, patients undergoing laparoscopic colon resection have less postoperative pain, fewer wound infections, shorter time to return of bowel function, and shorter hospital stays. There is no difference in reoperation rate or postoperative complications, but the procedure time is longer in laparoscopic procedures.[19] Of note, this difference in operative time between the 2 approaches has steadily decreased as further experience with minimally invasive techniques has accrued over time.

For these reasons, a laparoscopic approach should be preferred in the establishment of a fast-track pathway, provided the patient is suitable for laparoscopy. However, some groups have successfully implemented a fast-track pathway using both open and laparoscopic techniques, with similar outcomes in bowel recovery, hospital stay, morbidity, and mortality.[20] Thus, although the laparoscopic approach will likely yield more rapid return to normal activity and hospital discharge, an open surgical approach should not exclusively preclude inclusion in a fast-track protocol.

FLUID MANAGEMENT

Standard fluid management in colorectal surgery involves liberal fluid administration during both intraoperative and postoperative periods. However, this practice has been challenged recently because excess intravenous (IV) fluid is suspected to increase interstitial volume and total body weight, leading to ambulation difficulty, cardiopulmonary dysfunction, and impaired tissue oxygenation. These effects are suspected to contribute to anastomotic breakdown and wound infections.[21] For this reason, some institutions have adopted a protocol of fluid restriction in the perioperative management of colorectal procedures.

Several randomized clinical trials have addressed the issue of fluid administration in surgical patients. Two trials of patients undergoing colorectal surgery comparing "standard" and "restricted" fluid administration found fewer complications in fluid-restricted patients,[22,23] whereas another found no difference in complications, discharge time, and diet advancement.[24] An additional trial comparing "restricted" with "excess" fluid administration found no difference in hospital stay or complications, but fluid-restricted patients had less hypoxia and improved pulmonary function.

Unfortunately, the specific definition of "standard," "excess," and "restricted" fluid administration is rather nebulous. A detailed description of perioperative fluid management is beyond the scope of this article, but in general, "standard" perioperative fluid management is divided into intraoperative and postoperative periods. Intraoperatively, insensible fluid losses are replaced 2 mL/kg/h and third-space losses are replaced 1 to 3 mL/kg/h for minor surgical trauma (eg, hernia repair) and up to 6 to 8 mL/kg/h for major surgical trauma (including colon resection procedures). Patients who are nil per os (NPO) preoperatively without hydration have a fluid deficit at the start of the procedure, which is replaced according to maintenance fluid rates. In patients receiving bowel preparations, this deficit may be even greater. Blood loss is replaced at 3 mL of crystalloid for every 1 mL of blood lost. Postoperatively, maintenance fluid is administered at 4 mL/kg/h for the first 10 kg of body weight, 2 mL/kg/h for the next 10 kg, and 1 mL/kg/h for each kg beyond 20 kg. Vital signs are monitored, with a urine output goal of 0.5 to 1 mL/kg/h.[25] Fluid administration is then altered as clinically necessary.

Owing to the differences in fluid administration in different trials, 1 meta-analysis[26] defined "standard" fluid management using calculated estimates of fluid requirements based on the patient weight, length, and type of procedure. A range was defined as the mean value ±10%. Fluid "restriction" was any amount more than 10% beneath the low limit of this range, and "excess" fluid administration was any amount more than 10% above the upper limit. This study failed to find any significant differences in mortality, anastomotic leakage, or wound infection, but overall morbidity was decreased when intraoperative fluids were restricted. Decreases in morbidity were also found in patients using intraoperative esophageal Doppler-guided fluid management, although this method is experimental and not in widespread use.

Although it is impossible to devise a universal fluid administration protocol that is satisfactory for all patients, the avoidance of excessive fluid administration is a prudent strategy, with fluid boluses reserved for clinical indications of hypovolemia. This strategy will decrease perioperative third spacing, likely facilitate a more rapid hospital discharge, and would thus be advocated in a fast-track protocol. It is imperative that any fluid administration protocol be developed in conjunction with the anesthesia team because the intraoperative fluid volume given seems to have the greatest effect on morbidity. Furthermore, the patient's specific health status should be considered, and fluid restriction should be used with caution or avoided completely in patients with renal dysfunction, diabetes mellitus, history of alcohol overconsumption, and inflammatory bowel disease. Similarly, a careful approach should ensue in patients who may not tolerate bolus fluid administration well, such as those with underlying congestive heart failure, although admittedly, both strategies involve inherent risks in this population.

PAIN MANAGEMENT

Pain management is another significant element of surgical perioperative care and is best accomplished through cooperation between patients, nurses, anesthesiologists, pain specialists, and surgeons. There are several methods available for pain control, but most patients who undergo colorectal surgery receive either patient-controlled opioid analgesia (PCA) techniques or indwelling continuous epidural analgesia (CEA) with opioid or local anesthesia infusion for pain control. PCA has the benefit of providing systemic delivery of opioids, which acts on opiate receptors in the brain and body, and yields immediate pain relief. It also allows patients to self-titrate to their individual pain level, and its use is associated with high levels of patient satisfaction.[27] However, disadvantages include systemic opioid effects including respiratory depression, sedation, nausea and vomiting, and prolongation of postoperative ileus.

Continuous epidural anesthesia, also known as neuraxial anesthesia, has the benefit of delivering a combination of local and opioid analgesia directly to the dorsal horn of the spinal cord, thus delivering pain relief without systemic opioid effects.[28] Negative side effects of CEA include pruritis, urinary retention, and arterial hypotension, often necessitating additional fluid administration. CEA also requires placement of a catheter in the epidural space, an additional invasive procedure that can be associated with rare complications of neuraxial bleeding or hematoma (approximately 1 in

150,000 cases).[29] CEA may be used safely in conjunction with pharmacologic deep venous thrombosis (DVT) prophylaxis, and practice guidelines for proper use are available from the American Society of Regional Anesthesia.[29]

Several trials have investigated the potential benefits of PCA and CEA in patients undergoing colorectal surgery with regard to pain control, resumption of diet, resolution of ileus, and hospital discharge. Most trials have found a benefit with CEA for the end points pain control, diet resumption, and ileus resolution but have failed to demonstrate a decrease in hospital stay.[30,31] One study demonstrated a higher rate of prolonged ileus[32] in CEA patients while showing superior pain control, diet advancement, and resolution of ileus with spinal anesthesia. Two different meta-analyses[33,34] and one systematic review[35] found significant improvement in pain control with CEA compared with PCA. Only 1 meta-analysis found improvement in ileus resolution with CEA,[33] although it was also associated with a higher incidence of urinary retention, pruritis, and hypotension.

Although a definitive decrease in hospital stay has yet to be demonstrated, CEA use does improve pain control when compared with PCA, and there is reasonable evidence to suggest that it hastens resolution of ileus and helps diet advancement. We would advocate for CEA use in fast-track pathways in patients without contraindications. Superiority of CEA seems to be greatest in the first 2 to 3 postoperative days (PODs), so routine removal of CEA after POD 2 or 3 may be a useful strategy in a fast-track pathway.[30,32] If not anticipated, waiting for catheter removal could actually delay discharge by an additional day, thereby nullifying any benefit achieved by earlier resumption of diet and resolution of ileus.

Other modalities of pain control include local control by wound infiltration with local anesthesia. This is an easy step with low morbidity and may help decrease doses of CEA or PCA required to achieve adequate pain control. Nonsteroidal antiinflammatory drugs (NSAIDs) such as ibuprofen (Motrin) or ketorolac (Toradol) are also useful in controlling postoperative pain and have the added benefit of not worsening postoperative ileus. Ketorolac is parenterally administered and particularly useful in the immediate postoperative period. It acts through prostaglandin inhibition and has a similar time to onset as IV morphine but has longer duration (6–8 h) and minimal central nervous system effects of respiratory depression, sedation, nausea, and vomiting. Side effects include inhibition of platelet aggregation, gastrointestinal (GI) ulceration, and renal toxicity and so should be avoided or used cautiously in patients with increased risk of bleeding or renal dysfunction. Acetaminophen can also be used and is available in both oral and IV formulation. It is particularly useful as an adjunct to oral narcotic pain medication. Because many oral preparations already contain acetaminophen, the total daily dose should be monitored to avoid liver toxicity.

DIET ADVANCEMENT

A central tenet of a fast-track protocol is diet advancement to the patient's preoperative regimen. All patients considered for fast-track management should have a functional nonobstructed GI tract immediately before their colorectal procedure. Gastric drainage tubes have been shown to increase pulmonary complications, delay bowel function, and increase length of stay without any difference in anastomotic breakdown and so should not be used without evidence of ileus or obstruction.[36] If they are used intraoperatively for technical purposes, they should be removed as soon as the surgery is completed.

Specific protocols for advancement of diet vary, and no protocol will be perfect for all patients and procedures. Early enteral feeding has been studied extensively, and multiple trials[37–40] and a meta-analysis[41] have shown it to be safe and possibly beneficial for patient recovery from colorectal surgery. Most fast-track protocols allow at least some liquids immediately after surgery, some with addition of protein shakes for added nutrition. Patients will then advance to their regular diet by POD 2 to 3, some with a soft or blenderized diet in between, whereas other protocols allow for discharge when tolerating a full liquid diet. The addition of alvimopan (Entereg), a highly selective μ-receptor antagonist, has been shown to improve recovery of intestinal function without adversely affecting postoperative analgesia[42] and may be useful in a fast-track protocol.[43,44]

DRAINAGE

Anastomotic drainage is a long-standing controversial topic, and many studies have been conducted investigating its merits. Meta-analyses of trials in this topic have failed to show a benefit for routine drainage,[45,46] and routine anastomotic drainage is not typically part of a fast-track pathway. However, if clinically indicated, drain placement should not interfere with a standard fast-track protocol.

READMISSIONS

Readmission after discharge after colorectal surgery has been a significant drawback to adoption of fast-track pathways. Several studies comparing fast-track to conventional pathways have demonstrated higher readmission rates for patients in the fast-track group when compared with the conventional group.[3–5,8] Importantly, despite the increased readmissions, the total hospital days are still lower for patients managed by fast-track pathways. It is generally difficult to predict readmissions after colorectal surgery,[47] and most readmissions occur after POD 5 to 7, indicating that a longer hospitalization may not have prevented the readmission.[3,5] However, a slightly higher readmission rate should be anticipated when adopting a fast-track protocol. It is prudent to notify patients of this preoperatively and verify that patients are reliable, have good social support structure, and are able to return to the hospital should concerns or complications arise.

SCIP MEASURES

SCIP is a widely publicized initiative by the Center for Medicare and Medicaid Services (CMS) and Centers for Disease Control (CDC) to reduce the number of postoperative complications.[44] Targeted events include surgical site infections (SSI), adverse cardiac events, DVT and thromboembolism, and postoperative pneumonia. All applicable measures currently recommended and recorded through SCIP can be incorporated into a fast-track protocol.

- SSI prevention—Appropriate hair clipping, appropriate antibiotic administration within 1 hour before skin incision and discontinued within 24 hours, and immediate postoperative normothermia (T >98.6°F within 1 hour of leaving operating room).
- Adverse cardiac events—Patients on preoperative beta-blockade should be continued throughout the operation and perioperative period.
- DVT—Appropriate thromboembolism prophylaxis (low-dose unfractionated heparin 5000 units twice or thrice daily or low-molecular-weight heparin combined with intermittent pneumatic compression or graduated compression stockings).

PROTOCOL MODIFICATIONS

No perioperative management protocol is perfect for all patients. The guidelines presented in this article are simply meant to act as a framework to standardize the postoperative management, minimize complications, and decrease hospital stays, and protocol deviations are expected. Each patient should be closely followed throughout his or her hospitalization, and protocol changes should be made for proper clinical indications. For example, patients with more severe pain may require an epidural or PCA for a longer time and those with nausea and abdominal distension may have prolonged ileus and will thus require longer hospitalization. The fast-track protocol should not usurp good clinical judgment. Even accounting for protocol deviations and hospital readmissions, the overall number of hospital days will likely decrease when a fast-track protocol is instituted.

SUMMARY

Fast-track protocols were developed to use current evidence to streamline perioperative management for patients undergoing colorectal surgery, decrease complications, reduce hospital resource use, and improve the overall quality of care. Most fast-track protocols include careful patient selection and preoperative planning, avoidance of bowel preparation, avoidance of excessive fluid, laparoscopic approach to surgery, multimodal pain management, early ambulation, and rapid diet advancement. Despite the faster return to normal function and discharge, a higher readmission rate is expected, although the overall hospital days are still fewer than with standard management techniques.

Sample fast-track pathway

Preoperative

Medical risk stratification and workup.

Lesion marked with tattoo, if possible.

Bowel preparation for small lesions or anticipating intraoperative colonoscopy.

Review the surgical procedure, plan of care, and milestones with patients, their families, and the anesthesia and nursing teams.

NPO after midnight before surgery.

Place epidural catheter for postoperative pain control.

Appropriate DVT and antibiotic administration.

Intraoperative

Prefer laparoscopic approach when feasible and safe.

Place Foley catheter for bladder drainage.

Appropriate antibiotic and thromboembolism prophylaxis.

Avoid excessive fluid; boluses for clinical indications.

Proper blood glucose level control.

Remove orogastric tube placed for technical purposes at the end of case.

No routine drainage unless clinically indicated.

POD 0

Maintenance IV fluids.

Return to normothermia within 1 hour of leaving operation room.

Restricted liquid diet (30–60 mL/h).

Begin ambulation out of bed to chair.

Begin incentive spirometry.

POD 1

Unrestricted liquid diet.

Heplock IV when tolerating liquids (>500 mL intake).

Monitor urine output for 0.5 mL/kg/h; bolus if clinically indicated.

Continue incentive spirometry and ambulation out of bed in hallway.

Discontinue bladder catheter.

Discontinue prophylactic antibiotics within 24 hours.

Consider scheduled acetaminophen or NSAIDS (ketorolac, ibuprofen) or for pain control if indicated.

POD 2

Advance to soft or regular preoperative diet.

Continue ambulation, incentive spirometry, and other perioperative care.

Schedule epidural catheter removal in the early morning.

Start oral pain regimen.

POD 3 to 4

Remove epidural catheter.

Discharge home if afebrile with stable vital signs, tolerating diet, urinating spontaneously, and pain controlled on oral regimen and if the patient is amenable to discharge.

REFERENCES

1. Kehlet H. Fast-track colorectal surgery. Lancet 2008;371:791–3.
2. Kehlet H, Wilmore DW. Evidence-based surgical care and the evolution of fast-track surgery. Ann Surg 2008;248:189–98.
3. Jakobsen DH, Sonne E, Basse L, et al. Convalescence after colonic resection with fast-track versus conventional care. Scand J Surg 2004;93:24–8.
4. Feo CV, Lanzara S, Sortini D, et al. Fast track postoperative management after elective colorectal surgery: a controlled trial. Am Surg 2009;75:1247–51.
5. Basse L, Thorbøl JE, Løssl K, et al. Colonic surgery with accelerated rehabilitation or conventional care. Dis Colon Rectum 2004;47:271–8.
6. Muller S, Zalunardo M, Hubner M, et al. A fast-track program reduces complications and lengths of hospital stay after open colonic surgery. Gastroenterology 2009;136:842–7.
7. Wichmann MW, Eben R, Angele MK, et al. Fast-track rehabilitation in elective colorectal surgery patients: a prospective clinical and immunological single-centre study. ANZ J Surg 2007;77:502–7.
8. Khoo CK, Vickery CJ, Forsyth N, et al. A prospective randomized controlled trial of multimodal perioperative management protocol in patients undergoing elective colorectal resection for cancer. Ann Surg 2007;245:867–72.
9. Wind J, Polle SW, Fung Kon Jin PH, et al. Systematic review of enhanced recovery programmes in colonic surgery. Br J Surg 2006;93:800–9.

10. Barkun A, Chiba N, Enns R, et al. Commonly used preparations for colonoscopy: efficacy, tolerability and safety – a Canadian Association of Gastroenterology position paper. Can J Gastroenterol 2006;20:699–710.

11. Guenaga KF, Matos D, Wille-Jorgensen P. Mechanical bowel preparation for elective colorectal surgery [review]. Cochrane Database Syst Rev 2011;(9):CD001544.

12. Pineda CE, Shelton AA, Hernandez-Boussard T, et al. Mechanical bowel preparation in intestinal surgery: a meta-analysis and review of the literature. J Gastrointest Surg 2008;12:2037–44.

13. Slim K, Vicaut E, Launay-Savary MV, et al. Updated systematic review and meta-analysis of randomized clinical trials on the role of mechanical bowel preparation before colorectal surgery. Ann Surg 2009;249:203–9.

14. Englesbe MJ, Brooks L, Kubus J, et al. A statewide assessment of surgical site infection following colectomy: the role of oral antibiotics. Ann Surg 2010;252: 514–20.

15. Society of American Gastrointestinal and Endoscopic Surgeons. Guidelines for laparoscopic resection of curable colon and rectal cancer. 2005. Available at: http://www.sages.org/publication/id/32/.

16. Vlug MS, Wind J, Hollmann MW, et al. Laparoscopy in combination with fast track multimodal management is the best perioperative strategy in patients undergoing colonic surgery: a randomized clinical trial (LAFA-study). Ann Surg 2011;254: 868–75.

17. Clinical Outcomes of Surgical Therapy Study Group. A comparison of laparoscopically assisted and open colectomy for colon cancer. N Engl J Med 2004; 350:2050–9.

18. Kuhry E, Schwenk W, Gaupset R, et al. Long-term results of laparoscopic colorectal cancer resection. Cochrane Database Syst Rev 2008;(4):CD003432.

19. Schwenk W, Haase O, Neudecker JJ, et al. Short term benefits for laparoscopic colorectal resection. Cochrane Database Syst Rev 2008;(4):CD003145.

20. Basse L, Jakobsen DH, Bardram L, et al. Functional recovery after open versus laparoscopic colonic resection: a randomized, blinded study. Ann Surg 2005; 241:416–23.

21. Holte K, Sharrock NE, Kehlet H. Pathophysiology and clinical implications of perioperative fluid excess. Br J Anaesth 2002;89:622–32.

22. Abraham-Nordling M, Hjern F, Pollack J, et al. Randomized clinical trial of fluid restriction in colorectal surgery. Br J Surg 2012;99:186–91.

23. Brandstrup B, Tønnesen H, Beier-Holgersen R, et al. Effects of intravenous fluid restriction on postoperative complications: comparison of two perioperative fluid regimens. A randomized assessor-blinded multicenter trial. Ann Surg 2003;238: 641–8.

24. MacKay G, Fearon K, McConnachie A, et al. Randomized clinical trial of the effect of postoperative intravenous fluid restriction on recovery after elective colorectal surgery. Br J Surg 2006;93:1469–74.

25. Morgan GE, Mikhail MS, Murray MJ. Fluid management and transfusion. In: Morgan GE Jr, Mikhail MS, Murray MJ, editors. Clinical anesthesiology. 4th edition. vol. 29. New York: The McGraw-Hill Companies; 2005. p. 690–707.

26. Rahbari NN, Zimmermann JB, Schmidt T, et al. Meta-analysis of standard, restrictive and supplemental fluid administration in colorectal surgery. Br J Surg 2009; 96:331–41.

27. Morgan GE, Mikhail MS, Murray MJ. Pain management. In: Clinical anesthesiology. 4th edition. vol. 18. p. 359–411.

28. Kleinman W, Mikhail M. Spinal, epidural, and caudal blocks. In: Clinical anesthesiology. 4th edition. vol. 16. p. 289–323.
29. Horlocker TT, Wedel DJ, Rowlingson JC, et al. Regional anesthesia in the patient receiving antithrombotic or thrombolytic therapy. American Society of Regional Anesthesia and Pain Medicine evidence-based guidelines (Third edition). Reg Anesth Pain Med 2010;35:64–101.
30. Carli F, Trudel JL, Belliveau P. The effect of intraoperative thoracic epidural anesthesia and postoperative analgesia on bowel function after colorectal surgery: a prospective, randomized trial. Dis Colon Rectum 2001;44: 1083–9.
31. Taqi A, Hong X, Mistraletti G, et al. Thoracic epidural analgesia facilitates the restoration of bowel function and dietary intake in patients undergoing laparoscopic colon resection using a traditional, nonaccelerated, perioperative care program. Surg Endosc 2007;21:247–52.
32. Levy BF, Scott MJ, Fawcett W, et al. Randomized clinical trial of epidural, spinal, or patient-controlled analgesia for patients undergoing laparoscopic colorectal surgery. Br J Surg 2010;98:1068–78.
33. Marret E, Remy C, Bonnet F. Meta-analysis of epidural analgesia versus parenteral opioid analgesia after colorectal surgery. Br J Surg 2007;94:665–73.
34. Werawatganon T, Charuluxananan S. Patient controlled intravenous opioid analgesia versus continuous epidural analgesia for pain after intra-abdominal surgery [review]. Cochrane Database Syst Rev 2005;(1):CD004088.
35. Levy BF, Tilney HS, Dowson HM, et al. A systematic review of postoperative analgesia following laparoscopic colorectal surgery. Colorectal Dis 2010;12: 5–15.
36. Verma R, Nelson RL. Prophylactic nasogastric decompression after major abdominal surgery [review]. Cochrane Database Syst Rev 2007;(3):CD004929.
37. Zhou T, Wu XT, Zhou YJ, et al. Early removing gastrointestinal decompression and early oral feeding improve patients' rehabilitation after colorectostomy. World J Gastroenterol 2006;12:2459–63.
38. Dag A, Colak T, Turkmenoglu O, et al. Randomized controlled trial evaluating early versus traditional oral feeding after colorectal surgery. Clinics 2011;66: 2001–5.
39. Han-Geurts IJ, Hop WC, Kok NF, et al. Randomized clinical trial of the impact of early enteral feeding on postoperative ileus and recovery. Br J Surg 2007;94: 555–61.
40. Reissman P, Teoh TA, Cohen SM, et al. Is early oral feeding safe after elective colorectal surgery? Ann Surg 1995;222:73–7.
41. Andersen HK, Lewis SJ, Thomas S. Early enteral nutrition within 24h of colorectal surgery versus later commencement of feeding for postoperative complications [review]. Cochrane Database Syst Rev 2011;(2):CD004080.
42. Curran MP, Robins GW, Scott LJ, et al. Alvimopan. Drugs 2008;68:2011–9.
43. Barletta JF, Asgeirsson T, El-Badawi KI, et al. Introduction of Alvimopan into an enhanced recovery protocol for colectomy offers benefit in open but not laparoscopic colectomy. J Laparoendosc Adv Surg Tech A 2011;21:887–91.
44. Jones RS, Brown C, Opelka F. Surgeon compensation: "Pay for performance," the American College of Surgeons National Surgical Quality Improvement Program, the Surgical Care Improvement Program, and other considerations. Surgery 2005;138:829–36.
45. De Jesus CE, Karliczek A, Matos D, et al. Prophylactic anastomotic drainage for colorectal surgery [review]. Cochrane Database Syst Rev 2008;(4):CD002100.

46. Urbach DR, Kennedy ED, Cohen MM. Colon and rectal anastomoses do not require routine drainage: a systematic review and meta-analysis. Ann Surg 1999;2:174–80.
47. Azimuddin K, Rosen L, Reed JF III, et al. Readmissions after colorectal surgery cannot be predicted. Dis Colon Rectum 2001;44:942–6.

Intraoperative Adjuncts in Colorectal Surgery

Husein Moloo, MD, MSc[a], David A. Etzioni, MD, MSHS[b],*

KEYWORDS

- Intraoperative adjuncts colorectal surgery • Omentoplasty • Intraabdominal drains
- Proximal diversion • Adhesion prevention • Wound closure technique

KEY POINTS

- More than 250,000 colorectal resections are performed annually in the United States, and 24% to 35% of these will develop a complication.
- The clinical and economic burden of these complications is enormous, and colorectal operations have been specifically highlighted as a leading cause of potentially preventable surgical morbidity.
- Approximately 3% of all laparotomies are done for small bowel obstruction and the need for resection during this surgery is associated most with previous colorectal surgery.
- Admissions for bowel obstruction (whether surgery is involved or not) cost over a billion dollars every year in the United States and similar high costs are seen in other countries.

INTRODUCTION

More than 250,000 colorectal resections are performed annually in the United States, and 24% to 35% of these will develop a complication.[1–4] The clinical and economic burden of these complications is enormous, and colorectal operations have been specifically highlighted as a leading cause of potentially preventable surgical morbidity.[4] This article focuses on intraoperative adjuncts that can be used in an attempt to improve outcomes after colon and rectal resections. Specifically, the evidence is reviewed regarding: (1) drains after pelvic surgery, (2) proximal diversion, (3) omental wrapping, (4) antiadhesion barriers and (5) wound closure technique.

DRAINS AFTER PELVIC SURGERY

A closed suction drain placed in the pelvis after a pelvic dissection has intuitive purpose. The most obvious purpose is to prevent deep organ space infection by

---

[a] Division of General Surgery, The Ottawa Hospital, Ottawa Hospital Research Institute, University of Ottawa, 737 Parkdale Avenue, Room 335, Ottawa, Ontario K1Y1J8, Canada; [b] Department of Surgery, Mayo Clinic College of Medicine, Mayo Clinic Arizona, 5777 East Mayo Boulevard, Phoenix, AZ 85054, USA
* Corresponding author.
E-mail address: etzioni.david@mayo.edu

Surg Clin N Am 93 (2013) 33–43
http://dx.doi.org/10.1016/j.suc.2012.09.007
0039-6109/13/$ – see front matter © 2013 Elsevier Inc. All rights reserved.

surgical.theclinics.com

minimizing the amount of fluid which stagnates in the pelvis, forming a potential medium for bacterial growth. Additionally, in cases of anastomotic dehiscence, a drain may help with early detection of leakage, as well as provide effective control and preclude the need for additional operative or percutaneous procedures.[5] On the other hand, there are potential problems associated with drain placement. A drain may conversely allow the entrance of bacteria, or be a source of mechanical problems related to its placement. The presence of a negative pressure drain in proximity to an anastomosis may actually contribute to the likelihood of leaks. Finally, there is evidence that a drain generally does not detect a neighboring anastomotic leak.[6]

In reviewing the accumulated evidence regarding the use of drains after pelvic surgery, it is critical to have a clear picture of which endpoints are salient. Deep space organ infection is likely the most important complication that is potentially prevented by the use of drains; however, an equally important endpoint is anastomotic leakage. Mortality is always an important endpoint to consider, but probably not pertinent to a discussion regarding the utility of drains. This is because the mechanisms by which a drain (or no drain) leads to mortality would almost universally be reflected in the complications of pelvic infection or anastomotic leakage.

In analyzing the effectiveness of pelvic drainage, it is important to restrict the review to only the results of randomized trials. A significant bias would be introduced by including cohort studies in which drains were used on a discretionary basis. Outside of surgeons who routinely use drains, operations in which a surgeon decided a pelvic drain was necessary are likely more complex and inherently more risky than those where a similar surgeon elected not to use a drain. Additionally, variability exists in multiple other factors surrounding drains, including type (ie, closed vs open), method of management (ie, irrigation vs none), and endpoint before removal (ie, time, volume).

There is a paucity of trials performed to date examining the putative benefits of drainage for pelvic surgery. Three studies, with a combined sample size of 291 subjects examined the use of closed suction drains in preventing leaks among subjects with colorectal anastomoses below the sacral promontory.[7–9] None of these three studies found a significant difference in leak rates, but this is not surprising. If one assumes, for the sake of argument, that the baseline leak rate of pelvic anastomoses is 7%, and that pelvic drainage lowered (or raised) this risk by 20% (to 5.6% or 8.4%), then an adequately powered study would require thousands of subjects in each arm to detect this level of difference. Hence, the difficulty with attaining Class I data on which to base recommendations.

Given the scarcity of randomized trial data regarding the use of closed suction drains in pelvic surgery, a cursory review of the largest cohort studies seems in order. Peeters and colleagues[5] performed an analysis of subjects treated as part of the Dutch TME (total mesorectal excision) trial, including a total of 924 subjects. Drains were placed at the discretion of the attending surgeon. Pelvic drainage was associated with a lower rate of symptomatic leakage (9.6% vs 23.5%, 792 vs 132 subjects). Also, subjects with a drain needed surgical intervention less often for leaks (56 out of 76 vs 30 out of 31). In a similarly large study, Yeh and colleagues[10] analyzed 978 subjects undergoing elective anterior resection for rectal cancer. They found a significantly higher rate of anastomotic leakage (adjusted odds ratio 9.1) with drain use, although it should be noted that in this study an irrigation-suction drain was used. On subset analysis, closed suction drains (used in 125 of 878 subjects) had no difference in leakage rates compared with no drainage.

Based on this review of the literature, there is no clear benefit or detriment associated with the routine use of closed suction drains in pelvic surgery. Does the absence of a demonstrable benefit imply that drains should not be used? The answer to this is clearly no; the accumulated evidence is not sufficient to support this type of statement. Most research has focused on the association between drains and leakage; while little attention has been paid to the impact of drains on the risk of abscess formation. Until better research emerges to clarify the role of pelvic drainage, the use of closed-suction drains is discretionary and based on surgeon preference.

PROXIMAL DIVERSION

The use of proximal diversion above a high-risk anastomosis is an exercise in surgical judgment. Proximal diversion has the potential to minimize clinical leaks, as well as facilitate nonsurgical management when leakage does occur. This benefit is diminished by the risks inherent in a second operation. The decision to divert (or not) depends on an accurate assessment of (1) the risk of clinical leakage in an undiverted patient, (2) the extent to which proximal diversion diminishes this risk, and (3) the clinical burden of the stoma, including quality of life issues, dehydration, rehospitalization, and the morbidity of a second operation to reverse the stoma, and so forth.

A significant body of evidence has been accumulated to guide surgeons in this assessment. Tan and colleagues[11] performed a meta-analysis of studies examining the use of defunctioning stomas in rectal cancer surgery, published in the *British Journal of Surgery* in 2009. They analyzed a total of 25 studies, of which four were randomized trials. Taken together, the four randomized trials (total of 358 subjects) had an overall risk ratio for leakage of 0.39 (95% CI, 0.23–0.66) for subjects with versus without a diversion. The risk of reoperation was lowered by 0.29 (95% CI, 0.16–0.53), also in favor of subjects with a stoma. The mortality rate was lower (risk ratio 0.64), but this finding did not reach statistical significance in a pooled analysis (95% CI, 0.17–2.38). Their meta-analysis of nonrandomized studies also found a reduced rate of leakage and reoperation in a pool of 7693 subjects. The investigators gave an unqualified recommendation for ostomy creation at the time of low anterior resection for rectal cancer.

Proximal diversion can be accomplished in one of two ways, ileostomy or colostomy, each with a different profile of clinical considerations. One Cochrane review, performed by Guenaga and colleagues[12] in 2007, examined randomized trial data regarding the use of these two methods. A total of five trials met their inclusion criteria, analyzing the outcomes of 334 subjects. Prolapse was more common among subjects with colostomy, but there was no other significant difference between the two groups. The study did note significant heterogeneity between studies in their analysis of rates of prolapse and, therefore, concluded that the two approaches should be considered equivalent. Also, rehospitalization was not formally analyzed. It is the authors' subjective experience that rates of this complication are higher among patients with a diverting ileostomy due to problems with fluid status. In a similar study published in 2009, Rondelli and colleagues[13] meta-analyzed 12 studies (five randomized trials) comparing outcomes with diverting loop ileostomy versus loop colostomy as a temporary fecal diversion. Their study found higher rates of overall complications with a loop colostomy, but also significantly higher likelihood of issues relating to hydration with a loop ileostomy. Diverting loop ileostomy and diverting loop colostomy are each appropriate in certain patient populations. Importantly, there may be technical challenges in the formation of a diverting loop colostomy that limit its use in certain patients. Patients who are sensitive to the specific complication of dehydration (eg, borderline renal function, difficulty with oral intake) may be better candidates for a loop colostomy than a loop ileostomy.

One of the problems in comparing the literature regarding the decision of whether or not to divert is the lack of follow-up data for subjects who are diverted. In addition to those who, for a number of reasons, never undergo a stoma takedown, the surgeon must weigh the morbidity and mortality of a potential future ostomy closure. These are not minor procedures. Each of the large series examining outcomes from these types of operations documents a distinct rate of bowel obstruction, leakage, and reoperation. Chow and colleagues,[14] in a systematic review that analyzed more than 6000 ileostomy reversals, found an overall morbidity rate of 17.3%, including a mortality rate of 0.4%. A recent single-institutional study of 944 subjects from the Mayo Clinic in Rochester found an overall morbidity rate of 21.5%, including a reoperation rate of 3.9% and a mean length of stay of 5.2 days.[15] When combined with that of the original operation, the outcomes of the original diversion with that of the stoma takedown are greater than what is reported.

Some specific attention has been paid to the technique used to close a diverting loop ileostomy: handsewn versus stapled side-side anastomosis. One single-institution randomized trial evaluated this question in 141 subjects, and found higher rates of postoperative bowel obstruction in the handsewn arm (14% vs 3%), but no significant differences in other complications or duration of operation.[16] In one large review of ileostomy closures, 315 subjects had a stapled closure compared with 629 undergoing some type of handsewn closure.[15] Subjects with stapled closures had lower overall morbidity, quicker return of gastrointestinal function, and shorter lengths of stay.[15] The question of whether stapled or hand-sewn closures are superior is the focus of a planned multicenter randomized trial, the German HASTA (Hand-suture versus stapling for closure of loop ileostomy) trial, with a targeted accrual of 334 subjects.[17] Until other results point to the contrary, a stapled anastomosis seems to be superior.

Based on the accumulated evidence, which types of pelvic anastomoses have a risk of leakage which is sufficient to warrant proximal diversion? Stated alternatively, how many ostomies should be formed to prevent one clinical anastomotic leak (number needed to treat)? If one assumes a leakage rate from an ostomy closure of 3%, then the ostomy reversal by itself performed 15 to 20 times would have an approximately 50% chance of a leak (**Table 1**). A number needed to treat of 15, therefore, would incur ≈0.5 leaks from ostomy closures while preventing one anastomotic leakage, thereby reducing the number of overall leaks by 50%.

Table 1										
Number needed to treat with proximal diversion to prevent one leak										
Baseline Risk of Leak	20%	16.7	14.3	12.5	11.1	10.0	9.1	8.3	7.7	7.1	6.7
	18%	18.5	15.9	13.9	12.3	11.1	10.1	9.3	8.5	7.9	7.4
	16%	20.8	17.9	15.6	13.9	12.5	11.4	10.4	9.6	8.9	8.3
	14%	23.8	20.4	17.9	15.9	14.3	13.0	11.9	11.0	10.2	9.5
	12%	27.8	23.8	20.8	18.5	16.7	15.2	13.9	12.8	11.9	11.1
	10%	33.3	28.6	25.0	22.2	20.0	18.2	16.7	15.4	14.3	13.3
	8%	41.7	35.7	31.3	27.8	25.0	22.7	20.8	19.2	17.9	16.7
	6%	55.6	47.6	41.7	37.0	33.3	30.3	27.8	25.6	23.8	22.2
	4%	83.3	71.4	62.5	55.6	50.0	45.5	41.7	38.5	35.7	33.3
	2%	166.7	142.9	125.0	111.1	100.0	90.9	83.3	76.9	71.4	66.7
	—	30%	35%	40%	45%	50%	55%	60%	65%	70%	75%
	Relative risk reduction from proximal diversion										

Using this estimate as a starting point, which anastomoses should be diverted? Published rates of leakage from nondiverted colorectal anastomoses vary widely, but they were as high as 24.4% in one recent meta-analysis of rectal cancer subjects.[11] A broad range of risk factors have been identified that correlate well with risk of leak, including primarily the height of the anastomosis and preoperative radiation treatment. Given the relative risk reduction of 61% that is apparent in the meta-analysis by Rondelli and colleagues,[13] and an number needed to treat of 15, any anastomosis which has a 12% or higher likelihood of leakage should be diverted.

This approach is a gross over-simplification of the factors which should be considered by a surgeon in determining whether or not to construct a proximal diverting ostomy. The decision is inherently stochastic, but there is the potential to be unduly liberal or conservative with the use of diversion. A more liberal use of ileostomies, recommending diversion when the perceived leak is greater than 5% has been recommended. For a patient with a 5% risk of leak, this translates to approximately 30 ileostomies that would be needed to prevent one leak.[15] Although, initially, this may suggest an inappropriate high rate of diversion, it is important to consider the alternative. In other words, any clinician who believes this to be unnecessarily risk-averse needs to consider the consequences of diverting too infrequently. The clinical consequences of leakage can be catastrophic relative to the clinical burden of a temporary diversion.

OMENTOPLASTY

The omentum is used by many surgeons to place over their anastomoses in the hope that placing a blanket and "tucking in the anastomosis" will help seal off a leak. This thought may be based on the traditional Graham patch repair of duodenal ulcers or laboratory studies that have shown that the omentum patches defects in the anastomosis and provides scaffolding for granulation tissue that results in an intact lumen.[18] This potential benefit has been demonstrated in clinical studies.[18] Potential downsides related to the omental flap consist of necrosis, stenosis of the anastomosis, and obstruction.[18,19] Fortunately, there is some level one evidence to guide the surgeon in the use of omentoplasty.

Three randomized controlled trials have addressed the potential benefit of omental wrapping question.[18] The largest trial was by Merad and colleagues[8] encompassing 712 subjects. In addition, there is a well done systematic review and meta-analysis by Hao and colleagues[20] that synthesizes the results from these studies. There was no difference found in rates of overall anastomotic leakage, radiologic leakage, reoperation, wound abscess, generalized or localized peritonitis, extraabdominal complications, or mortality. Interestingly, based on one study,[18] length of stay was significantly shorter in the omentoplasty group. Clinical anastomotic leakage was also significantly lower in the omentoplasty group based on all three studies. This finding should be interpreted carefully, however, because Hao and colleagues[20] point out that this subjective outcome was not consistently defined across studies and that there was inadequate allocation concealment and blinding. The objective outcome of radiologic leakage may be a more useful outcome to consider. Additional, well-designed studies are needed to answer this question but, based on existing evidence, anastomotic leak rate and outcomes do not seem to be significantly altered by omentoplasty.

In abdominoperineal resections, omentum may be useful for filling the dead space in the pelvis leading to improved perineal healing. Retrospective studies examining these potential advantages seem to show benefit for omentoplasty,[18] but there is no higher level evidence to support this as yet.

ANTIADHESION BARRIERS
Pathophysiology

Adhesions form postoperatively because of trauma to the peritoneum. The body, in an attempt to heal this creates an inflammatory response that results in a fibrinous exudate. If there is complete fibrinolysis, there is no adhesion; if fibroblasts persist, then a fibrous adhesion results.[21,22] Plasmin is responsible for degrading fibrin; tissue plasminogen activator and urokinase-like plasminogen activator convert plasminogen to plasmin and are, therefore, important to the fibrinolytic process. Conversely, plasminogen activator inhibitors block fibrinolysis and lead to greater adhesion formation.[18]

Clinical Significance

Colorectal surgery causes adhesions; both upper and lower midline wounds have over a 90% chance of creating adhesions.[18] Adhesions are the leading cause of small bowel obstruction which can lead to admission and potentially surgery. In addition, adhesions can lead to fertility issues and difficulty at reoperation.

Approximately 3% of all laparotomies are done for small bowel obstruction[18] and the need for resection during this surgery is associated most with previous colorectal surgery.[18] Admissions for bowel obstruction (whether surgery is involved or not) cost over a billion dollars every year in the United States and similar high costs are seen in other countries.[23–26] Subsequent procedures can be made more challenging due to adhesions. Operative time and morbidity are increased due to intestinal injury. Accessing the abdominal cavity at a subsequent procedure can also be difficult owing to adhesions and can increase operative time[18] and morbidity due to intestinal injury.[18]

Surgical Technique

First, the approach of laparotomy compared with laparoscopy should be considered. Laparoscopy is thought to decrease adhesion formation due to the decrease in trauma to the peritoneum.[18] There have been two randomized prospective studies that compared postoperative obstructions with respect to laparoscopy versus laparotomy for colorectal surgery.[18] In both studies, there was no difference in the rate of postoperative obstruction. In Taylor's study,[27] which followed up subjects in the CLASICC trial, the highest rate of obstruction was seen in subjects who required a conversion. Other technical considerations, besides operative approach, relate to gentle tissue handling, good hemostasis, and avoidance of closure of peritoneum. There are two randomized trials in the gynecologic literature that would support this,[18] as well as avoidance of starch powdered gloves.[28,29]

Hydroflotation

The idea of separating peritoneal surfaces from each other during the initial phase of healing to prevent adhesions from forming is the main idea behind hydroflotation. Crystalloid solutions, such as Ringer lactate, have been instilled in the peritoneal cavity in hopes of providing this. In reality, these solutions are absorbed within 24 hours and, likely due to this short duration of being present, have not been shown to reduce adhesions.[18]

Chemical Fluid Instillation

At the present time, icodextrin 4% (Adept) is the only chemical that is approved for this indication by the Food and Drug Administration (FDA). One liter of the solution is instilled and left in the abdomen at the end of a case with the hope that it will separate damaged peritoneal surfaces from other structures during the initial postoperative period when adhesion formation will occur. A trial in the gynecologic literature involved 402 subjects that were randomized intraoperatively after laparoscopic adhesiolysis[18] to either instillation of Adept or Ringer lactate solution. At a second laparoscopy done 4 to 8 weeks after, adhesions were found to be significantly less and fertility was found to be significantly better in the Adept group.

Recently, a randomized controlled trial involving 180 subjects who underwent laparotomy for bowel obstruction and who were followed to determine whether the use of Adept would lead to a decrease in incidence, extent, and severity of adhesions.[30] Interestingly, incidence of small bowel obstruction was lower in the Adept group, but there was no difference in need for laparotomy for small bowel obstruction with a mean follow-up of 3.5 years. In addition, there was no significant difference found in the severity of adhesions.

Another agent that had been proposed is a 0.5% ferric hyaluronate (Intergel). A randomized controlled trial examining colorectal subjects was designed and the sample size calculation was 200. After 32 subjects were enrolled, the study was terminated owing to unacceptably high postoperative complications relating to a statistically significant higher rate of anastomotic leak and postoperative ileus in the Intergel group.[18] At this time, it is not available for use in the US market for colorectal procedures.

Gels

SprayGel is a sprayable gel (as its name implies) that lasts for 5 to 7 days and then is absorbed. It is a more viscous solution compared with Adept, with the idea that this will provide an improved barrier to adhesion formation. A small randomized trial was done examining planned loop ileostomy closure.[31] SprayGel was compared to a group without any antiadhesive barrier. The investigators concluded adhesions and operative time were significantly reduced with use of SprayGel (n = 19 SprayGel, n = 21 control group).

Another randomized trial involving 66 subjects was performed by gynecologists comparing adhesion formation with second look laparoscopy after laparoscopic or open uterine myomectomy using SprayGel in the intervention group. This study also found decreased adhesion extent and tenacity. Despite these studies, and others showing some efficacy, SprayGel has been removed from the market because of late onset postoperative pain and foreign body reaction. At this time there are no other gels available for adhesion prevention.

Barriers

The most commonly used mechanical barriers are films of hyaluronic acid on a carboxymethylcellulose frame (Seprafilm; Genzyme Corporation, Cambridge, MA, USA), oxidized cellulose (Interceed; Ethicon Division of Johnson and Johnson, Arlington, TX, USA) and nonabsorbable meshes. One of the main proposed advantages is that a fixed barrier is created for a known duration. The disadvantage is that it is only effective where applied. If approaching a case laparoscopically, a barrier such as Seprafilm can also be technically challenging to apply, and Seprafilm currently has no FDA indication for use in laparoscopy.

Seprafilm has been the focus of multiple studies. A Cochrane review was published in 2009[32] summarizing the results of seven randomized controlled trials,[18] with the two largest enrolling 1791 and 1701 subjects.[33,34] Overall, the findings were a decreased incidence, extent, and severity of adhesions with the use of Seprafilm. There was no difference found in rates of obstruction or operation. There was also a risk of leak identified if Seprafilm was wrapped around the anastomosis.[32] The investigators concluded, "In the absence of an ideal or alternative agent of proven efficacy in general surgical patients, hyaluronic acid/carboxymethylcellulose (HA/CMC) may be considered in the prophylaxis of intra peritoneal adhesions." Clinically, the main advantage to patients would be related to reoperative surgery, but there does not seem to be a lower incidence of obstruction and subsequent need for operative intervention.

Interceed has mostly been studied in the gynecologic literature, whereas its presence in colorectal arena seems limited. A Cochrane review examining barrier agents for prevention of adhesions after gynecologic surgery[35] found that adhesion formation was reduced significantly after laparoscopy and laparotomy; however, improved fertility rates were not seen. One trial in the review compared Gore-Tex (Gore & Associates, Newark, Delaware, USA) to Interceed and found that there were decreased pelvic sidewall adhesions with Gore-Tex mesh. This trial was done in women with bilateral pelvic sidewall adhesions noted during abdominal wall reconstruction. Gore-Tex or Interceed was placed randomly on the left or right sidewall and a second-look laparoscopy was done to check severity of adhesions. Because of the need for suturing in a solid mesh, risk of infection and potential need for removal, it has been used minimally in colorectal surgery.

Wound Closure

In closing midline wounds, the layers to consider are the fascia, subcutaneous fat, and skin. Many studies have been done looking at optimal fascial wound closure for laparotomy incision. Five systematic reviews and 14 trials were reviewed in a literature review by Diener and colleagues[36] in 2010. Essentially, based on the outcomes of nearly 8000 subjects, the optimal closure is a continuous running technique with slowly absorbable suture material in the elective setting, whereas in the emergency setting the results were inconclusive. Another conclusion of this study is that no further trials should be conducted for determining optimal midline wound closure in the elective setting because there have multiple studies examining this question (involving many individuals) and that the optimal closure seems well-defined after synthesizing the results from these trials.

One interesting study has challenged the conventional 1 cm wide sutures that are taken on the fascia. Millbourn and colleagues[37] randomized 737 subjects to either a group with wound closures with fascial bites of at least 10 mm or a group with closures with bites between 5 and 8 mm away from the fascial edge (using polydiaxanone sutures [PDS] suture). The underlying hypothesis was that a stitch length to wound length ratio of at least four leads to decreased hernia rates.[38,39] The study found that there was a significantly lower surgical site infection rate (5.2% vs 10.2%) and incisional hernia rate (5.6% vs 18%) in the group with smaller bites.[37] The STITCH trial is another randomized trial that will examine this question and is currently recruiting subjects with a planned sample size of 576.[40] If these results are consistent with Millbourn and colleagues'[37] trial, it may challenge the current dogma that exists regarding wound closure.

With respect to the subcutaneous layer, closure is usually considered in patients who are obese. Cardosi and colleagues[41] randomized 225 subjects with 3 cm or more of adipose fate in vertical midline wounds into three groups: suture approximation of Camper fascia, closed suction drainage, or no intervention (control group). There was no difference found in wound complications or disruption. In another randomized controlled trial by Paral and colleagues[42], 415 subjects were randomized to either subcutaneous fat suturing or no intervention. No difference was seen with respect to infectious or noninfectious complications. Overall, it would seem the extra time spent on suturing subcutaneous fat does not lead to improved outcomes.

Skin is usually approximated with the use of staple or suture. Twenty randomized controlled trials (seven of which were from general surgery) were summarized by Iavazzo and colleagues,[43] comparing suture closure to staples. Included in studies were 2111 subjects ranging in size from 15 to 182. Not surprisingly, time for closure was significantly less with staples. Interestingly, the wound infection rate was lower (12 studies, 1529 subjects; odds ratio, 2.06; 95% CI, 1.20–3.51) in the staple group, whereas five studies demonstrated more pain with stapled closure. Nonsignificant results were found regarding cosmesis and subject satisfaction. Skin staples, mostly because of lower infection rate and faster time for wound closure, would seem to be the optimal choice.

Tissue adhesives are a relatively newer method of skin closure that avoids the use of a sharp needle and does not require removal. In 2010, a Cochrane review examined tissue adhesives in the closure of surgical wounds.[44] In total, results from 1152 subjects from 14 randomized trials were considered. Despite the purported advantages of adhesives, sutures were found to have a lower rate of dehiscence and were also faster to use.

SUMMARY

There are many beliefs that surgeons hold to that have been passed on from mentors with whom they have trained. Some of this becomes part of the idiosyncratic method that each surgeon applies to his or her cases; the portion of the case where the "art" of surgery can be observed. However, this "art" should not become dogma and new techniques should not be assumed to be better bases on novelty. As can be seen from the multiple studies presented in this article, surgical approaches should be examined with proper methodological rigor so that patient care continuously improves.

REFERENCES

1. Alves A, Panis Y, Mathieu P, et al. Postoperative mortality and morbidity in French patients undergoing colorectal surgery: results of a prospective multicenter study. Arch Surg 2005;140(3):278–83 [discussion: 284].
2. Ragg JL, Watters DA, Guest GD. Preoperative risk stratification for mortality and major morbidity in major colorectal surgery. Dis Colon Rectum 2009;52(7): 1296–303.
3. Etzioni DA, Beart RW Jr, Madoff RD, et al. Impact of the aging population on the demand for colorectal procedures. Dis Colon Rectum 2009;52(4):583–90 [discussion 590–1].
4. Schilling PL, Dimick JB, Birkmeyer JD. Prioritizing quality improvement in general surgery. J Am Coll Surg 2008;207(5):698–704.
5. Peeters KC, Tollenaar RA, Marijnen CA, et al. Risk factors for anastomotic failure after total mesorectal excision of rectal cancer. Br J Surg 2005;92(2):211–6.
6. Urbach DR, Kennedy ED, Cohen MM. Colon and rectal anastomoses do not require routine drainage: a systematic review and meta-analysis. Ann Surg 1999;229(2):174–80.
7. Brown SR, Seow-Choen F, Eu KW, et al. A prospective randomised study of drains in infra-peritoneal rectal anastomoses. Tech Coloproctol 2001;5(2):89–92.
8. Merad F, Hay JM, Fingerhut A, et al. Is prophylactic pelvic drainage useful after elective rectal or anal anastomosis? A multicenter controlled randomized trial. French Association for Surgical Research. Surgery 1999;125(5):529–35.

9. Sagar PM, Hartley MN, Macfie J, et al. Randomized trial of pelvic drainage after rectal resection. Dis Colon Rectum 1995;38(3):254–8.

10. Yeh CY, Changchien CR, Wang JY, et al. Pelvic drainage and other risk factors for leakage after elective anterior resection in rectal cancer patients—A prospective study of 978 patients. Ann Surg 2005;241(1):9–13.

11. Tan WS, Tang CL, Shi L, et al. Meta-analysis of defunctioning stomas in low anterior resection for rectal cancer. Br J Surg 2009;96(5):462–72.

12. Guenaga KF, Lustosa SA, Saad SS, et al. Ileostomy or colostomy for temporary decompression of colorectal anastomosis. Cochrane Database Syst Rev 2007;(1):CD004647.

13. Rondelli F, Reboldi P, Rulli A, et al. Loop ileostomy versus loop colostomy for fecal diversion after colorectal or coloanal anastomosis: a meta-analysis. Int J Colorectal Dis 2009;24(5):479–88.

14. Chow A, Tilney HS, Paraskeva P, et al. The morbidity surrounding reversal of defunctioning ileostomies: a systematic review of 48 studies including 6,107 cases. Int J Colorectal Dis 2009;24(6):711–23.

15. Luglio G, Pendlimari R, Holubar SD, et al. Loop ileostomy reversal after colon and rectal surgery: a single institutional 5-year experience in 944 patients. Arch Surg 2011;146(10):1191–6.

16. Hasegawa H, Radley S, Morton DG, et al. Stapled versus sutured closure of loop ileostomy: a randomized controlled trial. Ann Surg 2000;231(2):202–4.

17. Loffler T, Seiler CM, Rossion I, et al. Hand-suture versus stapling for closure of loop ileostomy: HASTA-Trial: a study rationale and design for a randomized controlled trial. Trials 2011;12:34.

18. Dasari BV, McKay D, Gardiner K. Laparoscopic versus Open surgery for small bowel Crohn's disease. Cochrane Database Syst Rev 2011;(1):CD006956.

19. John H, Buchmann P. Improved perineal wound healing with the omental pedicle graft after rectal excision. Int J Colorectal Dis 1991;6(4):193–6.

20. Hao XY, Yang KH, Guo TK, et al. Omentoplasty in the prevention of anastomotic leakage after colorectal resection: a meta-analysis. Int J Colorectal Dis 2008;23(12):1159–65.

21. Dijkstra FR, Nieuwenhuijzen M, Reijnen MM, et al. Recent clinical developments in pathophysiology, epidemiology, diagnosis and treatment of intra-abdominal adhesions. Scand J Gastroenterol Suppl 2000;232:52–9.

22. van der Wal JB, Jeekel J. Biology of the peritoneum in normal homeostasis and after surgical trauma. Colorectal Dis 2007;9(Suppl 2):9–13.

23. Kossi J, Salminen P, Rantala A, et al. Population-based study of the surgical workload and economic impact of bowel obstruction caused by postoperative adhesions. Br J Surg 2003;90(11):1441–4.

24. Ray NF, Denton WG, Thamer M, et al. Abdominal adhesiolysis: inpatient care and expenditures in the United States in 1994. J Am Coll Surg 1998;186(1):1–9.

25. Tingstedt B, Isaksson J, Andersson R. Long-term follow-up and cost analysis following surgery for small bowel obstruction caused by intra-abdominal adhesions. Br J Surg 2007;94(6):743–8.

26. Wilson MS, Hawkswell J, McCloy RF. Natural history of adhesional small bowel obstruction: counting the cost. Br J Surg 1998;85(9):1294–8.

27. Taylor GW, Jayne DG, Brown SR, et al. Adhesions and incisional hernias following laparoscopic versus open surgery for colorectal cancer in the CLASICC trial. Br J Surg 2010;97(1):70–8.

28. Cooke SA, Hamilton DG. The significance of starch powder contamination in the aetiology of peritoneal adhesions. Br J Surg 1977;64(6):410–2.

29. van den Tol MP, Haverlag R, van Rossen ME, et al. Glove powder promotes adhesion formation and facilitates tumour cell adhesion and growth. Br J Surg 2001; 88(9):1258–63.

30. Catena F, Ansaloni L, Di Saverio S, et al. P.O.P.A. study: prevention of postoperative abdominal adhesions by icodextrin 4% solution after laparotomy for adhesive small bowel obstruction. A prospective randomized controlled trial. J Gastrointest Surg 2012;16(2):382–8.

31. Tjandra JJ, Chan MK. A sprayable hydrogel adhesion barrier facilitates closure of defunctioning loop ileostomy: a randomized trial. Dis Colon Rectum 2008;51(6): 956–60.

32. Kumar S, Wong PF, Leaper DJ. Intra-peritoneal prophylactic agents for preventing adhesions and adhesive intestinal obstruction after non-gynaecological abdominal surgery. Cochrane Database Syst Rev 2009;(1):CD005080.

33. Beck DE, Cohen Z, Fleshman JW, et al. A prospective, randomized, multicenter, controlled study of the safety of Seprafilm adhesion barrier in abdominopelvic surgery of the intestine. Dis Colon Rectum 2003;46(10):1310–9.

34. Fazio VW, Cohen Z, Fleshman JW, et al. Reduction in adhesive small-bowel obstruction by Seprafilm adhesion barrier after intestinal resection. Dis Colon Rectum 2006;49(1):1–11.

35. Wiseman DM, Trout JR, Diamond MP. The rates of adhesion development and the effects of crystalloid solutions on adhesion development in pelvic surgery. Fertil Steril 1998;70(4):702–11.

36. Diener MK, Voss S, Jensen K, et al. Elective midline laparotomy closure: the INLINE systematic review and meta-analysis. Ann Surg 2010;251(5):843–56.

37. Millbourn D, Cengiz Y, Israelsson LA. Effect of stitch length on wound complications after closure of midline incisions: a randomized controlled trial. Arch Surg 2009;144(11):1056–9.

38. Israelsson LA, Jonsson T, Knutsson A. Suture technique and wound healing in midline laparotomy incisions. Eur J Surg 1996;162(8):605–9.

39. Jenkins TP. The burst abdominal wound: a mechanical approach. Br J Surg 1976; 63(11):873–6.

40. Harlaar JJ, Deerenberg EB, van Ramshorst GH, et al. A multicenter randomized controlled trial evaluating the effect of small stitches on the incidence of incisional hernia in midline incisions. BMC Surg 2011;11:20.

41. Cardosi RJ, Drake J, Holmes S, et al. Subcutaneous management of vertical incisions with 3 or more centimeters of subcutaneous fat. Am J Obstet Gynecol 2006; 195(2):607–14.

42. Paral J, Ferko A, Varga J, et al. Comparison of sutured versus non-sutured subcutaneous fat tissue in abdominal surgery. A prospective randomized study. Eur Surg Res 2007;39(6):350–8.

43. Iavazzo C, Gkegkes ID, Vouloumanou EK, et al. Sutures versus staples for the management of surgical wounds: a meta-analysis of randomized controlled trials. Am Surg 2011;77(9):1206–21.

44. Coulthard P, Esposito M, Worthington HV, et al. Tissue adhesives for closure of surgical incisions. Cochrane Database Syst Rev 2010;(5):CD004287.

Unexpected Intra-operative Findings

Jason F. Hall, MD, MPH[a,b,*], Sharon L. Stein, MD[c,d]

KEYWORDS

- Reoperative abdominal surgery • Hostile abdomen • Damage control
- Presacral hemorrhage • Intestinal anastomosis

KEY POINTS

- Unexpected intraoperative findings are a commonly encountered; however, there is little peer-reviewed evidence on which to base management decisions.
- Modern cross-sectional imaging techniques often elucidate manyintra-abdominal findings. Careful review of any available preoperative imaging often assists the surgeon in anticipating challenges in difficult operations.
- Many intraabdominal collections can usually be temporized withnonoperative techniques such as image-guided percutaneous drainage allowing definitive surgical treatment after sepsis has resolved.
- Surgeons should be familiar with a number of different techniques to address commonly encountered unanticipated findings.

INTRODUCTION: INTRAOPERATIVE COMPLICATIONS AND FINDINGS

With advances in perioperative imaging and diagnostic studies, surgeons will have greater degrees of access to important surgical diagnoses before entering the operating theater. However, undiagnosed intraoperative findings and complications from surgery can still arise and cause challenges in decision making and treatment. Guidance on how to treat these intraoperative occurrences is difficult to find. For many topics there are few data and surgeons are left with only rare descriptions in the

Financial disclosure: J.H: The author has nothing to disclose. S.S: The author receives teaching support from Ethicon Endosurgery and Covidien.

[a] Department of Colon and Rectal Surgery, Lahey Clinic, 41 Mall Road, Burlington, MA 02139, USA; [b] Tufts University School of Medicine, 136 Harrison Avenue, Boston, MA 02110, USA; [c] Case Acute Intestinal Failure Unit, Inflammatory Bowel Disease Center of Excellence, Digestive Health Institute, Cleveland, OH, USA; [d] Division of Colon and Rectal Surgery, University Hospital/Case Medical Center, 11100 Euclid Avenue, LKS 5047, Cleveland, OH 44106, USA
* Corresponding author. Department of Colon and Rectal Surgery, Lahey Clinic, 41 Mall Road, Burlington, MA 02139.
E-mail address: jason.f.hall@lahey.org

Surg Clin N Am 93 (2013) 45–59
http://dx.doi.org/10.1016/j.suc.2012.09.008
0039-6109/13/$ – see front matter © 2013 Elsevier Inc. All rights reserved.

literature. The best advice often comes from senior colleagues with significant surgical experience. This article seeks to describe options for treatments using both available literature and the wisdom of senior surgeons to better prepare surgeons for handling unexpected intraoperative findings.

UNEXPECTED INTRAOPERATIVE FINDINGS

Because of the wide availability of cross-sectional imaging in the United States, it is unusual to operate without extensive preoperative intra-abdominal imaging. At our respective institutions, it is rare for patients to undergo elective or emergent surgery without having had imaging in the form of either a computed tomography (CT) or magnetic resonance imaging. Nevertheless, on occasion, patients have findings that were not suggested by the preoperative evaluation. Four of the more common intra-operative findings are abdominal abscess, Meckel diverticulum, right-sided diverticulitis, and endometriosis.

Abscess

Abscesses can be encountered in any case involving perforation of a hollow viscus. Preoperative diagnosis of sepsis of unknown origin should be addressed with preoperative imaging such as CT scanning. Abscesses can usually be managed with nonoperative techniques such as image-guided percutaneous drainage. This approach allows sepsis to resolve, patients to recover, and inflammation to dissipate before definitive operation. This approach is common in the management of diverticulitis, Crohn disease, and perforated appendicitis.[1–4]

When abscess cavities are encountered intraoperatively (**Fig. 1**A), the surgeon should attempt to control sepsis and provide adequate drainage. Initially, the abscess cavity should be unroofed. In most cases, full exposure of the abscess cavity will involve resection of the perforated segment of bowel. Often, the abscess cavity can be separated from other organs by using finger-fracture and other blunt dissection techniques, minimizing damage to adjacent loops of bowel (see **Fig. 1**B). These techniques are particularly helpful when the anatomic relationships are unclear.

In the setting of an infected field requiring bowel resection, diversion is considered the most conservative approach. However, several studies have demonstrated that an anastomosis can be performed safely provided the remaining bowel has a good vascular supply, the bowel is not significantly dilated, the infection is largely cleared, and the patient is an otherwise good candidate for anastomosis.[5,6]

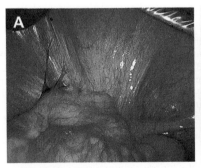 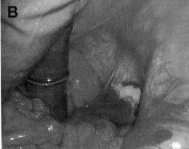

Fig. 1. (*A*) Walled-off abscess cavity from diverticulitis. (*B*) Abscess cavity following opening from finger-fracture technique. (*Courtesy of* Howard Ross, MD.)

Meckel Diverticulum

Meckel diverticulum is the most prevalent congenital abnormality found in the gastro-intestinal tract, occurring in 1.2% of individuals. Data on whether to resect an inciden-tally discovered Meckel diverticulum are sparce.[7] Zani and colleagues[7] recommend against a policy of routine resection to reduce the rate of postoperative complications. The authors did not observe an increase in long-term complications related to Meckel diverticula. In fact, they calculated that 758 Meckel diverticula would need to be resected to prevent one death. Other authors have suggested a selective approach to resection. Park and colleagues,[8] in a review of 1476 patients from the Mayo Clinic, found symptoms were more common in select conditions and recommended resec-tion of incidental Meckel diverticulum in patients younger than 50 years (odds ratio [OR] = 3.5; 95% confidence interval [CI], 2.5–4.8), in male patients (OR = 1.8; 95% CI, 1.3–2.4), in patients with diverticulum greater than 2 cm in length (OR = 2.2; 95% CI, 1.1–4.4), and when associated with intraluminal abnormalities (OR = 13.9; 95% CI, 9.9–19.6). These recommendations were based on a retrospective review of a single-center series instead of large prospective studies. As such, it is important to take into account all factors (condition of the patient, comorbidities, appearance of the diverticulum) when deciding how to proceed.

Right-Sided Diverticulitis

Right-sided diverticulitis is more common in the Far East than in Western countries.[9] Historically it was difficult to distinguish a patient with right-sided diverticulitis from appendicitis, but refinements in imaging have made this distinction relatively simple. In the absence of peritoneal signs, patients with right-sided diverticulitis may be treated with antibiotics. For patients who present with several attacks or complica-tions (perforation or abscess), resection is indicated. Fang and colleagues reviewed the outcomes of 85 patients treated for cecal diverticulitis.[10] Less than 40% (32 of 85) overall were treated successfully with antibiotics and bowel rest. Sixty-seven patients underwent laparotomy, of whom 47 patients (70%) were diagnosed preoper-atively with appendicitis. Of this subset, 24 underwent appendectomy, 9 underwent diverticulectomy, and 14 underwent right colectomy. Of those undergoing an appen-dectomy only, 7 had recurrent disease. Twenty patients with a preoperative diagnosis of diverticulitis underwent right colectomy with 2 deaths and 5 complications. The authors concluded that aggressive resection is warranted when the diagnosis of cecal diagnosis is known, especially in light of the higher recurrence with appendectomy only. Conversely, Thorson and Ternent suggested that right colectomy is the best surgical option when diagnosis is uncertain.[11] The aforementioned data suggest that ideally, this condition can be typically adequately treated nonoperatively with anti-biotics. However, if the diagnosis is encountered unexpectedly, it would seem prudent to proceed with right colectomy because it is associated with a definitive cure and low morbidity.

Endometriosis

Endometriosis is a common condition that affects 6% to 10% of women of child-bearing age.[12] Endometriosis commonly involves the adenexa, but it can also involve the gastrointestinal tract. Because endometriosis may involve small lesions scattered throughout the abdomen, preoperative diagnosis may not be known, with symptoms ranging from partial obstruction to chronic pain. When the gastrointestinal tract is involved, the most common sites include the rectosigmoid region (72%), the rectova-ginal septum (13%), small intestine (7%), cecum (3.6%), and appendix (3%).[13]

Magnetic resonance imaging seems to have the greatest sensitivity for preoperative diagnosis, but it may still miss small lesions.[14]

The surgical treatment of endometriosis aims to remove active disease. Often, involvement of the uterus, adnexa, and bowel requires a multidisciplinary team approach. Superficial areas on the pelvic wall or peritoneum can be vaporized with carbon dioxide laser, whereas those lesions involving rectal wall may be dissected using electrocautery. Sometimes a full-thickness disc excision can be performed and the rectal wall can be closed primarily. For larger lesions on the rectum or in the rectovaginal septum, a sleeve resection or low anterior resection may be required.[13] Lesions larger than 3 cm can be treated with small or large bowel resection and anastomosis. This approach is associated with lower rates of dysmenorrhea, dyspareunia, and recurrence.[15] Endometriosis of the appendix may present as intussusception and can be managed with an appendectomy or right colectomy. In situations in which the lesions cannot be distinguished from malignancy, an ileocecetomy or a segmental colectomy should be performed to ensure good margins.

SURGICAL CHALLENGES RELATED TO BOWEL LENGTH

A critical component of most abdominal surgery involving resection and reconstruction is the ability to move and manipulate tissue in a tension-free fashion. Surgeons may encounter difficulty in abdominal surgery if there is insufficient reach for the creation of an anastomosis or stoma. The colon can be tethered by both lateral and medial attachments and by attachments to the retroperitoneum. Ensuring that the mobilized colon has adequate blood supply to prevent ischemia is paramount. Although the small bowel may be mobilized more easily, difficulties can still exist–especially in an obese patient with significant subcutaneous fat, a patient with prior abdominal sepsis, or a patient with a foreshortened mesentery.

When mobilizing the colon for a coloanal anastomosis, the descending colon will generally be used for anastomosis. There are several important steps to ensuring adequate length for a technically sound anastomosis. Initially, the left-sided white line of Toldt is mobilized and the sigmoid and left colon are rendered midline structures. Care is taken to avoid the hypogastric nerves and nervi erigentes. For a coloanal anastomosis to be successful, complete mobilization of the splenic flexure is generally necessary. The omentum should be removed from the transverse colon, along with entering the lesser sac to mobilize the colon away from the stomach. High ligation of the inferior mesenteric artery and inferior mesenteric vein are performed at the sacral promontory, which results in the left colic artery being taken at its origin. To gain additional length, the inferior mesenteric vein is divided again as it dives under the pancreas close to the ligament of Treitz. All posterior attachments to the pancreas should be resected. Ensuring all these steps are performed will completely mobilize the left colon to maximize reach into the pelvis.

During this mobilization, there may be concern for adequate residual vascular supply to the left colon. This should be checked by assessing for adequate pulsatile flow before transecting the arc of Drummond at the site of colon resection. For cases with significant concern, use of a bulldog clamp to temporarily occlude the vascular supply while mobilization occurs can provide additional information and time to determine is any ischemic changes will occur. If the colon lacks pulsatile flow or there is any suggestion of inadequate supply, additional resection is necessary.

Additionally, if patients have had previous intra-abdominal operations, all of the operative notes should be reviewed in a detailed fashion to ensure that the vascular supply of the colonic conduit will not be compromised. If there are questions about the vascular supply of the colon, modern CT-angiography can provide a detailed overview of the vascular anatomy.

The adequacy of the conduit length can be judged by whether the conduit reaches the pubic symphysis. If the viable colon reaches the symphysis, it will generally reach the anus without tension. If the distal resected colon does not reach without tension, there are additional steps that may be taken. First, it is often helpful to reevaluate the initial steps detailed earlier to ensure they were done completely; often a few adhesions or bands may be holding the colon in place. Next, similar to extending the reach of an ileoanal pouch, the surgeon may score the mesentery without transecting additional vessels. If that fails to supply adequate reach, the mesentery can be divided up to the level of the left branch of the middle colic artery. In this situation, the conduit will be perfused exclusively by the arc of Drummond and a pulsatile vascular supply to the distal conduit should be verified.

If the surgeon still does not have adequate reach, the middle colic vessels can be transected. This should be done at the base of the mesentery to avoid damage to the collaterals supplying the colon conduit, namely the marginal artery of Drummond. If these maneuvers are not successful, the colon can be passed through a window in the mesentery of the terminal ileum. This avascular plane is generally located just proximal to the ileocolic artery. If the colon cannot be passed through the small bowel mesentery, then the hepatic flexure should be mobilized. The right and transverse colon can also be rotated counterclockwise into the patient's right abdomen reaching the pelvis by via the right paracolic gutter into the pelvis. Care must be taken when using this maneuver to not kink the vessels and cut off blood supply.

Other authors have devised a novel technique of anastomosis using an extra-anatomic route. In this situation the colon is passed through the retroperitoneal space below the duodenum toward the right ventral aspect of aortic bifurcation and into the pelvis. This procedure was performed in 10 patients and allowed coloproctostomy in 6 patients and coloanal anastomoses in 3 patients that would otherwise not be possible.[16]

Another situation when it may difficult to obtain adequate reach is in the creation of a stoma. This is particularly true in obese patients, and in emergency situations when the mesentery can be fibrosed and shortened. Preoperative marking with multiple alternative sites may help to optimize placement and postoperative care. The importance of preoperative consultation with enterostomal therapists is amplified in patients with multiple incisions. Unfortunately, this may be difficult to do in emergent cases, because they may be the least likely to see a stoma therapist or be marked preoperatively.[17]

Although end stomas are generally the easiest to mature, the thickness of the colon and colonic mesentery can be prohibitive for creating a small trephine. Techniques to create the stoma include widening the trephine and resuturing before maturation and the removal of addition fat and fascia. These maneuvers should be performed with caution because they may increase the risk of hernia. In obese patients, using the upper abdomen at the thinnest portion of abdominal wall may assist with providing adequate reach. The upper abdomen generally has a smaller amount subcutaneous and abdominal wall fat, thereby allowing the stoma to pass through the abdominal wall more easily.

Mobilization of the splenic flexure may aid in increasing reach to the abdominal wall. In addition, thinning of the vascular arcade without devascularization may be helpful. Just as in mobilization for a low anterior dissection, transection of the Inferior mesenteric artery (IMA), Inferior mesenteric vein (IMV), and lateral attachments can also facilitate reach. Mesenteric windows may also be created. As a last resort, up to 3 cm of distal bowel can be stripped of mesentery and will maintain adequate blood flow through submucosal circulation in most cases.[17]

In cases of an ileostomy or a colostomy, using a loop-end as described by Hebert may increase reach and decrease chances of a devascularized stoma.[18] This may be used in cases of small bowel stoma or colostomy, as described by Turnbull and Weakley.[19] The antimesenteric portion of the bowel is matured to the skin, and a drain or Penrose can be left at the distal staple line to prevent suture line "blowout."

In situations when the bowel itself is too friable for maturation, the Jones technique can be used. This involves bring several additional centimeters of bowel through the skin, wrapping it with clean gauze bandage, and maturing the stoma 5 to 7 days later. Some authors have advocated maturation of the difficult stoma before closure of an abdomen.[17] This allows for maturation with careful observation, preventing too much tension during maturation. It also prevents the surgeon from accepting an inadequate result, instead of reopening the abdomen.

In desperate situations, the stoma may be matured to the midline incision or the bowel drained via a large bore tube, similar to a duodenostomy drainage. Both of these techniques may have considerable consequences; however, given the situation, it may be the only alternative other than leaving the bowel in discontinuity. The stoma on the midline incision will have difficulty with pouching and use of a negative transcutaneous pressure device may help prevent damage to the skin. Using a large-bore tube may allow drainage distal to the tube and can also be easily clogged by effluent.

STAPLER WILL NOT PASS

The advent of the end-to-end anastomotic stapler, as demonstrated by Ravitch and Steichen in 1979, has facilitated the colorectal anastomosis and advanced the ability to uniformly create low rectal anastomoses.[20] Unfortunately, this technique is not without potential problems. Surgeons who perform circular anastomoses frequently will eventually face difficulty such as difficulty passing the stapler to the distal end of the rectum, malfunction during firing, or difficulty removing the stapler.

There are few data concerning management of a stapler that will not pass to the level of the desired anastomosis. Anecdotally, this occurs most frequently in cases of diverticulitis, often in the setting of Hartmann reversal. It may also occur secondary to a failure of the distal transection to be at the level of the true rectum; therefore, this should be confirmed. Initial maneuvers include advancing the stapler with direct or laparoscopic guidance. Often, the inexperienced assistant may fail to elevate his/her hands sufficiently to negotiate the sacral curve. Gentle "jiggling" of the stapler, similar to movement of a key in a lock, in a slow and steady manner, may also be of assistance. Caution is paramount during these procedures, as excessive force can result in serosal tears or proctotomy.

Additional reasons include intraluminal contents blocking the stapler to reach the end—especially in cases of urgent cases or those without bowel preparation. Saline irrigation or rectal washout may assist in dislodging retained feces or mucus that is occluding the lumen. Shlasko and colleagues[21] described the use of lidocaine lubrication with success. Use of a flexible or rigid proctoscope may also elucidate local anatomy, such as a distal stricture, that is the source of inability to pass. Countertension may be helpful; deferring transection of the top of the Hartmann until circular stapler placement has been verified may assist advancement and help demonstrate an appropriate transection site.

Often, further dissection of the rectum will be necessary. At times, this may be extramesenteric tissue, such as adhesions to the vagina, prostate, or sidewalls. If this fails to mobilize the rectum sufficiently, further resection may be necessary.

Alternative methods of anastomosis are also available to the surgeon. Zacharias and colleagues[22] demonstrated a reverse circular stapling technique in 2 patients. The anvil was placed in the distal rectum and closed with a pursestring; the stapler itself placed through a colotomy in the proximal colon. The colotomy was then closed after successful completion of the anastomosis. Other methods include a handsewn end-to-end or Baker end-to-side anastomosis, both of which can be performed even in laparoscopic cases through a small Pfannenstiel incision. After unsuccessful attempts at placing the stapler through the anus, the surgeon is cautioned to ensure that the distal rectum is clear of obstruction before completion of the case, via either flexible or rigid proctoscopy.

HOSTILE ABDOMEN

The goal of every operation is to identify the necessary pathologic conditions, avoid injury to the intra-abdominal contents, and adequately close the abdominal wall. These objectives can be particularly challenging to achieve in patients with a "hostile" abdomen.

A hostile abdomen is generally defined as one in which access to the pathologic condition of interest is impeded or difficult because of difficulty traversing the abdominal wall or massive intra-abdominal adhesions.[23] Patients who have undergone a damage control surgery, severe intra-abdominal infections, necrotizing pancreatitis, and anastomotic leaks are at high risk for a hostile abdomen.[24] Much of the literature of this topic is derived from data on patients with complex abdominal wall hernias and enterocutaneous fistulas.[23,25,26] In some studies, patients who were managed with delayed closure of an open abdomen were at high risk for developing enterocutaneous fistulas, most commonly colocutaneous fistulas (69%), and were associated with increased intensive care and hospital length of stay and hospital charges.[27]

Most surgeons advise waiting 3 to 6 months, or even longer, from the previous operation in the patient suspected to have a hostile abdomen. There are data suggesting that waiting only 4 to 5 weeks before operating is safe,[28] although the natural history of adhesions would suggest this is a time period when extensive dense adhesions may be present. Waiting longer intervals is theoretically improved because these highly vascularized and difficult adhesions are replaced with "softer" avascular ones that are typically more amendable to separating. Although laparoscopic approaches can be attempted, generally patients with hostile abdomen are approached with the open technique.

Adequate preoperative preparation is essential. Patients should be nutritionally replete, ambulating, and able to recover from a significant intra-abdominal operation. All previous operative notes should be reviewed thoroughly. Because these procedures can be arduous, the surgeon should prepare for a long procedure and make the necessary allowances for uninterrupted access to the operating theater. The importance of an unhurried and patient approach to these difficult cases cannot be overemphasized. Often, complications during these procedures can be directly related to surgeon fatigue or other scheduling pressures.

It is helpful to have an experienced assistant or fully trained surgeon available for intraoperative consultation. Considerations of possible complications should be discussed preoperatively; ureteric stents may be helpful to identify and prevent injury to the ureter; a gastroenterologist may elucidate pathologic conditions with intraoperative upper endoscopy or colonoscopy; preoperative consultation with a reconstructive plastic surgeon is helpful when significant abdominal wall reconstruction is anticipated; and consultation with an enterostomal therapist is helpful for marking multiple sites of possible stoma placement.

Adequate access to the entire abdominal cavity is needed to appropriate lyse all of the necessary adhesions. This access is generally best provided with a midline incision. When entering the abdomen, paramedian incisions should be avoided, because they or transverse incisions can destroy potential sites for a stoma and limit exposure.

Entering directly under an old incision is often challenging, because it is common for the intestines to adhere to the previous incision—especially when prior mesh has been used. It is often helpful to extend the previous incision to a "virgin" area of the fascia where no incision has been made. This maneuver will often provide a small window of access to the peritoneal cavity. Although external incision lines provide guidance, fascial incisions may extend several centimeters beyond the external scar. In laparoscopic cases, using a open Hassan or optical trocar technique in a location far from both prior incisions and prior dissection provides the best chance of safe entry. When entering through an old incision, we place the fascia on traction using Kocher clamps with an adequate amount of traction or countertraction on the omentum or small bowel adherent to the underside of the incision. Finger-fracturing of adhesions can often safely dissect areas and help to identify safe planes in filmy adhesions, although surgeons should be comfortable with sharp dissection.[28] Too much traction may cause serosal tears and bowel injuries. Sharp dissection with Mayo or Metzenbaum scissors or a scalpel is often the safest way of entering the abdomen. Electrocautery may be used in some cases with care. Hydrodissection may be helpful, especially in the setting of early reexplorations—squirting the field with a bulb syringe can help remove small amounts of blood, separate bowel loops, and ultimately identify the correct plane.

When dissection becomes difficult, varying the approach and approaching the area of adhesion from a different direction may help to elucidate the correct plane. When dissection is difficult, start with what is easy. Understanding the anatomy of the bowel, prior surgeries and location of mesentery will help prevent devascularization and identify correct planes.[28]

If an enterocutaneous fistula exists, one strategy is to leave the area of fistula for the last portion of dissection. Leaving a small amount of fascia or devascularized omentum on the bowel may be necessary to avoid injury to the intestine. On the other hand, when vital structures are involved, such as the ureter or iliac veins, it may be necessary to leave small amounts of bowel on the structure.[29] On the other hand, if there is concern for a malignancy, en bloc oncologic resection is standard.

If enterotomies are created, repairing them immediately, at least transiently, keeps from soiling the field. If they are not closed immediately, marking sutures can be placed on serosal tears. Final repair may be left until the dissection is complete, because multiple injuries over a short area of bowel may be better treated with resection than repair. Serosal tears are generally treated with Lambert seromuscular closure, whereas full-thickness enterotomies should be closed in 1 or 2 layers, depending on surgeon preference and technique.[30]

After completion of a difficult dissection, checking the field to ensure that no unrecognized injury remains is of utmost importance. Running the small bowel with meticulous detail to recognized previously unidentified injuries is a standard approach. Mesenteric hematomas are concerning for injuries and should be checked. In addition, placing the bowel under saline and injecting air through an enterotomy, stoma, or nasogastric tube advanced through the bowel may help identify injuries.[31]

PRESACRAL BLEEDING

Presacral bleeding is a serious and potential dangerous complication of pelvic surgery. The rate of presacral bleeding is estimated to be 3% to 9.4%.[32] Significant pelvic bleeding most frequently occurs when the surgeon intentionally or unintentionally extends dissection deep of the presacral fascia or lateral to the pelvic sidewalls. Radiation, retroperitoneal fibrosis, prior pelvic sepsis, and reoperative fields may also make differentiation of the planes and inadvertent injury more likely (N. Hyman, personal communication, 2012).[33] This is especially true in cases of Hartmann reversal. In cases of reoperative pelvic surgery and cancer recurrence, traditional planes may already have been dissected, and the surgeon may have no choice but to extend the dissection to obtain cancer-free margins.[31]

Although bleeding can come from several sources, the most common and difficult injury to manage is to the basivertebral veins. Several large basivertebral veins penetrate through the sacral foramina and extend into the presacral fascia. Often, these fragile veins are avulsed and retract into the sacral foramina when injured. Several factors contribute to the difficulty controlling bleeding from these vessels. The veins tend to be thin walled and fragile. In addition, they lack valves, allowing a vigorous flow when injured. Patient positioning in the Trendelenburg position during pelvic dissection can increase venous pressure to 2 to 3 times that of the inferior vena cava, creating a significant gradient for bleeding. Blood loss of up to 1000 mL/min has been recorded from a 2- to 3-mm presacral vein.[34] Limitation of space within the pelvis, including the continued presence of a bulky tumor, difficulty in visualization, and poor lighting may create additional hazards in treating the bleeding vessel.[29]

Injuries to the lateral sidewall and internal iliac vessels can also occur. In cases of reoperative surgery, the right common iliac vein is particularly difficult to deal with, in large part caused by its natural position of lying under the right common iliac artery. Techniques for ligation including transection, vein patch, and repair are well described in the vascular literature. Consultation with a vascular surgeon can be helpful in these cases. In presacral bleeding, vessel ligation is rarely helpful. Although bilateral hypogastric ligation and vascular embolization have been described to decrease bleeding from presacral sources, they are rarely helpful secondary to the complex interconnected nature of the pelvic plexus and bidirectional flow. In addition, this may lead to necrosis or ischemia of the perineum and bladder and is rarely successful or necessary to stop the bleeding.[34]

When the surgeon first encounters significant bleeding, several initial maneuvers are helpful. In most cases, the bleeding is from low-pressure venous systems and can be easily occluded with the use of a finger, sponge stick, or packing. This allows the surgical, nursing, and anesthesia team time to prepare for further blood loss. When confronted with massive bleeding, having the appropriate tools available is essential for successful treatment. Several different techniques to treat bleeding are described, but good lighting, excellent retraction, and a second suction are always helpful. Unfortunately, retraction and adequate exposure are often the most difficult parts in high-risk patients, commonly because of limited mobility and the presence of fibrotic scar tissue. Additionally, the surgeon needs to be aware that extensive suctioning can lead to a rapid loss of much blood. When possible, digital pressure to isolate the tear is preferred. Consideration of intraoperative blood salvage may be made. Calling for an experienced colleague is often appropriate. Anesthesia personnel should have time to ensure that the patient is appropriately resuscitated, blood is available, and access is adequate.

Often initial attempts to contain bleeding include cauterization. Several techniques have been described including increasing the current on the electrocautery, peripheral-to-central movement with longer than 2 minutes of cauterization, and use of Surgicel (Ethicon, Sommerville, NJ) to help seal the vessel. Argon beam anticoagulation has also been described in both open and laparoscopic cases.[35] Although some surgeons have good success with these techniques, caution is urged because they may cause further retraction of the source and increase bleeding.

The use of a sterile thumbtack was first described to stop presacral hemorrhage by Nivatvongs and colleagues[36] in 1985. A simple sterilized thumb tack, implanted into the sacrum can tamponade vessels and supply durable solution to bleeding. Literature describing the technique consists of primarily case series but is generally successful (N. Hyman, personal communication, 2012).[36,37] A commercially available occluder pin has been developed and described by Stolfi and colleagues[33,38] Firm placement and solid bone are necessary preconditions for success; failures occur from tack bending or failure to place completely.

Muscle welding has also been well described. Xu and Lin first described this technique in 1994.[39] A 1.5- to 2.0-cm^2 segment of the rectus abdominis muscle is harvested from the midline incision. This is held in place with forceps over the area of bleeding. Electrocautery is then applied on a high setting until the muscle has welded to the site, occluding the bleeding, requiring approximately 2 or more minutes in most studies.[40,41] Benefits of this method include readily available and low cost necessary components. Again, data on this technique are derived mostly from small case series. Remzi and colleagues[42] described creation of a rectus abdominus flap based on the inferior epigastric and rotated down into the pelvis. This technique is considerably more involved and has not been widely reported in the literature.

Multiple topical techniques have also been used with varying success in severe presacral bleeding. Various preparations of thrombin, collagen, and fibrin and have been used with some success in conjunction with a tack, muscle flap, packing, or electrocautery. Several studies have described the successful use of cyanoacrylate adhesive and hemostatic sponge in a small group of patients with good success.[43–45] During approximately 1 month, the cyanoacrylate dissolves into soluble polybutylcyanoacrylate and formic acid and is renally excreted. Cost of application is estimated at only $44 per application, and materials are often widely available in hospitals at which orthopedic surgeons practice.[45]

When the aforementioned methods fail, further attempts at definitive treatment are futile. In these cases, the patient should be packed and resuscitated with plans to return to the operating room in 24 to 48 hours. Bleeding is virtually always eliminated when the pelvis is tightly packed. It is important to ensure that the first packs make the turn toward the perineum at the level of the coccyx and are well placed. The pelvis is filled with packs well enough to occlude venous bleeding but allow arterial blood supply. Often, after resuscitation and 24 to 48 hours, no further treatment will be necessary. The packs are removed, the pelvis is checked for bleeding, and any additional procedures that were not completed secondary to bleeding at the first operation are performed. Hyman noted a 0% rebleed rate after packing (N. Hyman, personal communication, 2012). This technique requires a return trip to the operating room but often is the safest and most effective method.

Less widely practiced techniques of packing may prevent a return trip and include the use of space-occupying devices such as a bowel isolation bag, normal saline, or tissue expander placed through a perineal wound. Metzger described a technique of packing the abdomen with a bowel isolation bag, with the neck extending through the perineal wound. The bag is filled with gauze and then removed at the bedside 24 to 48 hours after surgery.[46] Cosman and Braley each described a similar technique using a breast implant or implant sizer. Fluid was slowly withdrawn during several days and the implant was removed through a perineal wound.[38,47] There are few data on the results of the aforementioned techniques, but avoiding a return trip to the operating room may be appealing.

DAMAGE CONTROL IN THE ELECTIVE SETTING

Damage control laparotomy is a technique popularized by trauma surgeons after massive intra-abdominal hemorrhage. The phrase's origin comes from the US Navy concept following vessel damage in which sailors perform all maneuvers necessary to keep the ship afloat at sea to reach the harbor where permanent repairs can be performed.[46] Ogilvie initially described the use of damage control laparotomy during World War II. In 1983 Stone described survival advantages associated with early control of hemorrhage followed by physiologic resuscitation before returning to the operating room for definitive operative repair.[47] In recent years damage control laparotomy has been used more widely in the management of several intra-abdominal conditions including acute pancreatitis, sepsis, vascular surgery, and colorectal surgery.

Surgeons occasionally encounter severe hemorrhage in elective settings. During colorectal surgery severe bleeding is most frequently encountered during challenging pelvic dissections. The management of massive pelvic hemorrhage is discussed earlier in this report. Less dramatic but voluminous blood loss can also be encountered during complex reoperative surgery. Often, these patients will be resuscitated with large amounts of crystalline and blood products. Ongoing blood loss and crystalloid resuscitation contribute to metabolic acidosis, hypothermia, and coagulopathy—the "triad of death." Large-volume resuscitation may lead to massive interstitial edema and can result in elevated intra-abdominal pressures and compartment syndrome.

Damage control laparotomy can be classified in 6 stages: (1) decision to perform damage control laparotomy, (2) control of hemorrhage and feculent contamination via a truncated laparotomy, (3) temporary closure of the abdomen, (4) resuscitation of patient in intensive care unit, (5) planned reoperation with definitive reconstruction, and (6) closure of the abdomen in multiple stages.

Several factors should be weighed when assessing the appropriateness of damage control laparotomy. These include the presence of hypovolemic or distributive shock, poor response to resuscitation, hypothermia, metabolic acidosis, coagulopathy, the presence of a major vascular injury that can only be controlled by packing, and the amount of work necessary to control contamination and complete reconstruction.

Once a decision to perform damage control laparotomy has been reached, this should be communicated to the anesthesiology and intensive care unit staff. Major vascular injuries should be controlled using clamps, shunts, or packing. Major bowel injuries should be closed with simple sutures or linear staplers. No definitive repairs or anastomoses should be performed. Typically, patients in these difficult situations are edematous and therefore the entire bowel is distended and swollen. This does not allow primary closure of the abdomen. Several strategies have been described to cover the intra-abdominal contents. These range from use of a sterile intravenous bags and x-ray cassettes to vacuum-assisted devices (**Fig. 2**).[48,49] Following

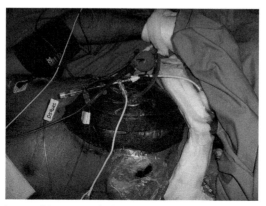

Fig. 2. Temporary closure. (*Courtesy of* Alec Beekley, MD.)

temporary closure of the abdomen, patients are transported to the intensive care unit for ongoing resuscitation. Rewarming can be accomplished through the administration of warmed fluids and blood products.

Once the affected patients have achieved hemodynamic stability, they are returned to the operating room for a definitive repair of the surgical pathologic conditions. All surgical packs should be counted and removed and a complete examination of the peritoneal cavity should be performed. Intestinal continuity can be reestablished and vascular injuries can be repaired if necessary.

Abdominal closure in patients undergoing damage control laparotomy is often complex. Often, it is often impossible to reapproximate the abdominal wall because of ongoing edema. Surgeons should resist the temptation to "raunch" the abdominal fascia together under tension. Patients undergoing this type of abdominal wall reconstruction are at high risk for the development of a ventral hernia. Forced fascial closure is associated with skin necrosis, fascial dehiscence, and fascial necrosis.[50] In these situations, we have chosen to slowly and progressively close the abdominal wall over a series of planned operations. Often final closure requires use of "biologic" mesh or absorbable prosthetic mesh for closure.

SUMMARY

Abdominal surgery is immensely rewarding because there are a wide variety of complex problems that surgeons are required to master. When surgeons are confronted with unexpected findings or complications, it is vital that they understand the basics of surgical technique but also have an armamentarium of "tricks of the trade" to help guide them in management.

ACKNOWLEDGMENTS

The authors would like to acknowledge the following master surgeons for their generous contribution of tricks and tips: Karim Alavi, David E. Beck, Richard P. Billingham, Theodore E. Eisenstat, Phillip Fleshner, Neil H. Hyman, Gerard Isenberg, Sang Lee, Feza Remzi, Anthony Senagore, and Michael Stamos.

REFERENCES

1. Soumian S, Thomas S, Mohan PP, et al. Management of Hinchey II diverticulitis. World J Gastroenterol 2008;14:716–9.
2. Golfieri R, Cappeli A. Computer tomography-guided percutaneous abscess drainage in coloproctology: review of the literature. Tech Coloproctol 2007;11: 197–208.
3. Ambrosetti P, Chautems R, Soravia C, et al. Long-term outcome of mesocolic and pelvic diverticular abscesses of the left colon: a prospective study of 73 cases. Dis Colon Rectum 2005;48:787–91.
4. Alvarez JA, Baldonedo RF, Bear IG, et al. Presentation, management and outcome of acute sigmoid diverticulitis requiring hospitalization. Dig Surg 2007; 24:471–6.
5. Constantinides VA, Tekkis PP, Athanasiou T, et al. Primary resection with anastomosis vs. Hartmann's procedure for nonelective surgery for acute colonic diverticulitis: a systematic review. Dis Colon Rectum 2006;49:966–81.
6. Aydin HN, Tekkis PP, Remzi FH, et al. Evaluation of the risk of a nonrestorative resection for the treatment of diverticular disease: the Cleveland Clinic diverticular disease propensity score. Dis Colon Rectum 2006;49:629–39.

7. Zani A, Eaton S, Rees CM, et al. Incidentally detected Meckel diverticulum: to resect or not to resect? Ann Surg 2008;247(2):276–81.
8. Park JJ, Wolff BG, Tollefson MK, et al. Meckel diverticulum: the Mayo Clinic experience with 1476 patients (1950–2002). Ann Surg 2005;241:529–33.
9. Nakaji S, Danjo K, Munakaata A, et al. Comparison of etiology of right-sided diverticula in Japan with that of left-sided diverticula in the West. Int J Colorectal Dis 2002;17:365–73.
10. Fang JF, Chen RJ, Lin BC, et al. Aggressive resection is indicated for cecal diverticulitis. Am J Surg 2003;185:135–40.
11. Thorson AG, Ternent CA. Cecal diverticulitis. In: Welch JP, Cohen JL, Sardella WV, et al, editors. Diverticular disease, management of the difficult surgical case. Baltimore (MD): Williams and Wilkins; 1998. p. 428–41.
12. Guidice LC. Clinical practice. endometriosis. N Engl J Med 2009;362:2389–98.
13. Saleem A, Navarro P, Munson JL, et al. Endometriosis of the appendix: report of three cases. Int J Surg Case Rep 2011;2:16–9.
14. Caramella T, Novellas S, Fournol M, et al. Deep pelvic endometriosis: MRI features. J Radiol 2008;89(4):473–9.
15. Hart RJ, Hickey M, Maouris P, et al. Excisional surgery versus ablative surgery for ovarian endometriomata. Cochrane Database Syst Rev 2008;(2): CD004992.
16. Ushigome T, Kawahara H, Watanabe K, et al. Colorectal anastomosis using retroperitoneal window after wide colorectal resection. Hepatogastroenterology 2011; 58:1983–4.
17. Orkin B, Cataldo P. Intestinal stomas. In: Wolf BG, Fleshman JW, Beck DE, et al, editors. The ASCRS textbook of colorectal surgery. New York: Springer Science + Business Media LLC; 2007. p. 625.
18. Herbert JC. A simple method for preventing retraction of an end colostomy. Dis Colon Rectum 1988;31:328–9.
19. Weakley FL, Turnbull RB Jr. Exclusion and decompression for toxic dilatation of the colon in ulcerative colitis. Proc R Soc Med 1970;63:73–5.
20. Ravitch MM, Steichen FM. A stapling instrument for end-to-end inverting anastomosis in the gastrointestinal tract. Ann Surg 1979;189:791–7.
21. Shlasko E, Gorfine SR, Gelernt IM. Using lidocaine to ease the insertion of the circular stapler. Surg Gynecol Obstet 1992;174:70.
22. Zachariah SK. Reverse transrectal stapling technique using the EEA stapler: an alternative approach in difficult reversal of Hartmann's procedure. J Surg Tech Case Rep 2010;(2):70–2.
23. Latifi R, Gustafson M. Abdominal wall reconstruction in patients with enterocutaneous fistulas. Eur J Trauma Emerg Surg 2011;37:241–50.
24. Leppaniemi A. The hostile abdomen – a systematic approach to a complex problem. Scand J Surg 2008;97:218–9.
25. Connolly TP, Teubner A, Lees PN, et al. Outcome of reconstructive surgery for intestinal fistula in the open abdomen. Ann Surg 2008;247:440–4.
26. Datta V, Engledow A, Chan S, et al. The management of enterocutaneous fistula in a regional unit in the United Kingdom: a prospective study. Dis Colon Rectum 2010;53:192–9.
27. Teixeira PG, Inaba K, Dubose J, et al. Enterocutaneous fistula complicating trauma laparotomy: a major resource burden. Am Surg 2009;75:30–2.
28. Hyman N, Nelson R. Intestinal complications. In: Wolf BG, Fleshman JW, Beck DE, et al, editors. The ASCRS textbook of colorectal surgery. New York: Springer Science + Business Media LLC; 2007. p. 643–52.

29. McCormick JT, Gregorcyk SG. Other intraoperative challenges. In: Whitlow CB, Beck DE, Margolin DA, et al, editors. Improved outcomes in colon and rectal surgery. 1st edition. London: Informa Health Care; 2009. p. 44–55.

30. Dietz DW, Bailey HR. Postoperative complications. In: Wolf BG, Fleshman JW, Beck DE, et al, editors. The ASCRS textbook of colorectal surgery. New York: Springer Science + Business Media LLC; 2007. p. 141–55.

31. Fazio VW. Introduction and overview: principles of reoperative pelvic surgery. In: Billingham RP, Kobashi KC, Peters WA, editors. Reoperative pelvic surgery. New York: Springer-Verlag; 2009. p. P1–4.

32. D'Ambra L, Berti S, Bonfante P, et al. Hemostatic step-by-step procedure to control presacral bleeding during laparoscopic total mesorectal excision. World J Surg 2009;33:812–5.

33. Perry WB. Management of perioperative hemorrhage. Clin Colon Rectal Surg 2001;14:49–56.

34. Wang QY, Shi WJ, Zhao YR, et al. New concepts in severe presacral hemorrhage during proctectomy. Arch Surg 1985;120(9):1013–20.

35. Kandeel A, Meguid A, Hawasli A. Controlling difficult pelvic bleeding with argon beam coagulator during laparoscopic ultra low anterior resection. Surg Laparosc Endosc Percutan Tech 2011;21:21–3.

36. Nivatvongs S, Fang DT. The use of thumbtacks to stop massive presacral hemorrhage. Dis Colon Rectum 1986;29:589–90.

37. Stolfi VW, Remzi FH, Oncel M, et al. Muscle tamponade to control presacral venous bleeding: report of two cases. Dis Colon Rectum 2002;45:1109–11.

38. Stolfi VM, Milsom JW, Lavery IC, et al. Newly designed occluder pin for presacral-hemorrhage. Dis Colon Rectum 1992;35:166–9.

39. Xu J, Lin J. Control of presacral hemorrhage with electrocautery through a muscle fragment pressed on the bleeding vein. J Am Coll Surg 1994;179:351–2.

40. Harrison JL, Hooks VH, Pearl RK, et al. Muscle fragment welding for control of massive presacral bleeding during rectal mobilization. Dis Colon Rectum 2003; 46:1115–7.

41. Ayuste E, Roxas MF. Validating the use of rectus muscle fragment welding to control presacral bleeding during rectal mobilization. Asian J Surg 2004;27: 18–21.

42. Remzi FH, Oncel M, Fazio VW. Muscle tamponade to control presacral venous bleeding. Dis Colon Rectum 2002;45:1109–11.

43. Losanoff JE, Richman BW, Jones JW. Cyanoacrylate adhesive in management of severe presacral bleeding. Dis Colon Rectum 2002;45:1118–9.

44. Chen Y, Chen F, Xie P, et al. Combined oxidized cellulose and cyanoacrylate glue in the management of severe presacral bleeding. Surg Today 2009;39(11): 1016–7.

45. Zhang CH, Song XM, He YL, et al. Use of absorbable hemostatic gauze with medical adhesive is effective for achieving hemostasis in presacral hemorrhage. Am J Surg 2012;203:e5–8.

46. Ogilvie WH. The late complications of abdominal war-wounds. Lancet 1940;2: 253–6.

47. Stone HH, Strom PR, Mullins RJ. Management of the major coagulopathy with onset during laparotomy. Ann Surg 1983;197:532–5.

48. Rutherford EJ, Skeete DA, Brasel KJ. Management of the patient with an open abdomen: techniques in temporary and definitive closure. Curr Probl Surg 2004;41:821–76.

49. Miller PR, Meredith JW, Johnson JC, et al. Prospective evaluation of vacuum-assisted fascial closure after open abdomen: Planned ventral hernia rate is substantially reduced. Ann Surg 2004;239:608–16.
50. Diaz JJ, Cullinane DC, Dutton DC, et al. The management of the open abdomen in trauma and emergency general surgery. J Trauma 2010;68:1425–38.

Complications of Colorectal Anastomoses
Leaks, Strictures, and Bleeding

Bradley Davis, MD[a],*, David E. Rivadeneira, MD[b]

KEYWORDS

- Anastomotic leak • Air leak test • Anastomosis • Stoma • Stricture • Bleeding

KEY POINTS

- Risk factors for anastomotic failure are categorized as surgeon-related, patient-related, and disease-related.
- Understanding the myriad of risk factors and the strength of the data helps guide a surgeon as to the safety of undertaking an operation in which a primary anastomosis is to be considered.
- In the absence of abandoning the goal of reuniting the cut ends of the bowel, a surgeon may choose to mitigate the risk of a leak by performing a proximal diverting stoma.
- Whether this risk can be modified by the use of adjuncts such as pelvic drains, omental wrapping, or tissue reinforcement remains unclear; however, the performance of a simple intraoperative air leak test allows a surgeon to assess if the anastomotic integrity has been compromised.
- Familiarity with the various approaches to stricture and bleeding at the anastomosis aids in optimizing patient outcomes with the least amount of morbidity should complications occur.

INTRODUCTION

In 1887, William Halsted wrote: "The death-rate attending enterorrhaphy has been large, and, in general, the operation, even in the hands of the most skillful surgeons, has been capricious in its results."[1] Although the modern surgeon enjoys considerably more success in the performance of an intestinal anastomosis compared with one belonging to a century ago, the results have never been perfect. Unreported studies have attempted to define the characteristics of the perfect anastomosis. Although the technique has largely been standardized and the importance of the anatomy elucidated, there remains an ever-present risk of failure with significant consequences to

[a] Department of Surgery, University of Cincinnati, 231 Albert Sabin Way, ML 0558, Cincinnati, OH 45267, USA; [b] Colon and Rectal Surgery, Saint Catherine of Siena Medical Center, Smithtown, NY, USA
* Corresponding author.
E-mail address: DAVISBD@UCMAIL.UC.EDU

Surg Clin N Am 93 (2013) 61–87
http://dx.doi.org/10.1016/j.suc.2012.09.014
0039-6109/13/$ – see front matter © 2013 Elsevier Inc. All rights reserved.

the patient. Death from intestinal resections was commonplace until the middle of the twentieth century when improvements in antisepsis and anesthetic techniques and the introduction of systemic antibiotic therapy all contributed to improved outcomes. While Halsted was demonstrating the importance of the correct placement of sutures in the intestinal wall, others were attempting to improve outcomes by purging the intestine of its fecal load, a variable thought to be directly responsible for the disruption of the intestinal anastomosis. The introduction of oral antibiotics and later systemic antimicrobials also had a significant effect on the outcomes of surgery for large- and small-bowel resections. The final major advance came with the introduction of the mechanical stapler, heralding the modern era of intestinal anastomosis. Much of the dogma surrounding the performance of an anastomosis was subsequently challenged, leading to the modification or abandonment of many of these techniques in twenty-first–century operating rooms.

The integrity of any anastomosis results from a complex interaction between the surgeon, the patient, and the disease process (**Table 1**). The surgeon is foremost responsible to ensure the execution of a technically perfect anastomosis. In addition, there are a host of preoperative and intraoperative decisions that come to bear that are ultimately the responsibility of the surgeon and, in the end, can mean the difference between success and failure.

SURGEON FACTORS

Surgeons learn from the beginning that the fundamental principles of a successful anastomosis entails anastomosing 2 ends of healthy bowel that have an adequate blood supply and lack any tension after union. Although these principles seem so rudimentary, reference to their criticality is difficult to find in the surgical literature.

Perfusion

Newer technologies have helped shed light on the effect of tissue ischemia on anastomotic integrity both in human and animal models. One such study by Myers and colleagues[2] describes the use of a tissue oxygen saturation ($TSaO_2$) probe to assess the $TSaO_2$ on either side of the large bowel and small bowel transected using staplers of various staple heights. The study used an adult swine model and demonstrated a significant reduction in mucosal $TSaO_2$ both at and 2 cm from the staple line. However, the serosa showed no such changes. These changes were independent of the staple line height, which did not seem to have an appreciable effect on tissue perfusion. In another study, the oxygen tension (PSO_2) on either side of an intestinal anastomosis was measured on dogs and compared with baseline measurements.[3] When the PSO_2 decreased to less than 30% of the baseline, anastomotic necrosis

Table 1 Factors influencing anastomotic integrity		
Surgeon Factors	**Patient Factors**	**Disease Factors**
Intestinal blood supply	Body mass index	Inflammatory bowel disease
Tension on the anastomosis	Anesthesia severity assessment	Metastatic carcinoma
Perioperative hypoxia	Age	Radiation therapy
Perioperative resuscitation	Smoking	Damage control surgery
Intraoperative blood loss	Nutritional status	Emergent surgery/peritonitis
Operative times	Alcohol use	Steroids
		Infraperitoneal location

occurred within 48 hours. In another study, rats that underwent large-bowel resection and immediate anastomosis were kept in either a hypoxic or a normoxic environment for 7 days.[4] Animals maintained in the hypoxic environment had a considerably lower anastomotic burst pressure when compared with normoxic controls. Sheridan and colleagues[5] examined the influence of serosal oxygen tension in a human trial using an electrode on either side of a colonic anastomosis. The tissue oxygen tension (ptO_2) on the proximal and distal sides was measured before any vascular ligation or mobilization of the colon. These results were then compared with measurements taken at the same location after the anastomosis. Fifty consecutive patients were assessed (28 anterior resections, 10 sigmoid resections, 5 left hemicolectomies, and 7 right hemicolectomies). The investigators reported 10 clinical leaks, with ptO_2 significantly lower perianastomotically in subjects with a leak (less than 20 mm Hg) when compared with those whose anastomosis was intact. Indirect evidence of the importance of the anastomotic blood supply comes from Zakrison and colleagues[6] who looked at the anastomotic leak rates in 223 patients admitted to an intensive care unit after 259 gastrointestinal anastomoses. They reported an overall leak rate of 9.9%; finding that the need for vasopressors in the immediate postoperative setting was associated with a higher leak rate (odds ratio [OR], 3.25; $P = .02$). Milan and colleagues[7] demonstrated that the colonic mucosal pH was the only predictor of success after left-sided resections in 90 consecutive patients. The leak rate was 22 times higher in patients with a mucosal pH less than 7.28 (a marker of anaerobic metabolism). Vignali and associates[8] used laser Doppler flowmetry to assess the rectal stump microperfusion in 55 consecutive patients who underwent rectal resections. Measurements were taken at baseline and after vascular pedicle ligation and transection of the bowel. Anastomotic leaks occurred in 14.5% of patients, with a linear correlation between decrease in rectal stump microperfusion and leak. Flow reduction was 6.2% in patients with no evidence of a leak and 16% in those with a leak ($P<.001$). These studies validate the timeless concept of the need for adequate blood supply to ensure the integrity of the colonic anastomosis, but there is no practical way to apply these techniques reproducibly in every operating room. This application may eventually be easier as new technologies find their way into operating rooms, allowing surgeons to easily and immediately assess the perfusion of tissue before performing intestinal anastomoses. Intraoperative fluorescence vascular angiography is one such tool that has been used in reconstructive and cardiac surgeries and has been shown to be effective in decreasing leak rates in colorectal anastomoses.[9] There is no reliable clinical indicator of adequate perfusion, and surgeons are often left to rely solely on their judgment to assess the patency of the blood supply. Although the color of the mucosa is not always a reliable indicator, the absence of mucosal bleeding at the point of transection should raise concerns about its adequacy. In general, there should be no doubt about the blood supply of a right colon anastomosis, as the mesentery of the small bowel is rarely limiting in terms of reach as long as great care is taken not to undermine the transection site when dividing the mesentery. This situation is also true of the transverse colon, assuming a patent marginal blood supply, which is assessed by demonstrating pulsatile blood flow after transecting the mesentery just before ligation. Should the mesentery fail to bleed, an alternate site of transection should be considered. For an anastomosis of the colon to the rectum the length of the mesentery can be restrictive. In an effort to ensure a tension-free union of the bowel, the inferior mesenteric artery (IMA) may have to be ligated along with the inferior mesenteric vein, which can be doubly ligated just distal to the duodenum if more length is needed. If a cancer resection is being performed, it may be desirable to ligate the IMA at its origin irrespective of reach to ensure an adequate nodal harvest. There is some controversy regarding the necessity of ligating the IMA flush to the aorta (high tie) when compared with preservation of the left colic branch (low tie). The oncological necessity of a high tie is predisposed on the fact that lymph nodes at the origin of the IMA can harbor malignant cells and recurrences following low tie are more frequent.[10] The impact of the high tie may be more important for advanced carcinomas,[11] and the effect of radiation may mitigate this benefit further. These benefits of a high tie have not been uniformly seen, and there is ongoing controversy about the oncological benefits of this technique.[12] The significance of the high tie as it pertains to the anastomotic leak rate is based on the blood supply to the conduit. If the descending colon or transverse colon is to be used as the proximal anastomosis, the impact of the high tie is mitigated, as there seems to be an adequate marginal blood supply to maintain tissue oxygen concentration in these patients. However, this may not be true with the sigmoid colon as the marginal blood supply off of the middle colic may not be adequate to perfuse such a long conduit.[13,14] If it is necessary to use the sigmoid colon as part of the colorectal or coloanal anastomosis then the left colic artery should be preserved.[15,16] An alternate hypothesis was proposed by Hall and colleagues[17] who measured the ptO_2 of the left colon before and after ligation of the IMA in 62 patients who underwent anterior resection. Baseline data demonstrated that the ptO_2 varied significantly between the sigmoid, the descending, and the transverse colon. After the IMA was ligated, the ptO_2 was significantly reduced in the sigmoid colon when compared with the left or transverse colon. This difference was observed irrespective of a high tie (proximal to the left colic artery takeoff) or low tie (distal to the left colic artery takeoff). These data suggest that it is the site of transection and not the site of arterial ligation that affects the integrity of the anastomotic blood supply. Although there is conflicting data if the IMA is to be ligated at any level, the surgeon should likely consider resecting the entire sigmoid colon. The toughest cases are those in which a patient has received preoperative radiation and requires a coloanal anastomosis. The point of transection is often determined by the extent of any radiation injury to the conduit and the need to perform an adequate lymphadenectomy. This condition often necessitates the removal of the sigmoid colon and the need to bring the descending colon all the way to the pelvis. A complete mobilization of the splenic flexure is required in these cases, with the dissection of the greater omentum off of the transverse colon at its fusion with the transverse mesocolon. In addition, the retroperitoneal attachments near the tail of the pancreas should be completely freed. To gain additional length, the inferior mesenteric vein is found just lateral to the ligament of Treitz and is not paired with the artery in this location. Ligating the vein at this location often adds several centimeters to the length of the conduit and is often necessary. Great care must be exercised in preserving the marginal blood supply during these maneuvers. Although all these techniques can be performed laparoscopically/robotically, they require a great deal of skill, and the learning curve is not as steep as other parts of this procedure. If the marginal blood supply is compromised because of inadvertent injury mobilizing the flexure or wandering too close the mesenteric border during ligation of the mesentery, the conduit becomes ischemic and very likely unusable. In general, if a transverse colon anastomosis is being fashioned, both the hepatic and splenic flexure should be mobilized so that the cut ends come together easily. Although no data exist to support the use of a hand-sewn technique in this setting, it is the authors' preference to perform an end-to-end colocolotomy. Alternatively, an end-to-end stapled anastomosis may be performed using an end-to-end stapler through a colotomy on either end or a linear staple line. A third technique has been described using a linear stapler to create a triangular anastomosis by deploying the stapler 3 separate times.

Tension

Many of the same techniques that the surgeon uses to ensure an adequate blood supply also facilitate a tension-free anastomosis as described earlier. The importance of tension on the integrity of an anastomosis has been poorly studied, as most experimental models of leaks rely on the assessment of bursting pressure and not stretch.[18] An exception in the more recent literature characterized the blood flow of various intestinal segments before and after the application of a tensile force after anastomosis. Shikata and Shida[19] found in an experimental model using dogs that the effects of tension on the submucosal blood flow was much better tolerated in the small bowel when compared with the colon. These data help to corroborate the clinical assertion that an anastomosis under tension is more likely to fail, as it is less likely that a small-bowel resection and anastomosis, given the laxity of the small-bowel mesentery, will leak when compared with a left-sided colonic resection that is more likely to be on stretch. Commonsense would indicate an anastomosis that is taught is in danger of failing for the additional reasons of mechanical forces that attempt to pull the newly anastomosed bowel away from each other.[20] Once the anastomosis has been performed, there may be a great deal of laxity between the proximal and distal bowel (ileocolic) or there may not be any (coloanal), and the surgeon relies on the intraoperative assessment to determine if the anastomosis will fail. As a general rule, if the cut edge of the conduit mesentery traversing over the pelvic brim is too tight to allow a finger to easily slip behind, the anastomosis may be under too much tension. Every effort should then be made to lengthen the conduit, even if this has already been attempted, as often reappraisal may identify a small adhesion to release. In general, if the mesentery is lax, there is likely little to no tension at the anastomosis.

Technique

Once the cut edges of the bowel have been attended to, the surgeon must decide how to reunite them. Although this debate may have once been relevant, there is little doubt that in the twenty-first century the surgeon's choices to what suture or stapler to use and how to use them makes little difference in the outcome. The question of hand sewn or stapled has been asked and answered many times, and few studies have ever shown superiority of one over the other when performed properly. The most recent Cochrane review,[21] which was published in 2012 and was an update of a previous meta-analysis,[22] analyzed the results of 1233 patients who underwent colorectal resections and anastomosis and found that the 2 techniques were equivalent for all relevant parameters including anastomotic leak rates, both clinically and radiographically. If a surgeon chooses to perform a hand-sewn anastomosis, even the choice of one technique over another has not been shown to be superior. In fact, the state of the art for intestinal suturing has essentially remained unchanged since Antoine Lembert first described the inverted suture for intestinal anastomosis. The choice of a single or double layer of suture has been the basis of a randomized trial by Burch and colleagues[23] who concluded that a single continuous layer of bowel apposition is quicker and has no adverse outcomes when compared with a double layer of interrupted suture. Although this study excluded anastomoses to the rectum, other investigators have demonstrated the reliability of the single-layer technique with a low rate of complications.[24,25] The choice of suture material has also been extensively reviewed, and although monofilament suture produces less of an inflammatory response, there is no evidence that this or any other aspect of a specific property of suture affects the success of an intestinal anastomosis.[26–30] The development of laparoscopic techniques for colorectal disease has been proved to have some short-term benefits and does not seem to be associated with a higher risk of anastomotic leak.[31] If a surgeon chooses to construct a colonic reservoir after proctectomy for rectal disease, there seems to be no benefit of a colonic J pouch over a transverse colo-plasty in terms of anastomotic integrity, and the results compare favorably with respect to leak rates versus a straight coloanal.[32,33]

Supplemental Oxygen

Perioperatively there are decisions that the surgeon can make that possibly mitigates the incidence of anastomotic failure. One such intervention is the use of supplemental oxygen in the perioperative period, with the hypothesis that increasing the oxygen saturation and its partial pressure in arterial blood improves the mucosal oxygen tension at the site of healing. In 1977, Kirk and Irvin[34] examined the influence of 50% inspired oxygen on the bursting strength of rats that had undergone a colonic anastomosis. This study was negative, and no benefit was noted in the bursting strength of the anastomosis when compared with control rats breathing air. However, investigators in Turkey demonstrated that the administration of hyperbaric oxygen during a left colon anastomosis and continued for 4 days postoperatively had signifi-cant benefit in the rat model. They showed that the bursting pressure and the hydrox-yproline content (a marker of collage content) of the submucosa in treated rats were significantly higher than in the controls.[35] This study has been replicated with similar results.[36,37] Human trials are limited with respect to the effects of supplemental oxygen on anastomotic healing, although there is a wealth of data on the benefits of this intervention on the prevention of surgical site infection. Investigators from Spain demonstrated that the use of 80% Fio_2 in the perioperative period in patients who underwent anterior resections of the rectum had significantly better tissue oxygena-tion at the anastomosis when compared with controls breathing 30% Fio_2.[38] Their study population included 45 patients, and there were no anastomotic complications in either group. Schietroma and colleagues[39] looked at the effect of supplemental oxygen in the perioperative period in patients who underwent elective infraperitoneal (IP) anastomoses for rectal cancer. Subjects were assigned to either 30% or 80% Fio_2 at the induction of anesthesia and maintained for 6 hours postoperatively. There was a 46% reduction in anastomotic complications ($P<.05$) for those patients receiving 80% Fio_2 when compared with those who received only 30%. There was no toxicity associated with the use of increased oxygen concentration. Although the evidence for supplemental oxygen is still in its infancy, the data would suggest that at a minimum they are equivalent and likely there may be some benefit. Owing to the ease and avail-ability of this intervention, surgeons performing left-sided, colorectal, and IP anasto-moses should consider its use to mitigate the risk of leak.

Resuscitation Strategies

Resuscitation strategies also affect anastomotic $TSaO_2$, with reports in the literature generally showing a decrease in overall postoperative complications with goal-directed and restrictive fluid strategies perioperatively.[40–42] Kimberger and colleagues,[43] using an experimental model of colorectal resections in pigs, suggested that the goal-directed approach is improved with the use of colloid instead of crystal-loid. In their study, the use of restrictive crystalloid administration had no effect on postoperative outcomes when compared with traditional resuscitation. Brandstrup and colleagues[44] evaluated the effects of a restrictive fluid strategy in a randomized controlled trial of 172 patients who underwent elective colorectal resections and found that patients in the restricted group (defined by perioperative maintenance of baseline weight) suffered significantly fewer overall ($n = 21$ vs 43 $P<.0001$) and major complications ($n = 8$ vs 19, $P<.026$). In this study, the restrictive strategy used a combination of colloid and crystalloid. Anastomotic leaks occurred in 1 patient in the restrictive group and 4 in the control group. These data were confirmed by Abraham-Nordling and colleagues[45] who assessed the use of a restrictive fluid strategy in a randomized controlled trial of 161 patients who underwent colorectal surgery to assess the effect on major surgical complications. Patients in the restricted fluid strategy group received a median of 3050 mL of crystalloid compared with 5775 mL of crystalloid in the control group. Overall, major surgical complications occurred in 5% versus 15% of the restrictive group when compared with controls ($P<.063$). However, there were only 7 anastomotic complications, and despite 6 occurring in the control group, this did not reach statistical significance. Contrary to these findings, Futier and colleagues[46] reported on 70 patients who underwent major abdominal surgery and reported that a restrictive fluid strategy (6 mL/kg/h) was associated with a higher rate of postoperative complications and anastomotic leaks when compared with a conservative approach (12 mL/kg/h). In sum, a restrictive fluid strategy perioperatively seems to be safe and may decrease the incidence of major and minor complications in patients undergoing elective colorectal surgery. However, its effect on anastomotic complications is less clear, and its implementation into everyday practice would seem more challenging than the simple use of supplemental oxygen.

Intraoperative Parameters

One final piece of this complex puzzle involving the surgeon's contribution to anastomotic failure is the intraoperative variables of blood loss and operative times. Most of these data come from retrospective databases of patients who underwent colorectal surgery who have been diagnosed postoperatively with an anastomotic leak. Because the incidence of leak is an uncommon, although widely varying, event in the literature (**Table 2**), this methodology can still be a powerful tool. However, the limitations of such wide-ranging studies can lead to erroneous conclusions. Nevertheless, several investigators have found in multifactorial analysis that excessive blood loss or blood transfusion and prolonged operative times are associated with a higher risk of anastomotic failure.[47–56] Further confounding the analysis, the definition of excessive blood loss and prolonged operating times differs in the literature. One representative study by Telem and colleagues[47] used 200 mL and 200 minutes, although this remains inconsistent. A more uniform finding entails any intraoperative transfusion is considered a risk factor for anastomotic leak, with the number of units not defined in most studies. The presence of one or more risk factors was shown to increase the incidence of anastomotic failure significantly over baseline, and in the study by Telem and colleagues[47] the presence of 3 risk factors (which in their study included operative times, blood loss, blood transfusion, malnutrition, and histologically positive margins) increased the OR of a leak to 21 (95% confidence interval [CI], 2.8–175.4), with a positive predictive value of 91%. In contrast, the absence of these risks was associated with an OR of a leak of 0.21 (95% CI, 0.16–0.5). More likely, blood loss and operative times represent a surrogate for a difficult operation, and the underlying pathophysiology can only be surmised, although ischemia and inflammatory mediators probably play a role. Surgeons should be mindful of these factors in deciding on the use of a protective stoma as a reliable way to decrease the clinical consequences, the reoperation rate, and the incidence of anastomotic leak in these difficult cases. **Table 2** summarizes the risk factors identified throughout the medical literature.[57–60]

Table 2
Summary of variables

	Type of Resection	Incidence of Anastomotic Leak (%)	Blood Loss (mL)	Operative Times (min)	Blood Transfusion (Risk Factor: Yes or No)	IP Anastomosis (Risk Factor: Yes or No)	Other Risk Factors
Schrock et al,[73] 1973	All	4.5		>300	Yes	Yes	Emergent surgery
Golub et al,[52] 1997	All	3.4	NS	NS	Yes	No	Low albumin, obstruction
Rullier et al,[66] 1998	Rectal	12		>240		Yes	Obesity, male gender
Sorensen et al,[70] 1999	All	15.9	>600	NS	Yes	Yes	Smoking
Alves et al,[55] 2002	All (excluded IP rectum)	6	NR	NR	Yes	NR	Emergent surgery, colocolic anastomosis
Makela et al,[54] 2003	Left sided	Not reported		>120	Yes	Yes	ASA classification >3
Law and Chu,[51] 2004	Rectal	5.6	>500			Yes	Male gender

Matthiessen et al,[83] 2004	Rectal	12	>2000	NS	Yes	Yes	Male gender
Choi et al,[61] 2006	Colonic	1.8					Emergent surgery, ASA classification >3
Lee et al,[56] 2006	Rectal	5			Yes	Yes	
Konishi et al,[48] 2006	Colorectal cancer	2.8	NR	>240	No	NR	Steroids
Suding et al,[53] 2008	All	3.6	NR	>220	NR	—	Steroids, Low albumin
Jestin et al,[50] 2008	Rectal	9.7	>600	>180	NR	Yes	Preoperative radiation, ASA classification >3
Eberl et al,[59] 2008	Rectal	10.4	NS	NS	NS	Yes	ASA classification >3
Buchs et al,[49] 2008	All	3.8	NS	>180	No	Yes	Obesity, ASA classification >3
Telem et al,[47] 2010	All	2.6	>300	>200	Yes	Yes	
Bertelsen et al,[58] 2010	Rectal	115	>600	NR	No	Yes	Male gender

Abbreviations: IP, infraperitoneal rectum; NR, not reported in the study; NS, not a significant risk factor.

PATIENT FACTORS

The surgeon is not the only variable in the complex interaction that results in anastomotic failure, as several patient-related factors have also been identified. Similar to the data describing risk in intestinal healing, the data on patient risk factors are not always consistent, and contradictory conclusions have often been made. For virtually every identified risk factor in this category, there is a report to refute the hypothesis. The weakest links seem to be in the category of smoking, alcohol consumption, age, and obesity, whereas the most consistent risk seems to be higher American Society of Anesthesia (ASA) classification and malnutrition/weight loss. **Table 3** summarizes these risks. A consistently higher ASA classification has been shown to increase the incidence of anastomotic complications, with a score of 3 or more usually defining a high-risk population (patient with severe systemic disease and definite functional impairment).[49,50,54,61] The patient's age at the time of surgery has also been shown to be a risk factor in some series, but no consistent cutoff has emerged.[62–64] Obesity is harder to quantify as a risk factor for elective colon surgery, especially in right-sided colectomies where it may be of no significance altogether.[65] However, several investigators have shown that in patients who underwent left-sided and more importantly rectal resections, especially in men, obesity increases the risk of anastomotic leaks.[65–68] Other modifiable patient risk factors include alcohol use and smoking, both of which have been shown to increase the risk of anastomotic leaks.[58,63,69–72] In the context of alcohol use, the quantity of problematic consumption is difficult to define and is fraught with the inaccuracies of self-reporting. However, in the study by Sorensen and colleagues,[53,54,63,70] patients who consumed more than 35 alcoholic drinks per week had a relative risk (RR) of anastomotic leak of 7.18 (95% CI, 1.2–43.01) when compared with patients who abstained. In the same study, smoking tobacco was associated with an RR of 3.18 (95% CI, 1.44–7.00) compared with nonsmokers. The nutritional status as defined by the serum albumin levels (varies between <3.5 and <3.0 g/dL) or the presence of preoperative weight loss greater than 10% has been reported to increase the risk of anastomotic failure in patients undergoing colorectal resections. Golub and colleagues[52] reported their experience in a retrospective review of 763 patients who underwent colorectal resections with an overall leak rate of 3.4%. The most common procedure was a right colectomy. Using a multivariate analysis they demonstrated that a serum albumin level of less than 3.0 g/dL was associated with an increased risk of anastomotic leak (OR, 2.73; 95% CI, 1.29–581; P<.009). In the study by Makela and associates,[54] strictly on left-sided resections, weight loss and malnutrition had an even more significant impact on the development of anastomotic leaks (OR, 13.22; 95% CI, 2.83–61.85; P<.0001).

Patient risk profiles are often difficult to modify and seem to have a much more variable impact on the failure of intestinal anastomosis than surgeon factors. The presence of multiple risk factors should alert the surgeon to the potential for complication development and perhaps lower the threshold for pursuing a diagnosis of a leak postoperatively in patients with softer indications. Smoking cessation, weight loss, and modification of alcohol use certainly benefits any patient undergoing surgery. However, whether this would result in an appreciable impact on postoperative leaks is unclear based on the variability of the data. On the other hand, an anorexic patient who has had weight loss might benefit from nutritional supplementation preoperatively (preferably enterally but in some cases parenterally) for at least 7 days before surgery. **Table 3** summarizes the patient-related risk factors in the literature.

Table 3
Patient-associated risk factors

	Type of Resection	Age	Obesity (Variably Defined)	Smoking	Alcohol Use	ASA ≥3	Malnutrition (Variably Defined)
Golub et al,[52] 1997	All	–	–	–	NR	+	+
Sorensen et al,[70] 1999	All	>63	–	+	+	NR	NR
Makela et al,[54] 2003	Left sided	NR	>27	–	Yes	+	+
Konishi et al,[48] 2006	All	–	–	NR	NR	–	–
Eberl et al,[59] 2008	Rectal	–	–	–	–	+	–
Suding et al,[53] 2008	All	–	–	–	NR	NR	+
Buchs et al,[49] 2008	All	–	+	NR	NR	+	NR
Asteria et al,[63] 2008	Rectal	>68	+	+	+	NR	+
Bertelsen et al,[58] 2010	Rectal	–	–	+	–	–	–

Abbreviations: +, positive risk factor; –, not a risk factor; NR, not reported.

DISEASE FACTORS

The final factor that contributes to anastomotic complications is the impact disease processes have on the healing of newly formed colorectal anastomoses.

Emergent Surgery

As a general rule, an anastomosis performed under emergent conditions has a greater propensity to leak.[55,61,67,73–76] Choi and colleagues[61] reviewed their series of 1417 patients who underwent colorectal resections for malignancy, all above the peritoneal reflection, with an anastomotic leak rate of 1.8%. Surgeries done emergently experienced a leak rate of 44%, although the overall numbers were low (11/25). The investigators did not differentiate the location of the leaks for their emergent cases, but the study cohort included all types of resections. This distinction is important, as generally surgeons are more reluctant to perform left-sided anastomoses in the context of an emergent procedure but are more willing to do so on the right. Biondo and colleagues[67] analyzed their experience with left-sided colonic emergencies and reported a leak rate of 5.7%. All patients ($n = 211$) in their cohort had primary resections and anastomosis for left-sided colonic emergencies (peritonitis, 106; obstruction, 98, and hemorrhage, 4), with on-table colonic lavage. Lee and colleagues[74] compared their results of left- versus right-sided colectomies in 243 patients who presented with an obstructing cancer (right sided, $n = 107$; left sided, $n = 136$). Most patients had a resection and primary anastomosis, although left-sided anastomoses were lavaged on table at the discretion of the surgeon. The overall leak rate was 6.1%, with no difference noted between left- and right-sided resections. There are not enough data to conclude that there is no difference in the risk associated with the site of the pathologic condition; however, given the data, it is safe to say that emergent colectomies are associated with a higher leak rate than those done electively. In the absence of shock and fecal peritonitis, the vast majority of patients can be considered for a primary anastomosis, right or left, when taken in the broader context of all other risk factors and the possibility that an on-table colonic lavage may reduce the risk of leak in emergent left-sided resections.

Infraperitoneal Location of Pathology

There are several compelling data that the anastomosis at highest risk of leak is the one situated below the peritoneal reflection.[49,50,55,56,59,61,62,66,75,77–80] The exception to this rule is the perineal proctectomy in which a hand-sewn coloanal anastomosis is created without the cover of a protective stoma with consistently good results.[81,82] This paradox demonstrates the complexity and the host of factors that may all contribute to anastomotic failure. Although perineal proctectomy has low associated leak rates (despite being a coloanal anastomosis), a similarly located anastomosis above the anal verge in the context of low rectal cancers is an independent risk factor for leak irrespective and independent of preoperative radiation and other surgery- and patient-related risks.[54,56,59,60] **Table 2** also shows the reported leak rates based on the type of resection along with the location of the anastomosis. As demonstrated, the incidence is consistently higher for rectal resections and almost uniformly associated with IP anastomoses. In the study by Sorensen and colleagues,[70] the reported anastomotic leak rate for 333 unselected consecutive patients was 15.9%. The RR of colorectal anastomotic leaks in a multivariate analysis was 11.06 (95% CI, 3.32–36.85) when compared with ileocolic and colocolonic anastomotic leaks. Among rectal resections alone, the distance from the anal verge is itself a consistent independent risk factor for leaks. Law and Chu[51] looked at leak rates after rectal surgery, comparing patients with a distal anastomosis (lower third of the rectum, $n = 396$) with patients whose anastomosis was in the middle or upper third of the rectum ($n = 226$). The over-all leak rate was low when compared with studies of rectal resections at 5.6%. The mortality was similar in both cohorts, despite a higher hazards ratio of 6.3 for leak in the low rectal group (95% CI, 3.4–46.7; $P<.0001$). Confounding many of these rectal cancer cohorts is the potential impact of previous radiation therapy on leak rates. The use of radiation therapy in Law and Chu's cohort was not stated, although they comment that it was not routine. Matthiessen and colleagues[83] reported on 436 patients who underwent rectal resections with an overall leak rate of 12%. Rectal cancer was the indication in 91% of the cases, and preoperative radiation was given in just 16%. The leak rate for anastomosis less than 6 cm from the anal verge was 24% compared with 13% for all others. In a multivariate analysis, anastomotic height was proved to be an independent risk factor ($P<.001$). In this same study, patients who had preoperative radiation therapy (most patients received short-course radiotherapy) had a leak rate of 31% compared with just 9% for those who were not treated. Radiation was also found to be an independent risk factor in a multivariate analysis ($P<.005$). The use of radiation has been shown in other studies to be an independent risk factor for leaks,[50,84] although this is not uniformly observed.[85]

Steroid, Immunomodulators, and Inflammatory Bowel Disease

The use of prednisone and other immunomodulators to treat inflammatory conditions can also have an effect on anastomotic leak rates, although the major risk factor for postoperative complications remains the routine use of oral or parenteral steroids.[48,52,53,55,86] The duration and extent of treatment likely affect the level of risk, although good data on the timing and safety of cessation are lacking. These effects may be mitigated in patients with inflammatory bowel disease, as it may be more critical that the associated inflammation and systemic effects of their disease be controlled.[87] However, the wealth of data on patients with Crohn disease (CD) and ulcerative colitis (UC) suggests that the use of steroids increases postoperative septic complications in general, with less evidence that the anastomotic leak rates are higher.[88–90] Immunomodulators also seem to be safe in this patient population, as does anti-TNF alpha therapy. Although data exist only for infliximab (IFX) and not the newer human monoclonal antibodies, there does not seem to be any substantial evidence in favor of stopping this treatment before elective colorectal surgery.[91–94] There remains uncertainty about the effect of anti-TNF alpha therapy in patients with UC undergoing restorative proctocolectomy. This treatment is relatively new, but the effect on postoperative complications and ileal J-pouch-anal anastomotic failure has been reported with different conclusions. Selvaseker and colleagues[95] studied 301 patients who underwent restorative proctocolectomy for medically refractory UC and analyzed the effect of preoperative IFX therapy on postoperative complications (IFX, $n = 47$; no IFX, $n = 254$). They found that IFX therapy was linked to increased occurrence of anastomotic leaks ($P<.02$) and infectious complications ($P<.01$). This study was performed before 2005; therefore, the use of IFX for the treatment of UC was off label, and bias certainly could have existed with respect to disease severity and overall health status of the patients in the study group. Mor and colleagues[96] were successful in eliminating this bias by reporting on disease severity and patient comorbidity. Their results supported the findings that IFX increased the occurrence of anastomotic leaks and infectious complications. These findings were refuted by 3 studies, which concluded that there was no such association between IFX therapy and postoperative pouch anal leaks or pelvic sepsis.[97–99] One of these studies (Ferrante and colleagues[98]) even concluded that the postoperative complications in their cohort were attributed to the use of steroid and not IFX.

Several factors have also been reported to increase the risk of anastomotic complications in patients undergoing resection for CD. These factors include histologically involved margin of resection,[47] intra-abdominal abscess or fistula at the time of surgery, malnutrition, and reoperative surgery for CD.[88,90] In addition, several investigators have suggested that a side-to-side anastomosis is associated with lower leak rates than an end-to-end anastomosis in CD, but the mechanics of why this occurs are not well understood.[100–102]

Evidence seems to support the tapering of steroids when possible in patients undergoing elective or urgent colorectal resections, but the cessation of immunomodulators and anti-TNF alpha therapy does not seem to be necessary. Because most surgeons are inclined to perform a stapled side-to-side anastomosis, its use in patients with CD seems particularly appropriate. Intra-abdominal sepsis should be controlled preoperatively when possible in all instances, which may prove particularly important in CD. The use of preoperative nutritional supplementation in patients with documented malnutrition is warranted whenever possible.

Malignancy

The previous section described the risk of anastomotic failure in low rectal cancer, but this was more related to the location of the IP anastomosis and not the primary pathologic condition itself. Malignancy has several potential issues that may contribute to variable leak rates. One such is the use of certain chemotherapeutics. There are some reports of the use of bevacizumab leading to an increased risk of anastomotic complications when used both before and after surgery. These complications typically occur in the early postoperative period, but case studies have demonstrated that there can be a delayed effect even as long as 30 months postoperatively.[103] It is reasonable therefore to wait a minimum of 6 weeks after the administration of bevacizumab before performing elective colorectal resections and to delay initiation of therapy for at least 28 days after surgery. In addition to the effect of drug therapy, metastatic colorectal cancer has been shown to be an independent risk factor for anastomotic leak, and surgeons should be vigilant to counsel the patient in need of a resection for stage IV disease regarding both the increased incidence and the profound impact of anastomotic failure.[71,104]

Trauma

The treatment of colonic injuries has undergone significant changes during the past century, evolving from a policy of mandatory colostomy use to that of primary repair or resection and anastomosis when possible. The American Association for the Surgery of Trauma (AAST) multicenter trial assessing the safety of primary repair or resection and anastomosis compared with diversion concluded that diversion was unnecessary in the absence of significant fecal contamination and shock.[105] The method of anastomosis does not seem to have an effect on the risk of leak in this setting.[106] The increase in the number of damage control techniques has also affected the development of anastomotic leaks. Ott and colleagues[107] performed a cohort-matched study on 174 patients with colonic injuries initially managed with resection and anastomosis in the setting of an open abdomen who underwent a damage control laparotomy. They identified a significantly higher leak rate among patients whose abdomens were left open compared with those whose abdomens could be primarily closed (27% vs 6%, $P = .002$). Leaks also occurred more frequently in patients requiring blood transfusions and after left-sided resections. Unfortunately, nearly all presumed risk factors have in some manner been associated with the development of anastomotic leak in the setting of trauma. There is a paucity of prospective data in this cohort to provide high-level evidence to base recommendations on, and surgeons are often left to rely on their experience and judgment in this scenario.

MITIGATING THE RISK OF ANASTOMOTIC FAILURE

A thorough knowledge of the risk factors associated with anastomotic failure is not enough to prevent leaks, and surgeons continue to look for ways to help mitigate this terrible complication. Bowel preparation, once thought to be essential to the success of a colorectal resection, has increasingly become irrelevant in modern surgery, although still widely practiced.[108] Oral and parenteral antibiotics essential for the control of postoperative surgical site infections do not seem to have a significant role in the prevention of anastomotic leaks. The medical industry has continued to improve on stapler technology, and there has been some interest in the use of materials to buttress the staple line in newly formed anastomoses. However, there has not been any success in human colorectal trials, whereas results in animal models are mixed.[109–112] Also on the fringe is the use of the omentum to biologically "buttress" or protect a newly formed anastomosis. Data are mixed, with some reports stating an advantage in terms of leak rates.[113–116]

Diverting Stoma

Perhaps the most effective intervention available to surgeons to decrease the incidence of anastomotic failure is the use of a protective stoma to divert the fecal flow away from the newly created anastomosis.[57–59,104,117–121] Although most of the literature on the use of protective stomas comes from studies in rectal surgery, the results should be applicable to all anastomoses. It has been suggested that a covering stoma only mitigates the clinical impact of anastomotic failure without preventing leaks,[83] despite multiple investigators and 3 recent meta-analyses, including the Cochrane review authored by Montedori and colleagues,[120] refuting this assertion. In this review of the published literature, the use of a diverting stoma in rectal cancer surgery resulted in both a decreased incidence of anastomotic leak (RR, 0.33; 95% CI, 0.21–0.53), as well as the need for urgent reoperation (RR, 0.23; 95% CI, 0.12–0.42).

Pelvic Drains

The use of pelvic drains after rectal resection was based on the assumption that blood and fluid naturally accumulate in the presacral space. It was thought that any infected collection would naturally point toward the suture line, with resultant disruption and leak.[122] Although several investigators have concluded that the use of closed-suction pelvic drains results in fewer anastomotic complications,[57,123] others have not.[124–127] Some reports conclude that the use of pelvic drains is associated with a higher leak rate, and their use have been identified as an independent risk factor for anastomotic disruption.[124,128,129] Jesus and colleagues[126] published a meta-analysis of the study of the use of pelvic drains and their effect on the anastomotic integrity. Of the 1140 patients reviewed encompassing 6 randomized controlled trials, there was a 5% leak rate in both groups. There was also no advantage in the numbers of patient requiring reintervention (6% vs 5%).

Air Leak Testing

An immediate test of an anastomotic integrity is to assess for an air leak, which is easily performed for colorectal and left-sided resections and may help prevent or identify anastomotic leaks.[130–132] Ricciardi and colleagues[132] reviewed the outcomes of 825 left-sided resections and found evidence that 8% of those tested showed positive results for an air leak. Postoperative leaks occurred in 7.7% of anastomoses that tested positive, in 3.8% of those that tested negative, and in 8.1% of those that were not tested ($P<.03$). Furthermore, the anastomotic leak rate was 12.1% when an anastomosis that initially showed positive results was suture repaired, so that they were air tight compared with 0% when they were completely redone or were diverted proximally (P = NS). Beard and colleagues[130] performed a randomized trial of 145 patients who underwent left-sided and rectal resections to intraoperative air leak testing or nothing. In the test group, air leaked from 25% of anastomoses, which were repaired. Clinically relevant anastomotic leaks occurred in 4% of the test group and in 14% in the no test group (P = .043). Although these benefits have not been uniformly demonstrated,[133] no investigators have shown that air leak testing is harmful, and likely never will. Owing to the potential benefit and the ease of performing this air test, surgeons should consider it as a routine part of their practice for left-sided and rectal resections. Because of the absence of data and the increased difficulty in anastomosis proximal to the splenic flexure, no recommendations can be made.

ANASTOMOTIC STRICTURE AND BLEEDING
Stricture

Anastomotic stricture after a colon anastomosis is a well-known but poorly defined complication. What may be a "small" narrowing to some is a tight stricture or even "wide open" to others. Furthermore, outside of symptoms or scheduled endoscopic follow-up, the anastomosis may not be evaluated for months or years. As such, it is difficult to determine the actual rate of stricture formation for colorectal anastomoses. Ambrosetti and colleagues[134] reviewed their experience in 68 patients who underwent elective laparoscopic sigmoid colectomy using a double-stapled colorectal anastomosis. They defined a stricture purely based on symptoms, identifying 22 patients (32%). Of these, only 12 patients (18%) eventually needed dilatation of their anastomosis. The investigators could not identify any risk factors that predisposed to stricture formation in their patient population. In a study of 179 patients (94 men) who underwent a colorectal anastomosis, Bannura and colleagues[135] defined stenosis as the inability to pass a rigid sigmoidoscope through the anastomosis. By using this criterion, a stricture was present in 21.1% of the cases. Unlike in the study by Ambrosetti and colleagues, male sex and evaluation within 4 months of surgery were independently associated with the development of a stenosis in stapled colorectal anastomosis. In 2012, Neutzling and colleagues[21] updated their Cochrane review that consisted of 9 randomized controlled trials with 1233 patients (622 stapled and 611 hand-sewn) who underwent a colorectal anastomosis. Although there were no other significant differences in evaluated metrics between the 2 methods, the investigators found that stricture was more common in a stapled anastomosis (risk difference [random-effects model] 4.6%; 95% CI, 1.2%–8.1%).

Treatment

Most strictures respond well to nonoperative means. In many cases, the simple passage of formed stool adequately distends the anastomosis and avoids the need for any further intervention. Depending on the location of the anastomosis, digital rectal examination with finger or Hegar dilators also aids in relieving distal strictures. Overall, dilation is a highly successful technique for the management of strictures and can be performed using either a rigid instrument or with the aid of pneumatic balloons. In a study of 256 consecutive patients who underwent low anterior resection,

Werre and colleagues[136] identified 21 patients (8.2%) with a stricture of the colorectal anastomosis. Stricture symptoms presented after a mean period of 7.7 months. Follow-up data were available for 15 of these patients. Because these were distal anastomoses, an endoscopic Savary dilation technique, with bougies of increasing diameters (10–19 mm), were used over a series of sessions. Normal defecation with complete resolution of symptoms occurred in 10 of the remaining 15 patients. In 5 patients, there was only partial improvement, but only 3 of them required reintervention. No complications occurred as the result of the dilations. A normal defecation pattern was never regained if more than 3 dilations were necessary.

In the study by Ambrosetti and colleagues,[134] dilation was performed in 12 patients with a median stenotic diameter of 7 mm at a mean time of 176 days postoperatively. Eight patients had only 1 session, 3 patients had 2 sessions, and 1 patient had 3 sessions. This study highlights the need for patient education to manage expectations regarding the oft-needed requirement for multiple treatments. There were no complications, and all patients were symptom-free after dilatation. Araujo and Costa[137] used pneumatic balloon dilatation in 24 symptomatic patients with benign colorectal anastomotic stricture using a through-the-scope balloon technique. In this series, dilation was successful in 22 (91.7%) patients, and there were no procedure-related complications. The mean number of sessions required was 2.3. The investigators were unable to identify a correlation between the number of dilation sessions and stricture recurrence. Several others have reported the successful use of dilation to treat symptomatic anastomotic strictures in greater than 95%, symptomatic relief in 70% to 100% of patients after the initial dilation, and 85% to 100% relief with subsequent sessions.[138–140] Failure to manage symptomatic stenosis with endoscopic techniques is correlated with previous radiotherapy, local recurrence of malignancy, and a prior large anastomotic dehiscence.[140]

For patients who fail pneumatic balloon dilatation of their symptomatic stricture, there exist a few additional options that may avoid the need for laparotomy or permanent stoma. A group from the United Kingdom studied the efficacy of self-expanding metallic stents and endoscopic transanal resection of strictures in managing high-grade benign colorectal anastomotic strictures after the failure of first-line therapies, demonstrating 90% satisfaction rates at a median follow-up of 29 months. Complications in this cohort included reoperation for bleeding, asymptomatic anastomotic perforation, and technical failure in an acutely angulated stricture.[141] Biodegradable stents have shown similar efficacy.[142] Other reported options that have proved successful include the use of electroincision (radial incisions of the scar) along with pneumatic balloon dilation,[143] circular and linear stapler re-resection of the stricture,[144] and dilation with concomitant corticosteroid injection.[145]

Bleeding

Bleeding after a gastrointestinal anastomosis is usually minor and self-limited. On occasion, a perforating vessel or trapped mesentery can result in symptomatic hematochezia and require intervention to control. When performing a stapled side-to-side anastomosis, the staple line should be inspected for evidence of pulsatile bleeding at the enteroenterostomy and controlled with a suture. After an end-to-end stapled anastomosis, evidence of significant bleeding may be harder to assess even with proctoscopic examination during the air leak test. Fortunately, clinically significant postoperative bleeding remains an uncommon entity. In a study involving 1389 colorectal procedures, clinically relevant bleeding from the colorectal anastomosis occurred in 7 patients (0.5%).[146] Although higher rates of bleeding (1.8%) have been reported,[147] the definition of what entails "significant bleeding" varies from study to study. Despite the low incidence of clinically significant bleeding after intestinal anastomoses, the early postoperative manipulation of a new anastomosis can be a harrowing experience. For that reason, some investigators advocate the routine use of endoscopy to evaluate the anastomotic line intraoperatively.[148] In this study, 338 patients who underwent a colorectal anastomosis were assessed. Immediate postanastomotic endoscopy was performed in 85 of these patients, with 5.9% requiring endoscopic intervention with a hemoclip as determined by the operative surgeon. Overall, the rate of clinically significant postoperative bleeding in both groups was similar, as was the need for postoperative intervention (2.8% in the nonendoscopy group vs 2.4% in the endoscopy group), making it difficult to make any recommendations.

Treatment

In most cases, the patient remains hemodynamically stable, and no intervention is required. The rate of transfusion requirement is routinely less than 5%.[147] In the review by Martinez-Serrano and colleagues,[146] bleeding in 6 of the 7 patients resolved with conservative treatment including endoscopy. Only 1 patient required surgical treatment, and there was no mortality and no anastomotic leaks in these 7 patients. Cirocco and Golub[147] reported nonoperative therapy to be successful in 14 of 17 patients (82%), using endoscopic electrocoagulation in 6 patients (43%) and blood transfusion alone in another 6 patients (43%). The investigators concluded that endoscopic electrocoagulation can be safely and effectively used on a newly created anastomosis to control unremitting anastomotic hemorrhage. Alternative endoscopic techniques include the use of submucosal injection of 10 mL adrenaline (1:200 000) in saline at the bleeding point, with good results.[149] The use of the endoscopic hemoclip has been well described in upper gastrointestinal procedures and in colonic diverticular bleeding; however, its application in postoperative anastomotic bleeding for colon or rectal anastomosis is lacking.[150,151] Anecdotally, the author (DR) has successfully used the endoscopic hemoclip to control bleeding at a colorectal anastomosis in the postoperative period. Finally, although rarely required, surgical exploration with oversewing of the anastomosis or resection may be needed for select recalcitrant cases.[152]

Bleeding is a rare event after intestinal anastomosis, and endoscopic techniques have largely replaced the need for laparotomy or other surgical interventions. It is advisable that the operative surgeon performs or be present when endoscopic manipulation of a newly created anastomosis is required.

SUMMARY

The intestinal anastomosis is an essential part of surgical practice, and with it comes the inherent risk of breakdown and leaks. In colorectal surgery, the consequences of such a leak is disastrous, as bacteria-laden stool accesses the peritoneal cavity, sometimes ending in lethal consequences. Risk factors for anastomotic failure are categorized as surgeon related, patient related, and disease related. Some of the risks are modifiable (malnutrition, smoking, and blood loss), whereas others are an inherent part of colorectal surgery (IP location of pathology, need for radiation, and emergency surgery). Understanding the myriad of risk factors and the strength of the data help guide a surgeon as to the safety of undertaking an operation in which a primary anastomosis is to be considered. In the absence of abandoning the goal of reuniting the cut ends of the bowel, a surgeon may choose to mitigate the risk of a leak by performing a proximal diverting stoma. Whether this risk is modified by the use of adjuncts such as pelvic drains, omental wrapping, or tissue reinforcement remains unclear; however, the performance of a simple intraoperative air leak test allows a surgeon to assess if the anastomotic integrity has been compromised. More importantly, it allows the surgeon the option of completely redoing it, repairing it, or diverting proximally with the expectation that the outcome will be better than if nothing is done or if the test is omitted. Similarly, familiarity with the various approaches to both stricture and bleeding at the anastomosis aids in optimizing patient outcomes with the least amount of morbidity should these complications occur.

REFERENCES

1. Halsted W. Circular suture of the intestine: an experimental study. Am J Med Stud 1887;94:436–61.
2. Myers C, Mutafyan G, Petersen R, et al. Real-time probe measurement of tissue oxygenation during gastrointestinal stapling: mucosal ischemia occurs and is not influenced by staple height. Surg Endosc 2009;23(10):2345–50.
3. Locke R, Hauser CJ, Shoemaker WC. The use of surface oximetry to assess bowel viability. Arch Surg 1984;119(11):1252–6.
4. Attard JA, Raval MJ, Martin GR, et al. The effects of systemic hypoxia on colon anastomotic healing: an animal model. Dis Colon Rectum 2005;48(7):1460–70.
5. Sheridan WG, Lowndes RH, Young HL. Tissue oxygen tension as a predictor of colonic anastomotic healing. Dis Colon Rectum 1987;30(11):867–71.
6. Zakrison T, Nascimento BA Jr, Tremblay LN, et al. Perioperative vasopressors are associated with an increased risk of gastrointestinal anastomotic leakage. World J Surg 2007;31(8):1627–34.
7. Millan M, Garcia-Granero E, Flor B, et al. Early prediction of anastomotic leak in colorectal cancer surgery by intramucosal pH. Dis Colon Rectum 2006;49(5): 595–601.
8. Vignali A, Gianotti L, Braga M, et al. Altered microperfusion at the rectal stump is predictive for rectal anastomotic leak. Dis Colon Rectum 2000;43(1):76–82.
9. Pineda C, Raju N. 2nd Biennial meeting of the Eurasian Colorectal Technologies Association (ECTA): Turin, Italy, 15-17 June 2011 ECTA president: F. Seow-Choen Congress President: M. Morino. Tech Coloproctol 2011;15(2):215–53.
10. Kanemitsu Y, Hirai T, Komori K, et al. Survival benefit of high ligation of the inferior mesenteric artery in sigmoid colon or rectal cancer surgery. Br J Surg 2006; 93(5):609–15.
11. Chin CC, Yeh CY, Tang R, et al. The oncologic benefit of high ligation of the inferior mesenteric artery in the surgical treatment of rectal or sigmoid colon cancer. Int J Colorectal Dis 2008;23(8):783–8.
12. Titu LV, Tweedle E, Rooney PS. High tie of the inferior mesenteric artery in curative surgery for left colonic and rectal cancers: a systematic review. Dig Surg 2008;25(2):148–57.
13. Rutegard M, Hemmingsson O, Matthiessen P, et al. High tie in anterior resection for rectal cancer confers no increased risk of anastomotic leakage. Br J Surg 2012;99(1):127–32.
14. Karanjia ND, Corder AP, Bearn P, et al. Leakage from stapled low anastomosis after total mesorectal excision for carcinoma of the rectum. Br J Surg 1994; 81(8):1224–6.
15. Lange MM, Buunen M, van de Velde CJ, et al. Level of arterial ligation in rectal cancer surgery: low tie preferred over high tie. A review. Dis Colon Rectum 2008;51(7):1139–45.

16. Buunen M, Lange MM, Ditzel M, et al. Level of arterial ligation in total mesorectal excision (TME): an anatomical study. Int J Colorectal Dis 2009;24(11): 1317–20.
17. Hall NR, Finan PJ, Stephenson BM, et al. High tie of the inferior mesenteric artery in distal colorectal resections–a safe vascular procedure. Int J Colorectal Dis 1995;10(1):29–32.
18. Nelsen TS, Anders CJ. Dynamic aspects of small intestinal rupture with special consideration of anastomotic strength. Arch Surg 1966;93(2):309–14.
19. Shikata J, Shida T. Effects of tension on local blood flow in experimental intestinal anastomoses. J Surg Res 1986;40(2):105–11.
20. Howes EL, Samuel HC. The healing of wounds as determined by their tensile strength. JAMA 1929;92(1):42–5.
21. Neutzling CB, Lustosa SA, Proenca IM, et al. Stapled versus hand-sewn methods for colorectal anastomosis surgery. Cochrane Database Syst Rev 2012;(2):CD003144.
22. Lustosa SA, Matos D, Atallah AN, et al. Stapled versus hand-sewn methods for colorectal anastomosis surgery. Cochrane Database Syst Rev 2001;(3):CD003144.
23. Burch JM, Franciose RJ, Moore EE, et al. Single-layer continuous versus two-layer interrupted intestinal anastomosis: a prospective randomized trial. Ann Surg 2000;231(6):832–7.
24. Sarin S, Lightwood RG. Continuous single-layer gastrointestinal anastomosis: a prospective audit. Br J Surg 1989;76(5):493–5.
25. Law WL, Bailey HR, Max E, et al. Single-layer continuous colon and rectal anastomosis using monofilament absorbable suture (Maxon): study of 500 cases. Dis Colon Rectum 1999;42(6):736–40.
26. Hastings JC, Winkle WV, Barker E, et al. Effect of suture materials on healing wounds of the stomach and colon. Surg Gynecol Obstet 1975; 140(5):701–7.
27. Trimpi HD, Khubchandani IT, Sheets JA, et al. Advances in intestinal anastomosis: experimental study and an analysis of 984 patients. Dis Colon Rectum 1977;20(2):107–17.
28. Munday C, McGinn FP. A comparison of polyglycolic acid and catgut sutures in rat colonic anastomoses. Br J Surg 1976;63(11):870–2.
29. Lord MG, Broughton AC, Williams HT. A morphologic study on the effect of suturing the submucosa of the large intestine. Surg Gynecol Obstet 1978; 146(2):211–6.
30. Koruda MJ, Rolandelli RH. Experimental studies on the healing of colonic anastomoses. J Surg Res 1990;48(5):504–15.
31. Tjandra JJ, Chan MK. Systematic review on the short-term outcome of laparoscopic resection for colon and rectosigmoid cancer. Colorectal Dis 2006;8(5): 375–88.
32. Ulrich AB, Seiler CM, Z'Graggen K, et al. Early results from a randomized clinical trial of colon J pouch versus transverse coloplasty pouch after low anterior resection for rectal cancer. Br J Surg 2008;95(10):1257–63.
33. Brown CJ, Fenech DS, McLeod RS. Reconstructive techniques after rectal resection for rectal cancer. Cochrane Database Syst Rev 2008;(2):CD006040.
34. Kirk D, Irvin TT. The role of oxygen therapy in the healing of experimental skin wounds and colonic anastomosis. Br J Surg 1977;64(2):100–3.
35. Hamzaoglu I, Karahasanoglu T, Aydin S, et al. The effects of hyperbaric oxygen on normal and ischemic colon anastomoses. Am J Surg 1998; 176(5):458–61.

36. Yagci G, Ozturk E, Ozgurtas T, et al. Preoperative and postoperative administration of hyperbaric oxygen improves biochemical and mechanical parameters on ischemic and normal colonic anastomoses. J Invest Surg 2006;19(4):237–44.
37. Sucullu I, Sinan H, Filiz AI, et al. The effects of hyperbaric oxygen therapy on colonic anastomosis in rats with peritonitis. J Invest Surg 2008;21(4):195–200.
38. Garcia-Botello SA, Garcia-Granero E, Lillo R, et al. Randomized clinical trial to evaluate the effects of perioperative supplemental oxygen administration on the colorectal anastomosis. Br J Surg 2006;93(6):698–706.
39. Schietroma M, Carlei F, Cecilia EM, et al. Colorectal intraperitoneal anastomosis: the effects of perioperative supplemental oxygen administration on the anastomotic dehiscence. J Gastrointest Surg 2012;16(2):427–34.
40. Noblett SE, Snowden CP, Shenton BK, et al. Randomized clinical trial assessing the effect of Doppler-optimized fluid management on outcome after elective colorectal resection. Br J Surg 2006;93(9):1069–76.
41. Rahbari NN, Zimmermann JB, Schmidt T, et al. Meta-analysis of standard, restrictive and supplemental fluid administration in colorectal surgery. Br J Surg 2009;96(4):331–41.
42. Donati A, Loggi S, Preiser JC, et al. Goal-directed intraoperative therapy reduces morbidity and length of hospital stay in high-risk surgical patients. Chest 2007;132(6):1817–24.
43. Kimberger O, Arnberger M, Brandt S, et al. Goal-directed colloid administration improves the microcirculation of healthy and perianastomotic colon. Anesthesiology 2009;110(3):496–504.
44. Brandstrup B, Tonnesen H, Beier-Holgersen R, et al. Effects of intravenous fluid restriction on postoperative complications: comparison of two perioperative fluid regimens: a randomized assessor-blinded multicenter trial. Ann Surg 2003; 238(5):641–8.
45. Abraham-Nordling M, Hjern F, Pollack J, et al. Randomized clinical trial of fluid restriction in colorectal surgery. Br J Surg 2012;99(2):186–91.
46. Futier E, Constantin JM, Petit A, et al. Conservative vs restrictive individualized goal-directed fluid replacement strategy in major abdominal surgery: a prospective randomized trial. Arch Surg 2010;145(12):1193–200.
47. Telem DA, Chin EH, Nguyen SQ, et al. Risk factors for anastomotic leak following colorectal surgery: a case-control study. Arch Surg 2010;145(4):371–6 [discussion: 376].
48. Konishi T, Watanabe T, Kishimoto J, et al. Risk factors for anastomotic leakage after surgery for colorectal cancer: results of prospective surveillance. J Am Coll Surg 2006;202(3):439–44.
49. Buchs NC, Gervaz P, Secic M, et al. Incidence, consequences, and risk factors for anastomotic dehiscence after colorectal surgery: a prospective monocentric study. Int J Colorectal Dis 2008;23(3):265–70.
50. Jestin P, Pahlman L, Gunnarsson U. Risk factors for anastomotic leakage after rectal cancer surgery: a case-control study. Colorectal Dis 2008;10(7):715–21.
51. Law WL, Chu KW. Anterior resection for rectal cancer with mesorectal excision: a prospective evaluation of 622 patients. Ann Surg 2004;240(2):260–8.
52. Golub R, Golub RW, Cantu R Jr, et al. A multivariate analysis of factors contributing to leakage of intestinal anastomoses. J Am Coll Surg 1997;184(4): 364–72.
53. Suding P, Jensen E, Abramson MA, et al. Definitive risk factors for anastomotic leaks in elective open colorectal resection. Arch Surg 2008;143(9):907–11 [discussion: 911–2].

54. Makela JT, Kiviniemi H, Laitinen S. Risk factors for anastomotic leakage after left-sided colorectal resection with rectal anastomosis. Dis Colon Rectum 2003; 46(5):653–60.
55. Alves A, Panis Y, Trancart D, et al. Factors associated with clinically significant anastomotic leakage after large bowel resection: multivariate analysis of 707 patients. World J Surg 2002;26(4):499–502.
56. Lee MR, Hong CW, Yoon SN, et al. Risk factors for anastomotic leakage after resection for rectal cancer. Hepatogastroenterology 2006;53(71):682–6.
57. Peeters KC, Tollenaar RA, Marijnen CA, et al. Risk factors for anastomotic failure after total mesorectal excision of rectal cancer. Br J Surg 2005;92(2):211–6.
58. Bertelsen CA, Andreasen AH, Jorgensen T, et al. Anastomotic leakage after anterior resection for rectal cancer: risk factors. Colorectal Dis 2010;12(1): 37–43.
59. Eberl T, Jagoditsch M, Klingler A, et al. Risk factors for anastomotic leakage after resection for rectal cancer. Am J Surg 2008;196(4):592–8.
60. Detry RJ, Kartheuser A, Delriviere L, et al. Use of the circular stapler in 1000 consecutive colorectal anastomoses: experience of one surgical team. Surgery 1995;117(2):140–5.
61. Choi HK, Law WL, Ho JW. Leakage after resection and intraperitoneal anastomosis for colorectal malignancy: analysis of risk factors. Dis Colon Rectum 2006;49(11):1719–25.
62. Jung SH, Yu CS, Choi PW, et al. Risk factors and oncologic impact of anastomotic leakage after rectal cancer surgery. Dis Colon Rectum 2008;51(6): 902–8.
63. Asteria CR, Gagliardi G, Pucciarelli S, et al. Anastomotic leaks after anterior resection for mid and low rectal cancer: survey of the Italian Society of Colorectal Surgery. Tech Coloproctol 2008;12(2):103–10.
64. Nesbakken A, Nygaard K, Westerheim O, et al. Audit of intraoperative and early postoperative complications after introduction of mesorectal excision for rectal cancer. Eur J Surg 2002;168(4):229–35.
65. Benoist S, Panis Y, Alves A, et al. Impact of obesity on surgical outcomes after colorectal resection. Am J Surg 2000;179(4):275–81.
66. Rullier E, Laurent C, Garrelon JL, et al. Risk factors for anastomotic leakage after resection of rectal cancer. Br J Surg 1998;85(3):355–8.
67. Biondo S, Pares D, Kreisler E, et al. Anastomotic dehiscence after resection and primary anastomosis in left-sided colonic emergencies. Dis Colon Rectum 2005; 48(12):2272–80.
68. Gendall KA, Raniga S, Kennedy R, et al. The impact of obesity on outcome after major colorectal surgery. Dis Colon Rectum 2007;50(12):2223–37.
69. Fawcett A, Shembekar M, Church JS, et al. Smoking, hypertension, and colonic anastomotic healing, a combined clinical and histopathological study. Gut 1996; 38(5):714–8.
70. Sorensen LT, Jorgensen T, Kirkeby LT, et al. Smoking and alcohol abuse are major risk factors for anastomotic leakage in colorectal surgery. Br J Surg 1999;86(7):927–31.
71. Richards CH, Campbell V, Ho C, et al. Smoking is a major risk factor for anastomotic leak in patients undergoing low anterior resection. Colorectal Dis 2012; 14(5):628–33.
72. Kim MJ, Shin R, Oh HK, et al. The impact of heavy smoking on anastomotic leakage and stricture after low anterior resection in rectal cancer patients. World J Surg 2011;35(12):2806–10.

73. Schrock TR, Deveney CW, Dunphy JE. Factor contributing to leakage of colonic anastomoses. Ann Surg 1973;177(5):513–8.
74. Lee YM, Law WL, Chu KW, et al. Emergency surgery for obstructing colorectal cancers: a comparison between right-sided and left-sided lesions. J Am Coll Surg 2001;192(6):719–25.
75. Platell C, Barwood N, Dorfmann G, et al. The incidence of anastomotic leaks in patients undergoing colorectal surgery. Colorectal Dis 2007;9(1):71–9.
76. Komen N, Dijk JW, Lalmahomed Z, et al. After-hours colorectal surgery: a risk factor for anastomotic leakage. Int J Colorectal Dis 2009;24(7):789–95.
77. Lipska MA, Bissett IP, Parry BR, et al. Anastomotic leakage after lower gastrointestinal anastomosis: men are at a higher risk. ANZ J Surg 2006;76(7):579–85.
78. Vignali A, Fazio VW, Lavery IC, et al. Factors associated with the occurrence of leaks in stapled rectal anastomoses: a review of 1,014 patients. J Am Coll Surg 1997;185(2):105–13.
79. Tagart RE. Colorectal anastomosis: factors influencing success. J R Soc Med 1981;74(2):111–8.
80. Pakkastie TE, Luukkonen PE, Jarvinen HJ. Anastomotic leakage after anterior resection of the rectum. Eur J Surg 1994;160(5):293–7 [discussion: 299–300].
81. Altomare DF, Binda G, Ganio E, et al. Long-term outcome of Altemeier's procedure for rectal prolapse. Dis Colon Rectum 2009;52(4):698–703.
82. Cirocco WC. The Altemeier procedure for rectal prolapse: an operation for all ages. Dis Colon Rectum 2010;53(12):1618–23.
83. Matthiessen P, Hallbook O, Andersson M, et al. Risk factors for anastomotic leakage after anterior resection of the rectum. Colorectal Dis 2004;6(6):462–9.
84. Buie WD, MacLean AR, Attard JA, et al. Neoadjuvant chemoradiation increases the risk of pelvic sepsis after radical excision of rectal cancer. Dis Colon Rectum 2005;48(10):1868–74.
85. Martel G, Al-Suhaibani Y, Moloo H, et al. Neoadjuvant therapy and anastomotic leak after tumor-specific mesorectal excision for rectal cancer. Dis Colon Rectum 2008;51(8):1195–201.
86. Ziegler MA, Catto JA, Riggs TW, et al. Risk factors for anastomotic leak and mortality in diabetic patients undergoing colectomy: analysis from a statewide surgical quality collaborative. Arch Surg 2012;147(7):600–5.
87. Tay GS, Binion DG, Eastwood D, et al. Multivariate analysis suggests improved perioperative outcome in Crohn's disease patients receiving immunomodulator therapy after segmental resection and/or strictureplasty. Surgery 2003;134(4):565–72 [discussion: 572–3].
88. Alves A, Panis Y, Bouhnik Y, et al. Risk factors for intra-abdominal septic complications after a first ileocecal resection for Crohn's disease: a multivariate analysis in 161 consecutive patients. Dis Colon Rectum 2007;50(3):331–6.
89. Post S, Betzler M, von Ditfurth B, et al. Risks of intestinal anastomoses in Crohn's disease. Ann Surg 1991;213(1):37–42.
90. Yamamoto T, Allan RN, Keighley MR. Risk factors for intra-abdominal sepsis after surgery in Crohn's disease. Dis Colon Rectum 2000;43(8):1141–5.
91. Canedo J, Lee SH, Pinto R, et al. Surgical resection in Crohn's disease: is immunosuppressive medication associated with higher postoperative infection rates? Colorectal Dis 2011;13(11):1294–8.
92. Colombel JF, Loftus EV Jr, Tremaine WJ, et al. Early postoperative complications are not increased in patients with Crohn's disease treated perioperatively with infliximab or immunosuppressive therapy. Am J Gastroenterol 2004;99(5):878–83.

93. Kunitake H, Hodin R, Shellito PC, et al. Perioperative treatment with infliximab in patients with Crohn's disease and ulcerative colitis is not associated with an increased rate of postoperative complications. J Gastrointest Surg 2008; 12(10):1730–6 [discussion: 1736–7].

94. Ali T, Yun L, Rubin DT. Risk of post-operative complications associated with anti-TNF therapy in inflammatory bowel disease. World J Gastroenterol 2012;18(3): 197–204.

95. Selvasekar CR, Cima RR, Larson DW, et al. Effect of infliximab on short-term complications in patients undergoing operation for chronic ulcerative colitis. J Am Coll Surg 2007;204(5):956–62 [discussion: 962–3].

96. Mor IJ, Vogel JD, da Luz Moreira A, et al. Infliximab in ulcerative colitis is associated with an increased risk of postoperative complications after restorative proctocolectomy. Dis Colon Rectum 2008;51(8):1202–7 [discussion: 1207–10].

97. Schluender SJ, Ippoliti A, Dubinsky M, et al. Does infliximab influence surgical morbidity of ileal pouch-anal anastomosis in patients with ulcerative colitis? Dis Colon Rectum 2007;50(11):1747–53.

98. Ferrante M, D'Hoore A, Vermeire S, et al. Corticosteroids but not infliximab increase short-term postoperative infectious complications in patients with ulcerative colitis. Inflamm Bowel Dis 2009;15(7):1062–70.

99. Gainsbury ML, Chu DI, Howard LA, et al. Preoperative infliximab is not associated with an increased risk of short-term postoperative complications after restorative proctocolectomy and ileal pouch-anal anastomosis. J Gastrointest Surg 2011;15(3):397–403.

100. Simillis C, Purkayastha S, Yamamoto T, et al. A meta-analysis comparing conventional end-to-end anastomosis vs. other anastomotic configurations after resection in Crohn's disease. Dis Colon Rectum 2007;50(10):1674–87.

101. Resegotti A, Astegiano M, Farina EC, et al. Side-to-side stapled anastomosis strongly reduces anastomotic leak rates in Crohn's disease surgery. Dis Colon Rectum 2005;48(3):464–8.

102. Choy PY, Bissett IP, Docherty JG, et al. Stapled versus hand-sewn methods for ileocolic anastomoses. Cochrane Database Syst Rev 2011;(9):CD004320.

103. Deshaies I, Malka D, Soria JC, et al. Antiangiogenic agents and late anastomotic complications. J Surg Oncol 2010;101(2):180–3.

104. Boccola MA, Lin J, Rozen WM, et al. Reducing anastomotic leakage in oncologic colorectal surgery: an evidence-based review. Anticancer Res 2010; 30(2):601–7.

105. Demetriades D, Murray JA, Chan L, et al. Penetrating colon injuries requiring resection: diversion or primary anastomosis? An AAST prospective multicenter study. J Trauma 2001;50(5):765–75.

106. Demetriades D, Murray JA, Chan LS, et al. Hand-sewn versus stapled anastomosis in penetrating colon injuries requiring resection: a multicenter study. J Trauma 2002;52(1):117–21.

107. Ott MM, Norris PR, Diaz JJ, et al. Colon anastomosis after damage control laparotomy: recommendations from 174 trauma colectomies. J Trauma 2011;70(3): 595–602.

108. Guenaga KF, Matos D, Castro AA, et al. Mechanical bowel preparation for elective colorectal surgery. Cochrane Database Syst Rev 2003;(2):CD001544.

109. Gaertner WB, Hagerman GF, Potter MJ, et al. Experimental evaluation of a bovine pericardium-derived collagen matrix buttress in ileocolic and colon anastomoses. J Biomed Mater Res B Appl Biomater 2010;92(1):48–54.

110. Hagerman GF, Gaertner WB, Ruth GR, et al. Bovine pericardium buttress reinforces colorectal anastomoses in a canine model. Dis Colon Rectum 2007; 50(7):1053–60.

111. Hoeppner J, Willa K, Timme S, et al. Reinforcement of colonic anastomoses with a collagenous double-layer matrix extracted from porcine dermis. Eur Surg Res 2010;45(2):68–76.

112. Fajardo AD, Chun J, Stewart D, et al. 1.5:1 meshed AlloDerm bolsters for stapled rectal anastomoses does not provide any advantage in anastomotic strength in a porcine model. Surg Innov 2011;18(1):21–8.

113. Goldsmith HS. Protection of low rectal anastomosis with intact omentum. Surg Gynecol Obstet 1977;144(4):584–6.

114. Lanter B, Mason RA. Use of omental pedicle graft to protect low anterior colonic anastomosis. Dis Colon Rectum 1979;22(7):448–51.

115. Agnifili A, Schietroma M, Carloni A, et al. Omentoplasty is effective in lowering the complications of ano-rectal resections. Minerva Chir 2004; 59(4):363–8 [in Italian].

116. Agnifili A, Schietroma M, Carloni A, et al. The value of omentoplasty in protecting colorectal anastomosis from leakage. A prospective randomized study in 126 patients. Hepatogastroenterology 2004;51(60):1694–7.

117. Matthiessen P, Hallbook O, Rutegard J, et al. Defunctioning stoma reduces symptomatic anastomotic leakage after low anterior resection of the rectum for cancer: a randomized multicenter trial. Ann Surg 2007;246(2):207–14.

118. Huser N, Michalski CW, Erkan M, et al. Systematic review and meta-analysis of the role of defunctioning stoma in low rectal cancer surgery. Ann Surg 2008; 248(1):52–60.

119. Tan WS, Tang CL, Shi L, et al. Meta-analysis of defunctioning stomas in low anterior resection for rectal cancer. Br J Surg 2009;96(5):462–72.

120. Montedori A, Cirocchi R, Farinella E, et al. Covering ileo- or colostomy in anterior resection for rectal carcinoma. Cochrane Database Syst Rev 2010;(5):CD006878.

121. Chude GG, Rayate NV, Patris V, et al. Defunctioning loop ileostomy with low anterior resection for distal rectal cancer: should we make an ileostomy as a routine procedure? A prospective randomized study. Hepatogastroenterology 2008;55(86–87):1562–7.

122. Gerber A. Editorial: the anastomosis should be made without tension. Surg Gynecol Obstet 1976;142(1):75–6.

123. Tsujinaka S, Kawamura YJ, Konishi F, et al. Pelvic drainage for anterior resection revisited: use of drains in anastomotic leaks. ANZ J Surg 2008;78(6):461–5.

124. Yeh CY, Changchien CR, Wang JY, et al. Pelvic drainage and other risk factors for leakage after elective anterior resection in rectal cancer patients: a prospective study of 978 patients. Ann Surg 2005;241(1):9–13.

125. Galandiuk S, Fazio VW. Postoperative irrigation-suction drainage after pelvic colonic surgery. A prospective randomized trial. Dis Colon Rectum 1991; 34(3):223–8.

126. Jesus EC, Karliczek A, Matos D, et al. Prophylactic anastomotic drainage for colorectal surgery. Cochrane Database Syst Rev 2004;(4):CD002100.

127. Merad F, Hay JM, Fingerhut A, et al. Is prophylactic pelvic drainage useful after elective rectal or anal anastomosis? A multicenter controlled randomized trial. French association for surgical research. Surgery 1999;125(5): 529–35.

128. Berliner SD, Burson LC, Lear PE. Use and abuse of intraperitoneal drains in colon surgery. Arch Surg 1964;89:686–9.

129. Smith SR, Connolly JC, Crane PW, et al. The effect of surgical drainage materials on colonic healing. Br J Surg 1982;69(3):153–5.
130. Beard JD, Nicholson ML, Sayers RD, et al. Intraoperative air testing of colorectal anastomoses: a prospective, randomized trial. Br J Surg 1990;77(10):1095–7.
131. Yalin R, Aktan AO, Yegen C, et al. Importance of testing stapled rectal anastomoses with air. Eur J Surg 1993;159(1):49–51.
132. Ricciardi R, Roberts PL, Marcello PW, et al. Anastomotic leak testing after colorectal resection: what are the data? Arch Surg 2009;144(5):407–11 [discussion: 411–2].
133. Schmidt O, Merkel S, Hohenberger W. Anastomotic leakage after low rectal stapler anastomosis: significance of intraoperative anastomotic testing. Eur J Surg Oncol 2003;29(3):239–43.
134. Ambrosetti P, Francis K, De Peyer R, et al. Colorectal anastomotic stenosis after elective laparoscopic sigmoidectomy for diverticular disease: a prospective evaluation of 68 patients. Dis Colon Rectum 2008;51(9):1345–9.
135. Bannura GC, Cumsille MA, Barrera AE, et al. Predictive factors of stenosis after stapled colorectal anastomosis: prospective analysis of 179 consecutive patients. World J Surg 2004;28(9):921–5.
136. Werre A, Mulder C, van Heteren C, et al. Dilation of benign strictures following low anterior resection using Savary-Gilliard bougies. Endoscopy 2000;32(5): 385–8.
137. Araujo SE, Costa AF. Efficacy and safety of endoscopic balloon dilation of benign anastomotic strictures after oncologic anterior rectal resection: report on 24 cases. Surg Laparosc Endosc Percutan Tech 2008;18(6):565–8.
138. Virgilio C, Cosentino S, Favara C, et al. Endoscopic treatment of postoperative colonic strictures using an achalasia dilator: short-term and long-term results. Endoscopy 1995;27(3):219–22.
139. Di ZH, Shin JH, Kim JH, et al. Colorectal anastomotic strictures: treatment by fluoroscopic double balloon dilation. J Vasc Interv Radiol 2005;16(1):75–80.
140. Pucciarelli S, Toppan P, Pilati PL, et al. Efficacy of dilatations for anastomotic colorectal stenoses: prognostic factors. Int J Colorectal Dis 1994;9(3): 149–52.
141. Forshaw MJ, Maphosa G, Sankararajah D, et al. Endoscopic alternatives in managing anastomotic strictures of the colon and rectum. Tech Coloproctol 2006;10(1):21–7.
142. Janik V, Horak L, Hnanicek J, et al. Biodegradable polydioxanone stents: a new option for therapy-resistant anastomotic strictures of the colon. Eur Radiol 2011; 21(9):1956–61.
143. Truong S, Willis S, Schumpelick V. Endoscopic therapy of benign anastomotic strictures of the colorectum by electroincision and balloon dilatation. Endoscopy 1997;29(9):845–9.
144. Nissotakis C, Sakorafas GH, Vugiouklakis D, et al. Transanal circular stapler technique: a simple and highly effective method for the management of high-grade stenosis of low colorectal anastomoses. Surg Laparosc Endosc Percutan Tech 2008;18(4):375–8.
145. Lucha PA Jr, Fticsar JE, Francis MJ. The strictured anastomosis: successful treatment by corticosteroid injections–report of three cases and review of the literature. Dis Colon Rectum 2005;48(4):862–5.
146. Martinez-Serrano MA, Pares D, Pera M, et al. Management of lower gastrointestinal bleeding after colorectal resection and stapled anastomosis. Tech Coloproctol 2009;13(1):49–53.

147. Cirocco WC, Golub RW. Endoscopic treatment of postoperative hemorrhage from a stapled colorectal anastomosis. Am Surg 1995;61(5):460–3.
148. Shamiyeh A, Szabo K, Ulf Wayand W, et al. Intraoperative endoscopy for the assessment of circular-stapled anastomosis in laparoscopic colon surgery. Surg Laparosc Endosc Percutan Tech 2012;22(1):65–7.
149. Perez RO, Sousa A Jr, Bresciani C, et al. Endoscopic management of postoperative stapled colorectal anastomosis hemorrhage. Tech Coloproctol 2007;11(1): 64–6.
150. Baron TH, Norton ID, Herman L. Endoscopic hemoclip placement for post-sphincterotomy bleeding. Gastrointest Endosc 2000;52(5):662.
151. Prakash C, Chokshi H, Walden DT, et al. Endoscopic hemostasis in acute diverticular bleeding. Endoscopy 1999;31(6):460–3.
152. Linn TY, Moran BJ, Cecil TD. Staple line haemorrhage following laparoscopic left-sided colorectal resections may be more common when the inferior mesenteric artery is preserved. Tech Coloproctol 2008;12(4):289–93.

Outcomes Following Proctectomy

Joshua I.S. Bleier, MD[a], Justin A. Maykel, MD[b],*

KEYWORDS

- Proctectomy • Function • Outcomes • Total mesorectal excision
- Sexual dysfunction • Urinary dysfunction • Treatment • Reconstruction

KEY POINTS

- Proctectomy often results in functional outcomes that can be significantly different from preoperative baseline status.
- A comprehensive understanding of normal anatomy and function, as well as the preoperative factors that may affect postoperative function, is crucial to guide an appropriate preoperative discussion outlining risk and options.
- Familiarity with operative technique and pitfalls and reconstructive options is necessary to optimize results.
- Common postoperative complications include derangements of defecatory, sexual, and urinary function.
- A rational approach to preoperative assessment and decision making will help maximize the potential for setting expectations as patients make critical decision that affect quality of life (QOL).

INTRODUCTION

Although successful removal of the rectum with reestablishment of gastrointestinal (GI) continuity is increasingly possible for pelvic surgeons, this article focuses on the consequences of proctectomy. For better comprehension, first the normal function of the rectum as well as the appropriate surgical techniques for proctectomy that have been specifically developed to minimize the risk of postoperative complications are discussed. Various options related to reconstruction and the functional issues seen after restoration of bowel continuity are also discussed. More specifically, the authors review bowel, urinary, and sexual changes after proctectomy, as well as the intraoperative pitfalls that may precipitate these. The authors also discuss management and the impact of new surgical techniques on function and outcome. Finally, the impact that all these factors have on patient QOL are reviewed.

Disclosures: None.
[a] Division of Colon and Rectal Surgery, Department of Surgery, Hospital of the University of Pennsylvania, 700 Spruce Street, #305, Philadelphia, PA 19106, USA; [b] Division of Colon and Rectal Surgery, Department of Surgery, UMass Memorial Medical Center, University of Massachusetts Medical School, 67 Belmont Street, Worcester, MA 01605, USA
* Corresponding author.
E-mail address: Justin.maykel@umassmemorial.org

Surg Clin N Am 93 (2013) 89–106
http://dx.doi.org/10.1016/j.suc.2012.09.012
0039-6109/13/$ – see front matter © 2013 Elsevier Inc. All rights reserved.

FUNCTION OF THE NORMAL RECTUM

In order to best understand the derangements that can occur after proctectomy, it is important to understand, at a basic level, the anatomy, normal function, and basic nervous innervation and reflexes of the rectum. This understanding will also help guide operative maneuvers designed to try to avoid some of these complications.[1]

Normal innervation of the rectum, anal canal, and sphincter complex is both autonomic and somatic. The sympathetic supply of the rectum arises from the L1–L3 lumbar branches of the spinal cord. The main sympathetic hypogastric plexus coalesces just below the sacral promontory around the root of the inferior mesenteric artery (IMA) to form the main hypogastric nerves. These nerves course laterally carrying postganglionic sympathetic fibers from the hypogastric plexus. At this level, the sympathetic nerves meet with the parasympathetic fibers to the rectum and anal canal, known as the *nervi erigentes*, which arise from S2–S4. These fibers join at the lateral side of the pelvis adjacent to the lateral stalks and pass laterally and anteriorly. In men, these fibers then continue on to the periprostatic plexus, which is situated on Denonvilliers fascia, between the seminal vesicles and the anterior mesorectal fascia (**Fig. 1**). Sexual function is closely regulated by these autonomic components. Erection

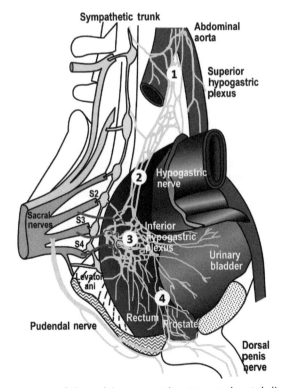

Fig. 1. Relational anatomy of the pelvic autonomic nerves and rectal dissection. Potential points of pelvic nerve injury during rectal injury include (1) damage to the superior hypogastric plexus from tension or high division of the IMA, (2) injury to the main trunks of the hypogastric nerve during retrorectal dissection, (3) injury to the inferior hypogastric plexus and *nervi erigentes* during mobilization of the lateral stalks, and (4) injury to the periprostatic plexus during dissection of Denonvillier fascia.

is primarily mediated by parasympathetic inflow, and ejaculation is primarily sympathetically mediated. Normal bladder function is also closely regulated by sympathetic function.

The external anal sphincter (EAS) is a skeletal muscle and is voluntarily controlled by the somatic nervous system, whereas the internal anal sphincter (IAS) is primarily autonomically mediated. Sympathetic inflow to the IAS is mediated by L5 and parasympathetic nerves derived from S2–S4. Motor control of the EAS is mediated by the inferior rectal branch of the pudendal nerve. Sensation to the anal canal is through the inferior rectal branch of the pudendal nerve, which may have a significant role in maintenance of continence.

The rectum is primarily a social organ, and its job is to store stool until a socially appropriate time for elimination. There are several reflex mechanisms for facilitating normal function. The rectoanal inhibitory reflex (RAIR) is the first mechanism involved in normal defecation. When fecal material enters the rectum and causes distention, there is a transient relaxation of the IAS. It is thought that this process allows a small amount of fecal material to come into contact with the upper anal canal, where specialized receptors sample the material to determine its consistency and state. If defecation is to be deferred, "receptive relaxation" of the rectal wall is triggered, allowing for increased distention and accommodation, without an increase in pressure. The RAIR is primarily dependent on intrinsic local innervation rather than a reflex arc mediated by the central nervous system. The reflex is often disrupted after low anterior resection (LAR) and is pathognomonically absent in Hirschsprung disease in which myenteric ganglia in the anal canal are missing; however, it is preserved even after transection of the hypogastric nerves and in the presence of spinal cord lesions.

At the same time as the RAIR is being triggered, the EAS and puborectalis contract to prevent inadvertent fecal loss. This reflex is termed the rectoanal excitatory reflex (RAER). The motor impulses mediating this contraction are likely transmitted through the pudendal nerve, because pudendal nerve block or damage may interfere with this reflex. Neuropathy identified on pudendal nerve terminal motor latency testing may portend derangements related to this reflex.

Intrinsic to the rectum's storage function is the compliance of a distensible rectum. As stool moves into the rectum, the receptive relaxation reflex allows progressive dilation of the rectum with a relatively blunted increase in wall tension. This process relies not only on normal innervation and sensation but also on healthy and compliant tissue.

Ultimately, for normal defecation to occur, movement of gas, liquid, or solid stool into the rectum initiates this complex series of reflex arcs. Distention of the rectum leads to initiation of the RAIR and movement of a small amount of fecal material into the upper anal canal. This process in turn stimulates external sphincter contraction via the RAER, as well as receptive relaxation, and distention of the rectal wall. If voluntary evacuation is called for, the puborectalis muscle relaxes, the anorectal angle straightens, and the combined abdominal wall and diaphragmatic muscles contract increasing the abdominal pressure, and the rectal contents are evacuated. Simply sitting or crouching aids in this entire process.

PREOPERATIVE FACTORS THAT MAY AFFECT POSTOPERATIVE FUNCTION

Given the complex interplay between the neural and anatomic mechanisms that govern normal rectal function, it becomes clearer how to identify preoperative factors that may affect postoperative function.

Radiation Therapy

For patients who have locally advanced rectal cancers, neoadjuvant radiation therapy is the standard of care to reduce local recurrence and potentially downstage the primary tumor and enhance resectability. However, radiation therapy can induce significant problems with normal function as a result of microvascular fibrosis. Early reports[2] did not bear out any functional effects on the residual rectum or its function, but the overwhelming majority of more recent data support significant functional morbidity as a result of radiation to the pelvis.[3–5] Radiation therapy not only affects the compliance of the residual rectum, which in turn, affects the critical aspect of distensibilty and capacitance, but also affects sphincter function.[3,5] Taken together, the radiation therapy may have significant deleterious effects on continence by affecting sphincter function and causing significant urgency by further limiting the capacitance of the residual rectum. When delivered postoperatively, radiation therapy can result in more significant bowel dysfunction because of the increased negative impact on the newly reconstructed, and intrinsically inferior, colonic reservoir. Owing to both the short-term and long-term toxic effects of adjuvant radiation therapy, neoadjuvant therapy is the currently preferred approach.[6]

Radiation therapy has also been shown to have a deleterious effect on sexual function postoperatively.[7] Compared with nonirradiated patients, men who receive radiation therapy encounter increased rates of ejaculatory and erectile disorders and women who receive the same note more pronounced sexual disorders.[4]

Prior Surgery

Patients who have had prior abdominal or pelvic surgery carry unique risks after proctectomy. In patients who have undergone prior colectomy, there may not be enough well-vascularized colon to allow for easy reanastomosis to the pelvic floor. Prior left or sigmoid colectomy may necessitate a proximal transverse to rectal anastomosis, or even an ileocecal transposition to reestablish GI continuity. In addition, loss of colon length may result in significant loss of absorptive surface area and the delivery of a large volume of liquid stool to the neorectum. This effect presents a particular challenge in patients with already compromised sphincter function after proctectomy. In addition, loss of the IMA vasculature may cause the available colon conduit to have marginal perfusion and increase the risk of anastomotic complications, or induce chronic ischemia and subsequent fibrosis or stenosis of the neorectal conduit.[8] In patients with prior pelvic surgery, either for benign disease or for inflammatory bowel disease, the mesorectal fascial planes may be obliterated, increasing the risk for pelvic autonomic nerve injury and subsequent compromise of bladder and sexual function. Finally, scarring in the lower retroperitoneum may place the ureters at risk in subsequent surgical procedures, and the astute surgeon should have a low threshold for the use of preoperative ureteral stenting to assist in ureteral identification and protection during surgery.

APPROPRIATE MESORECTAL DISSECTION—THE TME TECHNIQUE

Before the wide acceptance of total mesorectal excision (TME) popularized by Heald in the early 1980s and 1990s,[9] proctectomy was a highly morbid operation, resulting in significant blood loss, higher injury rates to pelvic autonomic nerves, and high local recurrence rates in oncologic resection. The principles of TME were developed based on rigid adherence to the known anatomic planes of dissection and preservation of the mesorectal fascial envelope. Because the dissection is based on intimate knowledge of pelvic anatomy, many of the pitfalls and complications related to rectal resection can be avoided. The basic principles of TME include careful dissection at the base of the IMA with avoidance of undue tension on the pedicle, because of the intimate association with the sympathetic hypogastric plexus. Injury to this plexus can result in urinary dysfunction (UD) and retrograde ejaculation. Careful entry into the areolar plane behind the IMA pedicle at the level of the sacral promontory guides a safe and relatively bloodless dissection posteriorly. In addition, careful dissection at this level allows for careful identification and preservation of the hypogastric nerves. Maintenance of dissection in this areolar plane laterally minimizes the risk of injury to the confluence of the sympathetic hypogastric fibers as they meet with the *nervi erigentes* in the lateral stalks of the rectum. Avoidance of deviation too posterolaterally at this level avoids disruption of the parasympathetic fibers and possible resultant sexual dysfunction (see **Fig. 1**). In addition to improving functional outcomes, proper TME technique has been shown to decrease the local recurrence and positive radial margin rate, owing to the lack of residual mesorectum left behind. Before TME, positive radial margin rates (one of the most important determinants of local recurrence risk) of 25% were not uncommon, as well as associated local recurrence rates as high as 40%.[10] After TME, rates of positive radial margins were reduced to approximately 7%, and local recurrence rates to as low as 5% to 7%, even in the absence of adjuvant radiation.[9]

More recently, the impact of minimally invasive techniques including laparoscopic and robotic-assisted proctectomy have been introduced and evaluated. Owing to the challenges and complexities of laparoscopic pelvic surgery, there is concern about the ability to perform a technically (oncologically) sound operation and preserve the pelvic nerves and the subsequent deleterious impact on postoperative outcomes including function.[11] Proponents of a minimally invasive approach counter that a magnified view of the pelvis may actually facilitate autonomic nerve preservation and optimization of postoperative outcomes.[12,13] The specific impact of robotic resection, with 3-dimensional view and fine motion control with 7 seven degrees of freedom, has not been rigorously studied. In 2012, Kim and colleagues[14] prospectively evaluated urinary and sexual function after laparoscopic ($n = 39$) and robotic ($n = 30$) TME for rectal cancer. When comparing the 2 surgical approaches, the investigators found earlier recovery of normal voiding and sexual function in patients undergoing TME after robotic resection. At least at this point in time, the study of minimally invasive options in the pelvis remains in its infancy, and formal recommendations await further experience with longer follow-up.

RECONSTRUCTION AND FUNCTION

Postoperative function after proctectomy can be significantly affected not only by preoperative and perioperative factors but also by the manner in which reconstruction is undertaken. In the setting of inflammatory bowel disease, reconstruction after proctectomy is usually limited to the surgical management of ulcerative colitis (UC). In general, restoration of GI continuity is ill advised after proctectomy for Crohn disease.[15] In the surgical management of familial adenomatous polyposis (FAP), total proctocolectomy is mandated, whereas reconstruction remains optional. Before the development of the ileal reservoir by Parks, end ileostomy was the gold standard for surgical management of patients with UC and FAP, whereas now, most patients choose restorative ileal J-pouch with pouch–anal anastomosis (IPAA). By introducing the concept of a neorectal reservoir, Parks revolutionized the concept of function after proctectomy.[16] Despite the creation of an adequate reservoir volume, there were still several functional deficits associated with the original description of the Parks pouch—mostly as a result of mucosal stripping of the distal rectal stump to the dentate line with hand-sewn ileoanal anastomosis. Despite maintenance of the sphincter mechanism, because stool consistency is always liquid or pastelike, daytime and nighttime seepage and incontinence were not infrequent. The double-stapled technique was developed to maintain the anal transition zone and its intrinsic neural pathways with the goal of preserving the physiology of the rectum and enhancing continence.[17] Although early reports showed no difference in function when comparing mucosectomy with the double-stapled technique,[18] most recent data from high-volume centers have shown convincing evidence of improved function with the double-stapled technique, with regard to daytime and nighttime seepage and continence.[19–21] This observation is believed to be due to maintenance of the sampling reflex (RAIR) afforded by preservation of a strip of the distal rectum and proximal anal canal. At present, this is the standard approach in the setting of UC, although mucosectomy and hand-sewn anastomosis still remains the option for most patients with FAP who require complete mucosal resection because of oncologic considerations.

Although there does not seem to be an overall difference on comparing men and women with regard to pouch function, women who have undergone an IPAA and have had a vaginal delivery are more likely to have nocturnal bowel frequency and seepage than women who have undergone an IPAA but have not had a vaginal delivery.[22] This observation should be a consideration regarding the mode of delivery after IPAA.

When proctectomy is undertaken for a rectal malignancy, reconstruction is generally performed using the proximal colon as conduit. As seen after proctectomy for UC, the loss of the rectal reservoir function causes significant postoperative urgency, frequency, and incontinence because of the lack of neorectal capacity. When reconstruction is done with a colorectal anastomosis, a constellation of symptoms known as "anterior resection syndrome" (ARS) develops, which is further discussed below. In order to address this problem, various operative techniques have been used to augment the neorectal capacity.

Straight colorectal or coloanal anastomosis (**Fig. 2**) is the standard by which these alternative techniques are judged because it is the modality most frequently performed to achieve adequate length to reach the pelvic floor for primary anastomosis. Initially, the 5-cm-long side-to-end or "Baker-type" anastomosis was used (**Fig. 3**), and this afforded an increase in neorectal volume via the blind loop of the efferent limb. As a result of the experience gained by ileal J-pouch reconstruction after total proctocolectomy, the colonic J-pouch was developed and initially described by Lazorthes and colleagues[23] and Parc and colleagues.[24] Typically 6 to 8 cm in length (**Fig. 4**), a colonic J-pouch can be constructed when there is adequate colonic length and pelvic volume to allow for its construction and placement. The other primary reconstructive alternative is coloplasty, which was described in 1999 by Z'graggen and colleagues,[25] in which an 8-cm longitudinal incision is made on the antimesenteric border of the conduit and then closed in a transverse manner (**Fig. 5**).

Since the development of these techniques, there have been numerous publications comparing overall outcomes and functions to each other and to straight coloanal anastomosis.[26,27] Although here have been no prospective randomized trials comparing all 4 techniques, numerous retrospective studies and trials have been published. Meta-analyses and Cochrane reviews have endeavored to accurately define the outcomes of these procedures relative to each other.[19,28–31] Initial experience with coloplasty suggested a higher leak rate, although most recent studies have not borne this out. Overall, reports indicate that within the first 12 to 24 months postoperatively, neorectal

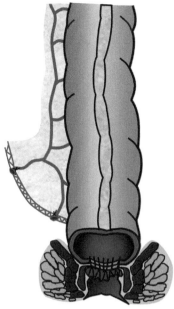

Fig. 2. Straight coloanal anastomosis.

function is best with the use of the colonic J-pouch when compared with coloplasty and straight anastomosis. There are some data to suggest, however, that creation of the pouch may be unnecessary and that side-to-end anastomosis (using the same total volume of neorectum without creating a common lumen) may offer equivalent functional results and no significant difference in complications.[32] This technique may also spare time and expense.[33] After 24 months, however, function among all the aforementioned options is essentially the same. The ability to create the colonic J-pouch is often limited by the lack of adequate length or a prohibitively narrow pelvis, especially in

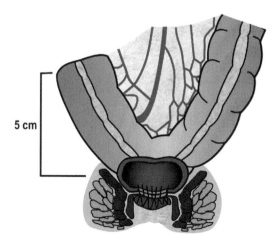

5 cm

Fig. 3. "Baker"-type side-to-end coloanal anastomosis. The blind limb is constructed to be approximately 5 cm in length.

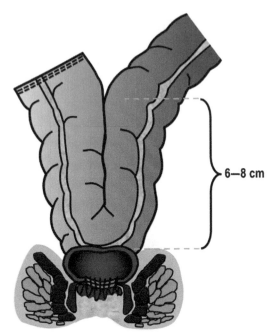

Fig. 4. Colon J-pouch. The typical colon J-pouch is constructed to be 6 to 8 cm in length.

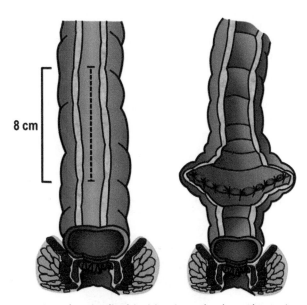

Fig. 5. Coloplasty: an 8-cm longitudinal incision is made along the antimesenteric taenia. The incision terminates 2 to 3 cm from the stapled end of the colon. The incision is then closed longitudinally.

men. The authors' preference is to perform a colonic J-pouch or Baker-type side-to-end anastomosis when technically feasible and reserve a straight coloanal anastomosis for the remaining cases. Alternative approaches such as transanal endoscopic microsurgery resection can be used in appropriately selected patients to preserve short-term and long-term anorectal function and QOL.[34]

SEXUAL FUNCTION POSTOPERATIVELY

Sexual dysfunction after proctectomy is frequently encountered in men, and likely underreported in women. As indicated earlier, before the development of the TME technique, rates of sexual dysfunction were as high as 75% in men. Sympathetic neuropathy caused by injury to the pelvic autonomic plexus at the sacral promontory causes ejaculatory difficulty, usually manifested as retrograde ejaculation. This difficulty can be avoided by minimizing traction on the IMA pedicle and trying to leave a 1-cm margin at the root of the IMA when dividing.[35] Parasympathetic injury either due to excessively lateral dissection along the lateral stalks or due to injury to the periprostatic plexus can cause impotence in up to 25% to 30% of men. With the anterior dissection in the TME, except when resecting an anteriorly based tumor, it is important to preserve the integrity of Denonvillier fascia that is invested by the periprostatic plexus, which can cause additional parasympathetic injury and impotence.[36] Before TME, postoperative impotence and retrograde ejaculation rates were observed in 25% to 75% of cases; however, careful adherence to TME principles have decreased this rate to 10% to 29% of cases.[1] Sexual manifestations of autonomic injury are much less pronounced in women but may cause vaginal dryness and dyspareunia. In addition, women have reported a loss of sexual desire and fear of fecal incontinence during intercourse after proctectomy and IPAA. On the contrary, in the setting of UC, men typically report improved sexual desire and function in the absence of any nerve damage after pelvic reconstruction.[37,38] As oncologic operations for rectal cancer may be more extensive, rates of sexual dysfunction have been shown to increase significantly after abdominal perineal resection (APR),[39,40] beyond the age of 65 years, after radiotherapy, and following intra-abdominal sepsis.[41]

Management of postoperative sexual function is multifactorial. Pilot studies of patients with neurogenic impotence after prostatectomy have shown that multidisciplinary treatment can demonstrate improvements in as soon as 6 to 12 months.[42] After proctectomy, pharmacologic treatment with phosphodiesterase inhibitors, such as oral sildenafil, has been shown to improve sexual function in 80% of patients compared with 17% with placebo.[43] Other, less-efficacious options include local intracavernous and intraurethral injections and vacuum constriction devices. Counseling of couples not only helps to reassure patients and their partners but also can enhance response to medical therapy.[35] Ultimately, in the event of failure of behavioral and pharmacologic therapies, placement of a penile prosthesis is effective but irrevocable and should be considered as a last resort.

BLADDER FUNCTION

Micturition is controlled by parasympathetic (contraction of the detrusor muscle), sympathetic (relaxation of the pelvic floor muscles and contraction of the trigone of the bladder), somatic (external sphincter muscle), and central nervous mechanisms.[44] Bladder dysfunction after pelvic surgery has been attributed to damage to the pelvic nerves, the sacral splanchnic (parasympathetic) nerves, the hypogastric (sympathetic) nerves, and the pelvic autonomic nerve plexus, with overall rates of dysfunction reported to range from 10% to 70%.[45–48] This variability in incidence may be explained by factors such as different degrees of preoperative symptoms, patient age, gender, length of follow-up, assessment instruments, and technical considerations, such as TME techniques, height of IMA/superior hemorrhoid vessel division, width of lateral node dissection, and nerve preservation technique.

As previously noted, the nerves that innervate the bladder course in close proximity to the rectum and its fascia propria. These nerves can be traumatized, damaged, or divided as a consequence of radiation and/or surgery. Injury to the sacral splanchnic nerves can also result in detrusor denervation and decreased sensitivity of the bladder with resultant urinary retention and overflow incontinence. The ligation of the IMA and dissection of the retrorectal space can cause damage to the superior hypogastric plexus and/or hypogastric nerves, causing reduced bladder capacity and urge incontinence. Anterolateral dissection in the "lateral ligament" area and division of Denonvillier fascia can damage the inferior hypogastric plexus and efferent pathways, resulting in urinary incontinence, voiding dysfunction, and bladder irritation (especially when injured bilaterally). Perineal dissection can indirectly damage the pudendal nerves, resulting in functional difficulties.[49]

In the immediate postoperative period, patients may have bladder dysfunction as a result of medications or inflammatory changes in the paravesical tissues or anatomic displacement of the bladder. This condition is typically managed with Foley catheter drainage/decompression, although it carries the concomitant increased risk of postoperative urinary tract infection. At 72 hours after proctectomy, the catheter can usually be removed and voiding proceeds normally. Approximately 40% of patients develop transient urinary retention, often requiring Foley catheter reinsertion.[50,51] Accordingly, the current Surgical Care Improvement Project guidelines exclude pelvic surgery from the requirement that Foley catheters are removed within 48 hours of surgery. The incidence of postoperative urinary retention seems to be higher in the elderly, generally men, and specifically higher in men with existing prostatic hypertrophy. However, there does not seem to be a significant difference when comparing APR with LAR.

Surgical technique plays a major role in preserving bladder function. The TME technique, coupled with nerve-preserving maneuvers, results in the most favorable outcomes. When conventional surgery is performed, and anatomic pelvic planes are not respected, permanent neurogenic bladder dysfunction can be seen in up to 10% of cases. In these cases, urodynamic studies identify significant signs of detrusor denervation including increases in bladder capacity, bladder compliance, residual volume, and an associated decrease in detrusor contraction pressure with increased volume of first sensation to void.[52] With meticulous dissection and preservation of the pelvic autonomic nerves, neurogenic bladder is not observed. The incidence of major UDs has decreased from 26% to 4% with the introduction of nerve-sparing mesorectal excision.[53] In Japan, autonomic nerve-preserving surgery for rectal cancer combines a radical lymphadenectomy along the aorta and iliac vessels with a sharp dissection along the presacral plane. Such extended lymphadenectomy has not been accepted outside of Japan because of unconvincing oncological results and fear of increased morbidity, such as bladder and sexual dysfunction. The laparoscopic approach may affect UD incidence, although recently, a study by Sartori and colleagues[54] suggests a very low incidence of UD when TME principles are followed. No sufficient data exists to comment on the impact of robotic dissection on bladder function. Intraoperative electrical stimulation of pelvic autonomic nerves and neuromonitoring may have a role in prevention or prediction of postoperative urinary[55] or fecal incontinence.[56] In the setting of inflammatory bowel disease, even when a "cancer surgery" is not performed and the dissection plane is kept close to the rectum, patients should be counseled regarding the risk of UD, including straining and sensation of incomplete emptying.[57] A recent study evaluating function in women after IPAA showed more severe UD and earlier onset of symptoms when compared with controls.[22]

Contradictory findings exist regarding the impact of radiation therapy on bladder function. Owing to variable regimens with regard to both dosage (short course vs long course) and timing (preoperative vs postoperative), it has been difficult to clearly delineate the impact of radiation therapy in relation to surgery. Most recently, Lange and colleagues[58] attempted to parse out the contribution of each treatment component (surgery and preoperative radiotherapy) to the development of long-term UD. QOL forms were available for 785 patients from the Dutch TME trial who were randomized to TME or TME with short-course preoperative radiation. The 5-year follow-up data showed that both new development and aggravation of UD occurs frequently after rectal cancer treatment. Postoperative urinary incontinence (38%) was associated with preoperative incontinence and female sex. Risk factors for difficulty in bladder emptying (31%) included preoperative difficulty, blood loss, and autonomic nerve damage. Preoperative radiation therapy did not seem to increase the risk of UD, highlighting the importance of surgical expertise and technique.

Treatment Options

Various treatment options exist in the management of postoperative UD. In the short-term, indwelling catheter can bypass issues due to incontinence and voiding dysfunction. If symptoms fail to improve with time, alternative options exist. It is prudent to consider formal urodynamic testing to aid in the diagnosis and implementation of a tailored treatment plan. Medications such as alpha-blockers function to relieve mechanical prostatic obstruction by relaxing the smooth muscle at the bladder neck and the prostatic capsule. 5-Alpha-reductase inhibitors only result in the reduction of prostatic size and therefore do not have a role in acute voiding dysfunction. Clean intermittent catheterization provides an alternative to prolonged indwelling catheter placement, which can cause local irritation, inconvenience, and risk of bladder infection. When catheters cannot be placed through the urethra, typically because of obstruction/stricture that cannot be successfully dilated, a suprapubic tube can be placed. If an enlarged prostate is the cause of retention, surgery may be considered when medication is not successful, and there are several types of surgical treatments available including transurethral resection of the prostate. Severe, persisting postoperative bladder dysfunction can be treated with stimulation of the sacral nerves using the Interstim (Medtronic Inc., Minneapolis, MN, USA) neuromodulation device, which is implanted into the buttocks with leads going into the S3 neural foramen. In severe recalcitrant cases, one has to consider urinary diversion with neobladder and urostomy construction.

ANTERIOR RESECTION SYNDROME

Regardless of the method used for rectal reconstruction, and potentially independent of the use of pelvic radiation therapy, 60% to 90% of patients undergoing proctectomy develop ARS.[59–62] To variable incidence and degrees, this syndrome of defecatory dysfunction is defined by a constellation of symptoms including frequency, urgency, fragmentation (incomplete evacuation and bowel movement "stacking"), and fecal incontinence. For many patients, ARS results in "toilet dependence," and this fear of leaving the home has an obvious major impact on QOL. Multiple causative factors are involved, including a loss of the reservoir function of the resected rectum with impaired capacity and compliance of the neorectum,[63] iatrogenic internal sphincter damage,[64] autonomic nerve injury,[65] effects of chemoradiation,[66] changes in the colonic motility after mobilization of the descending colon,[67] and pelvic floor disease predating surgery.[68,69]

It is imperative that the surgeon counsel the patient preoperatively regarding the functional expectations after rectal resection and reconstruction. Such proper and comprehensive education and counseling can better empower patients as they decide on the prudence of rectal reconstruction and the consequences of that decision. Although ARS is predominately a physical problem, it can have a major impact on body image and psychosocial aspects of life for patients, specifically surrounding confidence and normality.[59] In reality, it is the rare patient who wishes to opt for permanent stoma simply because of the *potential* of postoperative bowel dysfunction.

ARS Treatment

Although a host of treatment options exist, most patients struggle through a difficult 6- to 12-month transition period while they trial various approaches. Bowel function changes over time, and patients can experience "good days" and "bad days" without any obvious cause or inciting event. Support services, either from experienced providers or patient support groups, can provide counsel and often ease this transition period.

Standard options

Fiber Modification of the stool texture and consistency is the mainstay of treatment of ARS. Oral supplementation with insoluble dietary fiber products reliably makes the stools bulky, facilitating the evacuation process by maintaining soft cohesive feces. Avoiding loose stools that are difficult to retain or hard small piecemeal stools can be challenging.

Time ARS symptoms tend to improve with time. Waiting for improvement of symptoms during a 6- to 12-month adaptation period can be frustrating but can provide patients with hope.

Antidiarrheal agents Antidiarrheal agents such as loperamide, diphenoxylate, codeine, and dilute tincture of opium function by slowing GI transit. This slowing helps to prevent multiple small stools and provides patients with a simple "tool" that can be used to provide some control of bowel dysfunction.

Enemas Transanal irrigation has been objectively studied and found to be an effective treatment of ARS, resulting in a marked improvement of continence scores and QOL.[70]

Biofeedback

Biofeedback therapy, aimed at lowering the threshold for discrimination of a rectal sensation of distension and synchronizing voluntary contraction of the EAS in response to such distension, may be an effective treatment of patients with ARS. Using a biofeedback program Kim and colleagues[71] have shown improvements in fecal incontinence scores, number of bowel movements, use of antidiarrheal medication, and anorectal manometry values. After a successful course of rehabilitation, many patients show an improvement in objective incontinence scales, whereas others become symptom free.[72]

Sacral nerve stimulation

More recently, investigators have studied the utility of neuromodulation, delivered by the implantable sacral nerve stimulator, on ARS in the postoperative setting. The largest study prospectively evaluated 14 patients for a median of 12 months.[73] Of these patients 7 noted considerable improvement in incontinence, frequency, and QOL after sacral nerve stimulation implantation. A possible explanation for poor outcome in the other 7 patients is surgical damage to the nerve supply innervating the rectum and pelvic floor and pelvic fibrosis resulting from neoadjuvant treatment and surgery.

Diversion/colostomy

Although generally considered a "last resort," some patients become so frustrated with ARS that they opt for fecal diversion, which can be accomplished either with a colostomy or ileostomy. Technically, the creation of a left-sided colostomy can be challenging because the redundant sigmoid has already been resected. While taking extreme care to protect the blood supply to the neorectum (to prevent necrosis), complete splenic flexure mobilization generally provides adequate length for a descending colostomy. Ultimately, the prolapse and pouching dysfunction commonly seen with a transverse colostomy and the intrinsic fluid and electrolyte issues associated with an ileostomy are avoided.

Quality of life and the stoma—its impact on ARS

As we better understand anatomy and pathophysiology, while concurrently embracing technologic advances in anastomotic staplers and surgical techniques, sphincter-preserving and reconstructive procedures have become the preferred form of treatment for patients with either low-lying rectal cancers or inflammatory bowel disease. Patients actively seek out specialists who can offer any option other than a permanent stoma. In reality, when evaluated systematically, the preconception that restoration of bowel continuity offers superior QOL has been challenged. Published reports suggest that the QOL after LAR might even be worse than after APR.[74–77]

In 2005, a Cochrane review of the literature regarding QOL after LAR and APR was performed. A total of 11 studies met the inclusion criteria: 6 showed no difference in QOL, 1 study showed that a stoma slightly affected QOL, and 4 showed significantly poorer QOL for patients with stoma after APR. The investigators concluded "It is not possible to draw conclusions whether the QOL measures of stoma patients are poorer than for non-stoma patients. However, the results challenge the assumption that people with stoma generally fare less well than non-stoma patients."[78]

To better understand this discrepancy, Cornish and colleagues[79] performed a meta-analysis in 2007. The investigators included 1443 patients from 11 (3 prospective) studies that assessed QOL using validated tools. Their results showed no difference in general health preconceptions after rectal cancer excision by LAR or APR. Patients with permanent stomas did not show any difference in "body image" and, in fact, had improved psychological and emotional scores. The most plausible explanation is that the negative psychological attitudes toward a stoma were balanced by poor functional outcomes associated with a low colorectal/anal anastomosis. Perhaps the "finality" of treatment with a permanent procedure also contributes to improved emotional scores for APR patients. Long-term comparison remains in question because most studies follow-up patients for 1 year and perhaps patient perceptions would change over time. Interestingly, when patients undergoing APR were asked postoperatively if they would choose LAR or APR, 80% stated that they would choose APR again.[80]

While there exists an extensive literature evaluating QOL after total proctocolectomy and restorative IPAA, there are little data comparing reconstruction to end ileostomy. Camilleri-Brennan compared QOL after total proctocolectomy with end ileostomy (TPC I) to that of the general public and found that when the diseased colon and rectum were removed, the patients' QOL was restored to normal, despite the presence of a permanent ileostomy.[81] The investigators then compared IPAA to end ileostomy. A total of 19 patients undergoing IPAA were matched and compared with those undergoing TPC I. Objective QOL tools were used to compare the 2 groups. IPAA was associated with a better perception of body image, although the general QOL was similar in both groups.[82]

Understanding the challenges of ARS and its importance in the management of patients with low rectal cancers underscores the fact that ARS should be addressed during the initial discussions as patients choose between reconstruction and stoma options, and this can be challenging on multiple levels. It is difficult for the average patient to appropriately understand the functional changes of ARS along with its impact on QOL. It is hard enough for patients to comprehend the new diagnosis of rectal cancer. Their initial focus is on survival, not on the decision between reconstruction and permanent stoma. Armed with a more comprehensive perspective, an experienced surgeon may recognize a patient with a high risk of postoperative ARS/incontinence and counsel that patient toward a stoma, even though a sphincter-sparing resection and anastomosis would be technically feasible. Such a recommendation often scares and motivates a patient to seek a second opinion. Hospital-based education programs, enterostomal nurse consultation,[83] stoma models, patient support groups, and online education and support options may be useful aids for many patients as they ponder and make this critical decision.

SUMMARY

Proctectomy often results in functional outcomes that can be significantly different compared with preoperative baseline status. A comprehensive understanding of normal anatomy and function, as well as preoperative factors that may affect postoperative function, is crucial to guide an appropriate preoperative discussion outlining risk and options. Familiarity with operative technique and pitfalls as well as reconstructive options is necessary to optimize results. Common postoperative complications include derangements of defecatory, sexual, and urinary function. Management of these disorders can be complex and at times unsuccessful and require an understanding of the social and emotional factors involved. A rational approach to preoperative assessment and decision making will help maximize the potential for setting expectations as patients make critical decision that affects QOL.

REFERENCES

1. Wolff BG, Fleshman JW, Beck DE, et al. The ASCRS textbook of colon and rectal surgery. New York: Springer Science + Business media, LLC; 2007.
2. Birnbaum EH, Myerson RJ, Fry RD, et al. Chronic effects of pelvic radiation therapy on anorectal function. Dis Colon Rectum 1994;37(9):909–15.
3. Canda AE, Terzi C, Gorken IB, et al. Effects of preoperative chemoradiotherapy on anal sphincter functions and quality of life in rectal cancer patients. Int J Colorectal Dis 2010;25(2):197–204.
4. Marijnen CA, van de Velde CJ, Putter H, et al. Impact of short-term preoperative radiotherapy on health-related quality of life and sexual functioning in primary rectal cancer: report of a multicenter randomized trial. J Clin Oncol 2005;23(9): 1847–58.
5. Pollack J, Holm T, Cedermark B, et al. Long-term effect of preoperative radiation therapy on anorectal function. Dis Colon Rectum 2006;49(3):345–52.

6. Sauer R, Becker H, Hohenberger W, et al. Preoperative versus postoperative chemoradiotherapy for rectal cancer. N Engl J Med 2004;351(17):1731–40.
7. Bonnel C, Parc YR, Pocard M, et al. Effects of preoperative radiotherapy for primary resectable rectal adenocarcinoma on male sexual and urinary function. Dis Colon Rectum 2002;45(7):934–9.
8. Park MG, Hur H, Min BS, et al. Colonic ischemia following surgery for sigmoid colon and rectal cancer: a study of 10 cases and a review of the literature. Int J Colorectal Dis 2011;27(5):671–5.
9. Heald RJ, Ryall RD. Recurrence and survival after total mesorectal excision for rectal cancer. Lancet 1986;1(8496):1479–82.
10. Local recurrence rate in a randomised multicentre trial of preoperative radiotherapy compared with operation alone in resectable rectal carcinoma. Swedish rectal cancer trial. Eur J Surg 1996;162(5):397–402.
11. Jayne DG, Brown JM, Thorpe H, et al. Bladder and sexual function following resection for rectal cancer in a randomized clinical trial of laparoscopic versus open technique. Br J Surg 2005;92(9):1124–32.
12. Liang Y, Li G, Chen P, et al. Laparoscopic versus open colorectal resection for cancer: a meta-analysis of results of randomized controlled trials on recurrence. Eur J Surg Oncol 2008;34(11):1217–24.
13. Asoglu O, Matlim T, Karanlik H, et al. Impact of laparoscopic surgery on bladder and sexual function after total mesorectal excision for rectal cancer. Surg Endosc 2009;23(2):296–303.
14. Kim JY, Kim NK, Lee KY, et al. A comparative study of voiding and sexual function after total mesorectal excision with autonomic nerve preservation for rectal cancer: laparoscopic versus robotic surgery. Ann Surg Oncol 2012;19(8):2485–93.
15. Braveman JM, Schoetz DJ Jr, Marcello PW, et al. The fate of the ileal pouch in patients developing Crohn's disease. Dis Colon Rectum 2004;47(10):1613–9.
16. Parks AG, Nicholls RJ. Proctocolectomy without ileostomy for ulcerative colitis. Br Med J 1978;2(6130):85–8.
17. Heald RJ, Allen DR. Stapled ileo-anal anastomosis: a technique to avoid mucosal proctectomy in the ileal pouch operation. Br J Surg 1986;73(7):571–2.
18. Reilly WT, Pemberton JH, Wolff BG, et al. Randomized prospective trial comparing ileal pouch-anal anastomosis performed by excising the anal mucosa to ileal pouch-anal anastomosis performed by preserving the anal mucosa. Ann Surg 1997;225(6):666–76 [discussion: 676–7].
19. Remzi FH, Fazio VW, Gorgun E, et al. Quality of life, functional outcome, and complications of coloplasty pouch after low anterior resection. Dis Colon Rectum 2005;48(4):735–43.
20. Remzi FH, Church JM, Bast J, et al. Mucosectomy vs. stapled ileal pouch-anal anastomosis in patients with familial adenomatous polyposis: functional outcome and neoplasia control. Dis Colon Rectum 2001;44(11):1590–6.
21. Chambers WM, McC Mortensen NJ. Should ileal pouch-anal anastomosis include mucosectomy? Colorectal Dis 2007;9(5):384–92.
22. Cornish J, Wooding K, Tan E, et al. Study of sexual, urinary, and fecal function in females following restorative proctocolectomy. Inflamm Bowel Dis 2012;18(9):1601–7.
23. Lazorthes F, Fages P, Chiotasso P, et al. Resection of the rectum with construction of a colonic reservoir and colo-anal anastomosis for carcinoma of the rectum. Br J Surg 1986;73(2):136–8.
24. Parc R, Tiret E, Frileux P, et al. Resection and colo-anal anastomosis with colonic reservoir for rectal carcinoma. Br J Surg 1986;73(2):139–41.

25. Z'graggen K, Maurer CA, Buchler MW. Transverse coloplasty pouch. A novel neo-rectal reservoir. Dig Surg 1999;16(5):363–6.
26. Lazorthes F, Chiotasso P, Gamagami RA, et al. Late clinical outcome in a random-ized prospective comparison of colonic J pouch and straight coloanal anasto-mosis. Br J Surg 1997;84(10):1449–51.
27. Ho YH, Brown S, Heah SM, et al. Comparison of J-pouch and coloplasty pouch for low rectal cancers: a randomized, controlled trial investigating functional results and comparative anastomotic leak rates. Ann Surg 2002;236(1):49–55.
28. Heriot AG, Tekkis PP, Constantinides V, et al. Meta-analysis of colonic reservoirs versus straight coloanal anastomosis after anterior resection. Br J Surg 2006; 93(1):19–32.
29. Liao C, Gao F, Cao Y, et al. Meta-analysis of the colon J-pouch vs transverse col-oplasty pouch after anterior resection for rectal cancer. Colorectal Dis 2010;12(7): 624–31.
30. Pimentel JM, Duarte A, Gregorio C, et al. Transverse coloplasty pouch and colonic J-pouch for rectal cancer–a comparative study. Colorectal Dis 2003; 5(5):465–70.
31. Siddiqui MR, Sajid MS, Woods WG, et al. A meta-analysis comparing side to end with colonic J-pouch formation after anterior resection for rectal cancer. Tech Col-oproctol 2010;14(2):113–23.
32. Machado M, Nygren J, Goldman S, et al. Similar outcome after colonic pouch and side-to-end anastomosis in low anterior resection for rectal cancer: a prospective randomized trial. Ann Surg 2003;238(2):214–20.
33. Ho YH. Techniques for restoring bowel continuity and function after rectal cancer surgery. World J Gastroenterol 2006;12(39):6252–60.
34. Allaix ME, Rebecchi F, Giaccone C, et al. Long-term functional results and quality of life after transanal endoscopic microsurgery. Br J Surg 2011;98(11):1635–43.
35. Eveno C, Lamblin A, Mariette C, et al. Sexual and urinary dysfunction after proc-tectomy for rectal cancer. J Visc Surg 2010;147(1):e21–30.
36. Lindsey I, Guy RJ, Warren BF, et al. Anatomy of Denonvilliers' fascia and pelvic nerves, impotence, and implications for the colorectal surgeon. Br J Surg 2000; 87(10):1288–99.
37. Gorgun E, Remzi FH, Montague DK, et al. Male sexual function improves after ileal pouch anal anastomosis. Colorectal Dis 2005;7(6):545–50.
38. Larson DW, Davies MM, Dozois EJ, et al. Sexual function, body image, and quality of life after laparoscopic and open ileal pouch-anal anastomosis. Dis Colon Rectum 2008;51(4):392–6.
39. Hendren SK, O'Connor BI, Liu M, et al. Prevalence of male and female sexual dysfunction is high following surgery for rectal cancer. Ann Surg 2005;242(2): 212–23.
40. Havenga K, Enker WE, McDermott K, et al. Male and female sexual and urinary function after total mesorectal excision with autonomic nerve preservation for carcinoma of the rectum. J Am Coll Surg 1996;182(6):495–502.
41. Tekkis PP, Cornish JA, Remzi FH, et al. Measuring sexual and urinary outcomes in women after rectal cancer excision. Dis Colon Rectum 2009;52(1):46–54.
42. Canada AL, Neese LE, Sui D, et al. Pilot intervention to enhance sexual rehabil-itation for couples after treatment for localized prostate carcinoma. Cancer 2005; 104(12):2689–700.
43. Lindsey I, George B, Kettlewell M, et al. Randomized, double-blind, placebo-controlled trial of sildenafil (Viagra) for erectile dysfunction after rectal excision for cancer and inflammatory bowel disease. Dis Colon Rectum 2002;45(6):727–32.

44. Kinder MV, Bastiaanssen EH, Janknegt RA, et al. The neuronal control of the lower urinary tract: a model of architecture and control mechanisms. Arch Physiol Biochem 1999;107(3):203–22.

45. Moriya Y. Function preservation in rectal cancer surgery. Int J Clin Oncol 2006; 11(5):339–43.

46. Pollack J, Holm T, Cedermark B, et al. Late adverse effects of short-course preoperative radiotherapy in rectal cancer. Br J Surg 2006;93(12):1519–25.

47. Junginger T, Kneist W, Heintz A. Influence of identification and preservation of pelvic autonomic nerves in rectal cancer surgery on bladder dysfunction after total mesorectal excision. Dis Colon Rectum 2003;46(5):621–8.

48. Vironen JH, Kairaluoma M, Aalto AM, et al. Impact of functional results on quality of life after rectal cancer surgery. Dis Colon Rectum 2006;49(5):568–78.

49. Moszkowicz D, Alsaid B, Bessede T, et al. Where does pelvic nerve injury occur during rectal surgery for cancer? Colorectal Dis 2011;13(12):1326–34.

50. Marks CG, Ritchie JK. The complications of synchronous combined excision for adenocarcinoma of the rectum at St Mark's Hospital. Br J Surg 1975;62(11):901–5.

51. Cunsolo A, Bragaglia RB, Manara G, et al. Urogenital dysfunction after abdominoperineal resection for carcinoma of the rectum. Dis Colon Rectum 1990;33(11):918–22.

52. Havenga K, Maas CP, DeRuiter MC, et al. Avoiding long-term disturbance to bladder and sexual function in pelvic surgery, particularly with rectal cancer. Semin Surg Oncol 2000;18(3):235–43.

53. Kneist W, Heintz A, Junginger T. Major urinary dysfunction after mesorectal excision for rectal carcinoma. Br J Surg 2005;92(2):230–4.

54. Sartori CA, Sartori A, Vigna S, et al. Urinary and sexual disorders after laparoscopic TME for rectal cancer in males. J Gastrointest Surg 2011;15(4):637–43.

55. Kneist W, Junginger T. Long-term urinary dysfunction after mesorectal excision: a prospective study with intraoperative electrophysiological confirmation of nerve preservation. Eur J Surg Oncol 2007;33(9):1068–74.

56. Kneist W, Kauff DW, Gockel I, et al. Total mesorectal excision with intraoperative assessment of internal anal sphincter innervation provides new insights into neurogenic incontinence. J Am Coll Surg 2012;214(3):306–12.

57. Neal DE, Parker AJ, Williams NS, et al. The long term effects of proctectomy on bladder function in patients with inflammatory bowel disease. Br J Surg 1982; 69(6):349–52.

58. Lange MM, Maas CP, Marijnen CA, et al. Urinary dysfunction after rectal cancer treatment is mainly caused by surgery. Br J Surg 2008;95(8):1020–8.

59. Desnoo L, Faithfull S. A qualitative study of anterior resection syndrome: the experiences of cancer survivors who have undergone resection surgery. Eur J Cancer Care (Engl) 2006;15(3):244–51.

60. Ho YH, Low D, Goh HS. Bowel function survey after segmental colorectal resections. Dis Colon Rectum 1996;39(3):307–10.

61. Batignani G, Monaci I, Ficari F, et al. What affects continence after anterior resection of the rectum? Dis Colon Rectum 1991;34(4):329–35.

62. Kakodkar R, Gupta S, Nundy S. Low anterior resection with total mesorectal excision for rectal cancer: functional assessment and factors affecting outcome. Colorectal Dis 2006;8(8):650–6.

63. Carmona JA, Ortiz H, Perez-Cabanas I. Alterations in anorectal function after anterior resection for cancer of the rectum. Int J Colorectal Dis 1991;6(2):108–10.

64. Farouk R, Duthie GS, Lee PW, et al. Endosonographic evidence of injury to the internal anal sphincter after low anterior resection: long-term follow-up. Dis Colon Rectum 1998;41(7):888–91.

65. O'Riordain MG, Molloy RG, Gillen P, et al. Rectoanal inhibitory reflex following low stapled anterior resection of the rectum. Dis Colon Rectum 1992;35(9):874–8.
66. Dahlberg M, Glimelius B, Graf W, et al. Preoperative irradiation affects functional results after surgery for rectal cancer: results from a randomized study. Dis Colon Rectum 1998;41(5):543–9 [discussion: 549–51].
67. Lee WY, Takahashi T, Pappas T, et al. Surgical autonomic denervation results in altered colonic motility: an explanation for low anterior resection syndrome? Surgery 2008;143(6):778–83.
68. Lewis WG, Martin IG, Williamson ME, et al. Why do some patients experience poor functional results after anterior resection of the rectum for carcinoma? Dis Colon Rectum 1995;38(3):259–63.
69. DeMiguel M, Ortiz H, Garrido JR, et al. Anal incontinence in patients with rectal neoplasms previous to surgical intervention. Rev Esp Enferm Dig 1996;88(1): 29–34.
70. Rosen H, Robert-Yap J, Tentschert G, et al. Transanal irrigation improves quality of life in patients with low anterior resection syndrome. Colorectal Dis 2011; 13(10):e335–8.
71. Kim KH, Yu CS, Yoon YS, et al. Effectiveness of biofeedback therapy in the treatment of anterior resection syndrome after rectal cancer surgery. Dis Colon Rectum 2011;54(9):1107–13.
72. Pucciani F, Ringressi MN, Redditi S, et al. Rehabilitation of fecal incontinence after sphincter-saving surgery for rectal cancer: encouraging results. Dis Colon Rectum 2008;51(10):1552–8.
73. de Miguel M, Oteiza F, Ciga MA, et al. Sacral nerve stimulation for the treatment of faecal incontinence following low anterior resection for rectal cancer. Colorectal Dis 2011;13(1):72–7.
74. Camilleri-Brennan J, Steele RJ. Quality of life after treatment for rectal cancer. Br J Surg 1998;85(8):1036–43.
75. Camilleri-Brennan J, Steele RJ. Objective assessment of morbidity and quality of life after surgery for low rectal cancer. Colorectal Dis 2002;4(1):61–6.
76. Ortiz H, Armendariz P. Anterior resection: do the patients perceive any clinical benefit? Int J Colorectal Dis 1996;11(4):191–5.
77. Sprangers MA, Taal BG, Aaronson NK, et al. Quality of life in colorectal cancer. Stoma vs. nonstoma patients. Dis Colon Rectum 1995;38(4):361–9.
78. Pachler J, Wille-Jorgensen P. Quality of life after rectal resection for cancer, with or without permanent colostomy. Cochrane Database Syst Rev 2005;(2):CD004323.
79. Cornish JA, Tilney HS, Heriot AG, et al. A meta-analysis of quality of life for abdominoperineal excision of rectum versus anterior resection for rectal cancer. Ann Surg Oncol 2007;14(7):2056–68.
80. Zolciak A, Bujko K, Kepka L, et al. Abdominoperineal resection or anterior resection for rectal cancer: patient preferences before and after treatment. Colorectal Dis 2006;8(7):575–80.
81. Camilleri-Brennan J, Steele RJ. Objective assessment of quality of life following panproctocolectomy and ileostomy for ulcerative colitis. Ann R Coll Surg Engl 2001;83(5):321–4.
82. Camilleri-Brennan J, Munro A, Steele RJ. Does an ileoanal pouch offer a better quality of life than a permanent ileostomy for patients with ulcerative colitis? J Gastrointest Surg 2003;7(6):814–9.
83. de la Quintana Jimenez P, Pastor Juan C, Prados Herrero I, et al. A prospective, longitudinal, multicenter, cohort quality-of-life evaluation of an intensive follow-up program for patients with a stoma. Ostomy Wound Manage 2010;56(5):44–52.

Considerations and Complications in Patients Undergoing Ileal Pouch Anal Anastomosis

Todd D. Francone, MD[a],*, Brad Champagne, MD[b]

KEYWORDS

- Restorative proctocolectomy • Ileal pouch anal anastomosis (IPAA) • Complications
- Pouchitis • Pouch failure • Salvage pouch surgery • Pouch vaginal fistula
- Crohn disease of the pouch

KEY POINTS

- Restorative proctocolectomy with ileal pouch anal anastomosis remains the standard operative approach for patients with ulcerative colitis and for most patients with familial adenomatous polyposis.
- Most of the literature suggests an acceptable complication rate with good-to-excellent functional and acceptable quality of life.
- Pelvic sepsis and delayed onset of Crohn disease remain critical obstacles in understanding the long-term outcomes in patients who undergo ileal pouch anal anastomosis.
- Proper evaluation for underlying pathology, in addition to preoperative counseling and optimization of the patient's condition, adherence to meticulous surgical technique, and diligent postoperative care, contribute to improving surgical outcomes that result in the preservation of pouch function over time.

INTRODUCTION

Total proctocolectomy with ileal pouch anal anastomosis (IPAA) preserves fecal continence as an alternative to permanent end ileostomy in select patients with ulcerative colitis (UC) and familial adenomatous polyposis. The procedure is technically demanding, but consistently offers improved quality of life, low reoperation rates for complications, and high patient satisfaction.[1,2] When a meticulous operation is performed and surgical complications are expeditiously managed, successful outcomes are achieved. This article outlines both the early and late complications that can occur after IPAA. The workup and management of these potentially morbid conditions is emphasized.

a Department of Colon and Rectal Surgery, University of Rochester Medical Center, 601 Elmwood Avenue, Rochester, NY 14642, USA; b Department of Colon and Rectal Surgery, Case Western Reserve University Medical Center, Cleveland, OH 44120, USA
* Corresponding author.
E-mail address: todd_francone@urmc.rochester.edu

Surg Clin N Am 93 (2013) 107–143
http://dx.doi.org/10.1016/j.suc.2012.09.004
0039-6109/13/$ – see front matter © 2013 Elsevier Inc. All rights reserved.

ACUTE COMPLICATIONS
Hemorrhage

The clinical features of postoperative pouch bleeding vary depending on timing, severity, and patient factors. The diagnostic and therapeutic methods include observation, endoscopy, and reoperative abdominal surgery. Acute hemorrhage can occur during surgery or in the early postoperative period. Furthermore, bleeding may be intraluminal, intra-abdominal or both.

The incidence of hemorrhage after IPAA is approximately 1.5% to 3.5%.[2,3] Lian and colleagues[3] found no differences in gender distribution, pouch configuration, and anastomotic type between patients with and without bleeding. Those patients who had the staple line reinforced during the initial surgery had less bleeding but this did not reach statistical significance. Furthermore, they discovered that 66% of bleeding occurred within 7 days after surgery. Of the 47 patients who bled, 34 bled transanally: 9 from the ileostomy, 2 from both, and 2 abdominally.

Intraoperatively there are several described, yet poorly studied, maneuvers that may decrease bleeding during IPAA surgery. During construction of the pouch, the linear and circular suture lines may commonly bleed. Biologic staple line reinforcement, suturing the staple line, and waiting 1 minute after the linear staple line is closed before firing have been suggested to reduce this potential problem. None of these preferences have been substantiated with data, although all are worthwhile to consider in practice. Furthermore, after firing the stapler, the suture lines should always be inspected after a few minutes have passed. This delay allows the vasoconstrictive phase of wound healing to pass and small but potentially significant bleeding commonly occurs from the new anastomosis. Last, at the completion of the IPAA, it is prudent to routinely perform pouchoscopy. This may help identify and reduce the number of patients with clinically significant hemorrhage within 24 hours.

During the postoperative phase, minor limited bleeding can be expected; however, when hemorrhage persists and the patient is stable, irrigation of the pouch with a 1:200000 adrenaline solution is commonly the first method of treatment.[2] In a series of more than 1000 patients, this method controlled bleeding in 80% of cases.[2] This procedure may initially be performed on the ward; however, if bleeding persists or the patient has any signs of hemodynamic instability, the patient must be brought to the operating room.

In the operative theater, the room must be prepared for both a thorough endoscopic evaluation and potentially an abdominal approach. The pouch is initially inspected with a variety of lighted anoscopes, and flexible endoscopes. In a series of patients requiring postoperative endoscopy and clot evacuation, 53% had bleeding from the linear stapling line.[3] The specific bleeding point can routinely be identified and then cauterized or clipped (**Fig. 1**). When a specific area along the staple line is not detected but generalized oozing is found (**Fig. 2**), epinephrine enemas are the treatment of choice. Lian and colleagues[3] reported a 96% success rate in this setting with cauterization, clips, or epinephrine injection. Minor re-bleeding after these treatments should be expected. This can often be managed with an epinephrine enema on the ward.[3]

Clinically significant delayed pouch bleeding is uncommon. When this occurs, it should be assumed to be a sign of pelvic sepsis from a dysfunctional ileal-anal anastomosis until proven otherwise. Therefore, the threshold for bringing these patients back to the operating room or sending for further imaging is low. If the anastomosis is bleeding and appears to be disrupted, the bleeding points should be sutured and any collections should be addressed by drainage through the anastomosis. Typically, a penrose drain, mushroom or even Foley catheter can be placed transanally into the

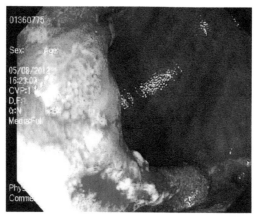

Fig. 1. Focal bleeding at ileal pouch–anal anastomosis.

cavity (**Fig. 3**). If the patient is diverted with a proximal ileostomy, the drain can be removed when any signs of pelvic sepsis resolve. This is discussed in the following section.

Intra-abdominal hemorrhage after IPAA requires immediate attention. The 2 most common locations of postoperative abdominal bleeding after IPAA are the mesentery and the pelvic sidewall.[4] The splenic flexure and region just lateral to the duodenum are also potential sites that require careful inspection during the primary dissection or any reoperation. The tip of the J pouch and the linear stapler line can also bleed externally into the abdominal cavity. If the bleeding site cannot be controlled and is coming from the pelvis, removal of the pouch may be required.[4] In these extreme cases, the pouch can be exteriorized as a left iliac fossa mucous fistula if re-anastomosis is considered unsafe. The last resort would be to pack the pelvis around the pouch and return to the operating room within 48 hours.

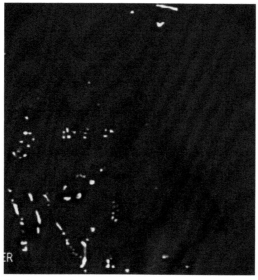

Fig. 2. Diffuse bleeding in J-pouch.

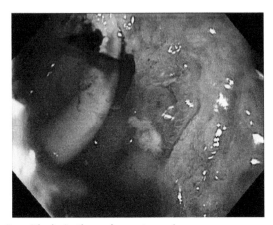

Fig. 3. Abscess cavity with drain through anastomosis.

In summary, the algorithm for the overall management of postoperative pouch bleeding is relatively straightforward. Early evaluation with endoscopy and clot evacuation offers both a diagnostic and therapeutic advantage. Cauterization for specific bleeding and the liberal use of epinephrine enemas for diffuse bleeding are highly successful measures, and an abdominal intervention or pouch excision is rarely required.

Abscess/Leak

Pelvic sepsis remains a major complication after IPAA. The overall incidence in the early postoperative period ranges from 5% to 19%.[5–7] Management strategies are diverse but include reoperation in approximately 24% to 63% of patients.[2,6] More specifically, in a series of 494 patients, Heuschen and colleagues[5] discovered that the overall incidence of pouch-related sepsis increased from 15% to 24% respectively within 1 and 3 years of surgery. The Mayo Clinic series reported an incidence of 73 (4.8%) of 1508 for pelvic sepsis after IPAA.[8] Fazio and colleagues[9] evaluated 1965 IPAA procedures performed for UC (60.7%), indeterminate colitis (27.9%), Crohn disease (3.8%), and familial adenomatous polyposis coli (0.7%). In this series, the rate of fistula formation was 7%, with anastomotic separation or pelvic abscess each occurring in 5% of patients.

Risk factors for the development of pelvic sepsis have been evaluated in a number of institutional series with varying results. Heuschen and colleagues[5] discovered that high-dose corticosteroid usage (systemic equivalent of 0.40 mg per day prednisolone) predisposed patients to sepsis after undergoing panproctocolectomy and IPAA. Similar conclusions were drawn by Cohen and colleagues[10] from a review of 483 patients. Whether steroids potentially impair healing of the anastomosis, decrease the ability to combat infection, or simply mark a subgroup of patients who are in poor clinical condition remains unknown. Patients with UC have been shown to be at greater risk for pelvic sepsis within the first 4 months after surgery than those with familial adenomatous polyposis. This may also be attributable to immunosuppression and delayed healing because of preoperative treatment with systemic corticosteroids.[5] Sagap and colleagues[11] performed a multivariate analysis of factors associated with pelvic sepsis that led to pouch failure. This study actually showed that preoperative use of steroids (defined here as patients who took steroids before proctocolectomy and IPAA) was associated with more pouch salvage in patients with septic complications. The association between steroid use and a greater rate of treatment success also did not appear to be diminished by looking at patients with or without anastomotic leak. Therefore, steroids may be associated with an increased risk for leak but then play a role in producing a much-reduced inflammatory reaction to sepsis. Our approach is to avoid IPAA formation and instead perform subtotal colectomy in patients who are acutely unwell and receiving high-dose corticosteroids. Finally, Crohn disease has been shown repeatedly to contribute significant morbidity from sepsis and result in significant pouch failure after IPAA.[12,13] It is therefore regarded as a relative contraindication for an IPAA procedure.

The location of an anastomotic leak after IPAA is variable but originates from vulnerable areas within the pouch (**Fig. 4**). These areas include the oversewn blind end of the ileum, the pouch-anal-anastomosis, and the parallel suture lines along the linear anastomosis. Heuschen and colleagues[14] excluded Crohn cases and demonstrated that presumed anastomotic leak with fistulae formation accounted for 76% of all septic events. Of these, the specific location of the fistula was isolated pouch-anal anastomotic (56%), pouch vaginal (13%), and proximal pouch (7%). The clinical presentation of pelvic sepsis after IPAA may be subtle or frankly apparent. Therefore, it is critical for the surgeon to carefully scrutinize any postoperative aberrations in patient symptoms or signs. An early expeditious diagnosis and treatment of ensuing pelvic sepsis may ultimately prevent long-term pouch failure. An early postoperative fever in a patient recovering from an IPAA operation should arouse suspicion of pelvic sepsis. A gentle digital examination may reveal an anastomotic defect or localized tenderness overlying an indurated or fluctuant mass. As with any abdominal surgery, an anastomotic leak that presents several days later may appear with an elevated white blood cell count and subsequent abscess.

Several imaging modalities for pelvic sepsis are available, depending on the severity and timing of the clinical manifestations. Before the refinement of nonoperative interventional techniques, patients with a palpable defect and minor symptoms would be treated in the operating room or with antibiotics alone. Currently, the benefits of preoperative imaging in stable patients for both diagnostic and therapeutic reasons must be recognized. Historically, fluoroscopic pouchography with water-soluble rectal contrast material was performed to identify the presence and origin of a leak (**Figs. 4** and **5**);

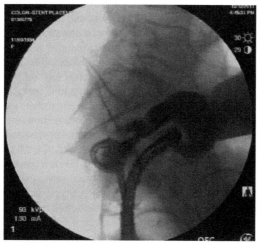

Fig. 4. Posterior J-pouch leak.

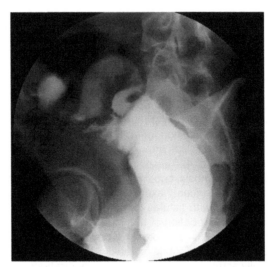

Fig. 5. Barium enema demonstrating "tip of the J" anastomotic leak.

however, computed tomography (CT) is significantly more sensitive than fluoroscopy in identifying abscesses, and may depict other possible causes of the patient's symptoms as well.[15] Furthermore, an initial fluoroscopic evaluation may make subsequent performance of CT problematic if marked enteric contrast enhancement persists. When CT is indicated, the amount of oral contrast material administered should be adequate to ensure opacification of the entire bowel, including the pouch. Water-soluble contrast material may also be injected directly into the pouch transrectally immediately before CT is performed; however, the surgery team or a very experienced radiologist should perform this maneuver to prevent iatrogenic trauma.

At our institution, we also consider magnetic resonance imaging (MRI) in patients with renal insufficiency and to monitor the course of a previously identified abscess in patients who require frequent imaging. Typically, the findings on CT or MRI appear as extraluminal fluid collections with air-fluid levels, well-defined enhancing walls, and a mass effect with displacement of the adjacent bowel (**Fig. 6**).[15] It is imperative for the surgeon to review the images when a leak or abscess is not reported. A minor leak may appear as a poorly defined fluid collection intercalated with the ileal mesentery, with irregular margins.[15]

When extravasated oral contrast material is visualized, the CT typically will aid in identifying the precise location of the leak (**Fig. 7**); however, if preparation with oral contrast material is inadequate, it can be challenging to distinguish fluid collections or abscesses from unopacified loops of ileum. In these cases, Broder and colleagues[16] explain that it may help to identify the suture lines and use them to track the pouch on serial images. If the source still remains nebulous an MRI with an experienced and knowledgeable clinical radiologist is useful. On MRI, extraluminal fluid collections have high signal intensity on T2-weighted MR images and low signal intensity with an enhancing rim on T1-weighted gadolinium-enhanced MR images.[16]

The successful treatment of pelvic sepsis after IPAA typically requires collaboration among the surgery team, the patient, and the interventional radiologist. CT-guided interventional techniques have broadened the spectrum of therapeutic options. These approaches are poorly studied specifically for IPAA, but have been widely investigated and recommended for the management of anastomotic leak and fluid collections after

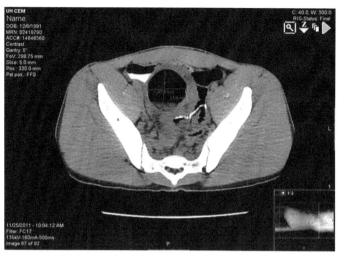

Fig. 6. Large para-pouch abscess showing displacement.

other colorectal resections. Pelvic fluid collections may be drained by a transgluteal or direct path through the pouch. Typically, an 18-gauge needle is used to access the fluid collection, and a 0.035-inch J-tip guide wire is threaded through the needle. A 12-F pigtail catheter is then advanced over the wire and into the fluid collection after serial tract dilation.[16] Judicious management of drainage catheters may improve clinical outcomes and minimize the need for further imaging. Ideally, the catheter should be flushed several times a day with small amounts of saline solution to maintain patency. Furthermore, transgluteal catheters are uncomfortable but premature removal of the catheter should be avoided because it may lead to reaccumulation of fluid in the abscess as a result of incomplete healing of the leakage site. Even after drainage has ceased or imaging has demonstrated resolution of the fluid collection, complete healing of the source of the leak, commonly a dehiscent suture line, may not have occurred. Broder and colleagues[16] recommend an evaluation for persistent leak before removing the catheter, by obtaining a fistulogram after gently infusing water-soluble contrast material directly into the catheter. They fill the residual cavity with contrast material to detect any persistent communication between the fluid

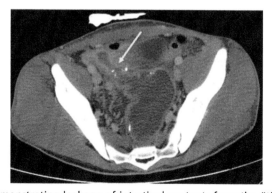

Fig. 7. CT scan demonstrating leakage of intestinal contents from the "tip" of a J-pouch.

collection and bowel. The investigators also suggest that orally or transrectally administered contrast material often follows the path of least resistance within the bowel lumen without extravasating through the leak and into the fluid collection, creating a false impression that the defect has completely healed. An abscess that persists despite repeated treatments with catheter drainage and antibiotics likely is the result of a continued leak and may require surgical intervention.[8]

Before the development of the aforementioned techniques, prompt examination under anesthesia (EUA) with endoscopy was the standard of care for the initial management of pelvic sepsis after IPAA. This procedure continues to play a role in management, but now is more of an adjunct to less invasive radiologic techniques. During EUA, anastomotic breakdown and early fistula formation can usually be directly visualized. The underlying area can be probed to determine the extent of any associated abscess cavity and suction applied to clear the contents. Larger defects may be amenable to digital examination and placement of a catheter through the defect for drainage and irrigation. A postoperative sinogram performed via the catheter may indicate when the cavity has collapsed. Furthermore, this evaluation will permit an endoscopic evaluation for both ischemia and a potential problem from the proximal suture or tip of the J pouch if they have not been detected on imaging.

Overall, management strategies remain very dependent on institution preference. Farouk and colleagues[8] found that operative peri-anal drainage was used in 6 (8%) of 73 cases, whereas Heuschen and colleagues[5] reported this approach in 33 (33%) of 131 cases. Despite this variability, there is consensus that laparotomy is reserved for cases in which CT-guided drainage or minor surgery have failed or for patients who deteriorate quickly with signs of generalized peritonitis. In the Mayo Clinic series, 40 (55%) of 73 patients were treated by laparotomy; 14 pouches were excised immediately, 2 as a result of ischemia, and the remainder for severe or persistent sepsis.[8] Laparotomy was ultimately required in 74 (56%) of 131 cases from Heuschen and colleagues.[14] Additionally, patients with a leak from the tip of the J pouch often require treatment with an abdominal approach. Kirat and colleagues[17] specifically reviewed the results of 27 patients with a leak from this location. Salvage surgery was performed in 25 patients by means of pouch repair (23) and new pouch creation (2). Twenty-four patients with salvage surgery have a functioning pouch after a mean follow-up of years.

In summary, the management of sepsis after IPAA, especially sepsis with abscess formation, follows the standard procedure of using less invasive techniques of percutaneous and transanal drainage procedures with broad-spectrum antibiotics before laparotomy. The effectiveness of this less invasive approach has been difficult to assess, considering that most series regarding IPAA complications include patients over a time period before and after these techniques were available. Major leaks require a proximal diverting loop ileostomy to be formed if one is not already in place. Consideration should be given to exteriorizing of the pouch if complete anastomotic disruption has occurred. With gross ischemia, one should resect the pouch and exteriorize the ileum.

MISCELLANEOUS
Small Bowel Obstruction

Small bowel obstruction (SBO) occurs in approximately 23% of patients undergoing IPAA.[18] Early SBO has been reported to account for approximately 44% of these obstructions.[18] Most cases of early SBO improved without surgery and early SBO has not been linked to late SBO. Most SBOs are related to adhesive disease.[2,19,20]

If adhesiolysis is indicated, care must be taken to prevent pouch damage that may otherwise go unrecognized and lead to pelvic sepsis. If laparotomy is performed before planned closure of the ileostomy, reversal of the stoma is appropriate if pouchography has demonstrated satisfactory healing of the IPAA.[21]

The afferent limb of the pouch may be also identified as the site of obstruction either as a result of adherence in the pelvis and creation of a flap valve by herniating behind the pouch, or as one point of an adhesional band that tracks to the abdominal wall often at the wound site of the closed ileostomy (**Fig. 8**).[22] Surgical options to correct an obstructed afferent limb include resection of the angulated bowel, mobilization of the pouch with small bowel fixation, or pouch excision. Investigators reporting this event have usually been able to free the offending limb and tack it to the abdominal wall.[22,23]

Although laparoscopic surgery has been shown to decrease abdominal adhesions, little difference, if any at all, has been demonstrated in the incidence of SBOs or the need for surgical intervention after IPAA creation. Fichera and colleagues[19] prospectively evaluated short-term and long-term outcomes between open and laparoscopic IPAA. When comparing the 2 groups, the incidence of SBO before or after closure of the ileostomy and need for surgical intervention to relieve bowel obstruction did not differ between laparoscopic and open groups. The incidence of late obstruction was seen in 12.7% of patients who underwent open restorative proctocolectomy (RPC) with IPAA; 4.7% required surgery. In comparison, 15.1% of patients who underwent laparoscopic RPC with IPAA presented with late obstruction; 9.6% required surgery ($P = .0660$).[19]

Inadequate length

The inability to perform IPAA without tension is an intraoperative dilemma rather than an acute complication, but deserves mentioning in this section. Cadaveric anatomic studies have shown that the tip of the pouch should ideally reach 2 to 6 cm beyond the lower margin of the symphysis pubis.[24] To have adequate mesenteric length, several techniques have been proposed: (1) preserving the ileocolic artery during the initial stage of right cotectomy[25]; (2) mobilizing the posterior attachment of the entire small bowel mesentery up to the third portion of the duodenum; (3) assessing

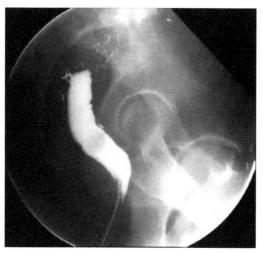

Fig. 8. Barium enema demonstrating afferent limb obstruction of J-pouch.

the most inferior point of the terminal ileum, generally located 15 to 20 cm from termination of the ileum[24]; and (4) dividing the peritoneum of the mesentery on both the anterior and posterior sides.[26] An S-shaped reservoir produces a gain in length of approximately 2 to 3 cm[24] but seems to have controversial functional outcomes.[27] Therefore, many surgeons prefer the J-pouch because of the inability to evacuate spontaneously with the S-pouch.

Understanding the most typical anatomy and possible anomalies of the superior mesenteric artery (SMA) distribution is essential to safely performing additional lengthening measures. If necessary, 1 to 3 distal ileal branches can usually be divided, providing an additional 2 to 4 cm of length.[24] However, a constant anastomotic loop between the terminal branches of the ileocolic artery and the SMA does not always exist. In these circumstances, this maneuver can be dangerous, considering that perfusion to the terminal ileum is exclusively provided from cecal vessels.[28,29] Martel and colleagues[30] suggest that the superior mesenteric pedicle (SMP) can be divided at a proximal level, at the point of origin of the last jejunal branch. This maneuver is safe if the ileocolic pedicle is preserved. The authors state that preoperative angiographic study is not necessary, but they recommend clamping of the SMP for at least 15 minutes before performing the division. Even if a minor complication of vascularization of the ileum is observed, this technique of mesenteric lengthening should be renounced. This technique provides regular lengthening of at least 5 cm for a J-pouch, each time sufficient, in our series, to reach the anus without hazardous stretching and interruption of terminal ileum blood flow. This maneuver is simple, even in patients with a fatty mesentery; vascular supply through the jejunal mesenteric arcades is efficient and safe.[30]

CHRONIC COMPLICATIONS AND LONG-TERM OUTCOMES OF THE IPAA
Chronic Pelvic Sepsis

The incidence of pelvic sepsis ranges from 3% to 40%[31–35] and remains the most critical postoperative morbidity after IPAA, particularly because it has been identified as a major predictor of pouch failure.[9,36] In the absence of failure, there is a high association of pelvic sepsis with poor functional outcome and long-term morbidity after IPAA.[9] As highlighted previously, this also signifies the importance of leak prevention and the need for rapid treatment once detected. Factors associated with increased risk for pelvic sepsis are listed in **Box 1**.

Inferior long-term pouch function in patients who have experienced a form of pelvic sepsis after IPAA is likely in part of the development of fibrosis and scarring of the pouch within the pelvis, which decreases pouch compliance and volume and, in

---

Box 1
Predictors of pelvic sepsis

Body mass index (BMI) >30[151,152]

Preoperative steroid use[5,153]

Infliximab[154,155]

Final pathologic diagnosis of ulcerative colitis (UC)/Indeterminate colitis[151]

Final pathologic diagnosis Crohn disease[151]

Intraoperative blood transfusion[151,156]

Postoperative blood transfusion[151,156]

turn, reduces function. A recent study by Kiely and colleagues[36] reported that patients with pelvic sepsis were more likely to experience some form of pouch dysfunction, with a greater degree of dietary, social, sexual, and work-related restrictions, as well as reduced quality of life (QoL). Long-term sequelae of chronic pelvic sepsis include a variety of pouch fistula to the vagina, anus, or perineum and anastomotic stenosis.

Pouch Vaginal Fistula

Recent evidence suggests that the incidence of pouch vaginal fistula (PVF) ranges between 2% and 6%[2,37–39] and older literature has reported incidence as high as 16%.[40–42] PVF is associated with major morbidity after IPAA and a relatively high incidence of pouch failure rates that range between 22% to 26%.[37,39,43] PVF most often arises from the anastomosis; however, it may also originate from the pouch body or cryptoglandular disease.[37,39] Management of PVF can be challenging with high recurrence rates of between 60% and 70%.

Numerous factors have been evaluated as risk factors for the development of PVF. The most consistently reported factors appear to be the presence of pelvic sepsis and a delayed diagnosis of Crohn disease. The distinction between postsurgical complications and Crohn disease is addressed later in this report; however, fistula development related to Crohn disease is a common development late after IPAA construction. If Crohn disease is suspected, a thorough investigation of the pouch is essential to help clarify the potential origin of the fistula. This type of investigation typically includes pouchoscopy, pouchogram with water-soluble contrast, and examination under anesthesia with potential injection of methylene blue or 1% hydrogen peroxide to help identify the tract.

The surgical approach for PVF depends on location. Patients with fistulas at or below the anastomosis are typically approached via a transanal[39] or transvaginal approach.[37] A combined approach has been used, but improved success rates have not been shown. Fistulas above the anastomosis, including those that arise from the efferent limb ("tip of the J"), are typically approached via the abdomen.

Reported success rates for initial local procedures are low and range between 30% and 40%, but have been shown to vary with approach.[37] Repair of a PVF often requires multiple procedures. In fact, Heriot and colleagues[37] showed nonsignificant trends of improved success rates with multiple transanal procedures and an overall success rate of 47%. This is consistent with other studies, including one from the Cleveland Clinic that reported pouch healing in 51.0% of patients to as high as 73.9%.[38,39,44] Predictors of success after pouch vaginal fistula surgery may include timing of PVF manifestation. Shah and colleagues[39] demonstrated better outcomes in PVF occurring within 6 months of IPAA construction when compared with those occurring after 6 months. This may be in part related to the fact that fistulas that occur after 6 to 12 months are possibly associated with Crohn disease, which is associated with higher failure rates after repair.

Recent studies have trialed collagen plugs with the addition of a button as an alternative to advancement flaps. The button potentially allows better fixation of the pouch and prevents early dislodgment. Reported success rates are substandard and one study reported no successes in 9 patients at a 2-year follow-up.[45] A similar study by Gonsalves and colleagues[46] yielded more promising results with closure of 4 of 7 PVFs; however, median follow-up was particularly short at 15 weeks.

PVF can be a destructive complication in female patients with IPAA. Several modalities have been trialed in the management of PVF with variable success rates, all of which were less than acceptable. In either case, local management should be the initial first step for low fistulas, but only after local sepsis has been controlled. This is typically achieved with the placement of seton drains before definitive surgery. In severe cases, proximal diversion may be required.

Stricture

Similar to other pouch complications, strictures of the IPAA commonly result in the setting of pelvic sepsis. Conversely, strictures may also develop in the absence of sepsis, specifically from anastomotic tension or ischemia, as well as less common causes, such as nonsteroidal anti-inflammatory drug (NSAID) use or Crohn disease. Strictures occur most commonly at the pouch anal anastomosis (pouch outlet) or at the junction of the afferent limb and pouch body (pouch inlet).[47] Although atypical, strictures can occur within the body of the pouch or at the site of a previous diverting loop ileostomy. Pouch-anal strictures are reasonably frequent with an incidence between 10% and 40%.[2,18,33,35,48,49] The manifestation of a stricture is often late, occurring between 6 and 9 months.[50] Patients often describe pouch function as poor and report symptoms of abdominal cramping, watery stools, straining, urgency, and a sensation of incomplete evacuation.[49] Multiple risk factors have been associated with the development of outlet strictures, including hand-sewn technique,[35,50] stapler size,[51] use of a defunctioning ileostomy,[48] mesenteric tension,[48,50] pelvic sepsis,[48,50] increased blood loss, and increased body mass index (BMI).[49]

Medical therapy may prove useful in select patients including those with strictures related to NSAID use or in the presence of Crohn disease. The presence a pouch outlet or afferent limb stricture should ignite a thorough investigation to rule out a delayed diagnosis of Crohn disease. If Crohn disease is diagnosed, strictures may respond to medical therapy with immunomodulator or biologic therapy. Additionally, patients with UC or ID with cuffitis will often respond to topical steroids, such as mesalamine enemas.[52]

In most cases, local management is sufficient for pouch outlet strictures and typically consists of self-dilations at home with graduated Hegar dilators or under general anesthesia.[48,50] Prudhomme and colleagues[50] suggested that nonfibrotic or "supple" strictures on digital rectal examination were more amenable to dilation with a 95% success rate compared with fibrotic strictures, which yield a 45% success rate. Length of the stricture also appears to predict response to local treatment; in particular, shorter strictures are more responsive to dilations. Differences in the type and length of the stricture may be partly related to surgical technique. In general, stapled IPAA are associated with shorter, weblike strictures, whereas mucosectomy with hand-sewn anastomoses produce longer, more fibrotic strictures.[48]

Although few data are available, successful endoscopic dilation of pouch outlet and inlet strictures has also been reported.[47,53] In a large series by Shen and colleagues,[47] 150 patients with IPAA and stricture were evaluated after endoscopic balloon dilation. Of the 646 strictures identified, pouch-inlet and pouch-outlet strictures were most common, followed by afferent limb strictures. Technical success with dilation was achieved in more than 97% of strictures and only 14 strictures were nonamenable to passage of the scope. These strictures were typically associated with sharp angulations or looping of the scope. Considering a median follow-up of 9.6 years, outcomes were favorable, with 80.0% of patients reporting improvement of symptoms and a pouch failure rate of 12.7%. Major complications were low, with only 6 adverse events in 3 patients, consisting of either bleeding, perforation, or both. Overall, balloon dilation was demonstrated to be fairly safe, although pouches with multiple strictures and acute angulations were technically more challenging.

Refractory strictures may require surgical intervention. Limited data are available for strictureplasty in the setting of pouch-anal strictures, but has been used in

Crohn-related strictures. An additional option includes excision of the strictured segment with advancement of an ileal mucosal advancement flap. According to Prudhomme and colleagues,[50] this procedure was reserved for short supple strictures that appeared as a "fibrous ring." Fazio and Tjandra[54] also reported transanal disconnection and advancement of the pouch for the treatment of low pouch anal anastomosis and PVF. Pouch excision or diverting loop ileostomy were rarely required.

Fertility

The bulk of current literature demonstrate a negative effect of IPAA on fertility.[55–58] Pregnancy may be at least 5 times less likely to occur compared with the general population. A meta-analysis by Rajaratnam and colleagues[58] demonstrated a statistically significant increase in relative risk of infertility of 3.91 (95% confidence interval [CI] 2.06–7.44) post-IPAA. A review by Cornish and colleagues[55] yielded similar findings and reported a weighted mean infertility rate of 12% before IPAA, which increased to 26% post-IPAA. The cause of this considerable increase is unknown; however, most investigators suspect a mechanical cause; in particular, dense pelvic adhesions scarring the ovaries and fallopian tubes into the pelvis. Various techniques have been attempted to reduce the effect of surgery on ovarian and tubal function. Procedures include oophoropexy, the technique of suturing the ovaries to the pelvic brim. On the downside, this may complicate retrieval of the ovaries if in vitro fertilization is necessary.[59] Interposition of an omental pedicled graft or placement of antiadhesion products, such as Seprafilm (Genzyme Corporation, Cambridge, MA), have also been used to keep the ovaries out of the pelvis and reduce adhesions.[60]

Given the apparent increase in infertility after IPAA and the predominance of young female patients undergoing the operation, other strategies to prevent or manage post-IPAA infertility should be considered. Preoperative considerations include delayed creation of an IPAA by construction of an ileorectal anastomosis after a total colectomy or subtotal colectomy with end ileostomy. Both procedures potentially expose patients to an increased risk of cancer, especially among those with familial adenomatous polyposis (FAP); however, as discussed later in this review, the removal of the rectum and creation of IPAA does not eliminate the risk of cancer. Rectal preservation is less often an option in UC patients, although IRA, in select cases where fertility is an issue, may be warranted.

Patients with IPAA who wish to conceive postoperatively should be referred to a fertility specialist. The most common treatments used in patients with IPAA are clomiphene and in vitro fertilization (IVF). Olsen and colleagues[57] reported a 30% pregnancy rate after IVF in female patients with IPAA compared with a 1.3% pregnancy rate in the reference general population. Success rates after infertility treatments are difficult to compare because of variations between studies and fertility programs. Further studies are required to determine the true success rates of fertility treatment following IPAA.

Pouch function and pregnancy

Overall, pouch function remains stable throughout pregnancy. Several studies have demonstrated an increase in stool frequency by 1.15 stools per day in the third trimester compared with the general population of pregnant women.[55] Studies have not demonstrated a difference in pouch function before and after pregnancy, although stool frequency and day and nighttime incontinence increased over time; this is a general observation seen with most patients with pouches. Similarly, pad usage and use of stool-regulating medications have not reported any change when comparing pregnancy with immediate postpartum status.[61]

Vaginal versus C-section delivery

Controversy remains concerning the preferred method of delivery in patients who received IPAA. The consensus among surgeons is to recommend C-section to avoid a decrease in pelvic muscle strength with pudendal nerve damage and direct injury to the sphincter or pouch. This was evident in a systematic review by Cornish and colleagues,[55] in which the incidence of C-section was significantly more than that of the general population. As one would expect, occult injuries to the anal sphincter occurred after vaginal delivery. Specifically, sphincter injuries have been reported to occur in as many as 35% of women who may not become symptomatic for years.[62] Additionally, adverse effects of perineal injury during vaginal delivery, leading to pouch excision, have been reported.[63] Conversely, C-section delivery is not without risk and is associated with the typical complications of abdominal surgery including formation of adhesions. As mentioned previously, vaginal delivery was not associated with the deterioration of pouch function over time; however, long-term results are not available. Remzi and colleagues[64] investigated the impact of childbirth on pudendal motor latency testing and electromyography. The study demonstrated normal tests after delivery in vaginal and C-section deliveries. Additionally, anal ultrasound demonstrated sphincter defects in 50.0% of those who had vaginal deliveries compared with 13.3% who did not. Nevertheless, the injuries were not noted to affect pouch function or patient QoL. Again, with a mean follow-up of only 4.9 years, effects on long-term function and QoL are unknown, which makes recommendations regarding mode of delivery unsubstantiated.[64]

POUCH DYSFUNCTION
Pouchitis

It is generally accepted that pouchitis refers to an idiopathic, nonspecific acute inflammation of the ileum, although a concise definition of pouchitis is lacking. Consequently, the incidence of pouchitis is variable throughout the literature, ranging between 16% and 48%, and is considered one of the most common complications after restorative proctocolectomy and IPAA. Further, incidence has been shown to increase over time after surgery[1,33] with approximately 40% of patients reporting at least one episode at 10 years after IPAA construction to as high as 70% 20 years after surgery.[33]

Pouchitis occurs in patients with UC or FAP, although it is more common after construction for UC,[32,65] especially those with associated sclerosing cholangitis.[66] In a meta-analysis performed by Lovegrove and colleagues,[65] a substantial increase in the risk of pouchitis was seen in patients with UC (30.1%) compared with those with FAP (5.5%) (odds ratio 6.44; 95% CI 3.21–12.93; $P<.001$). Although the incidence of pouchitis is clearly elevated in patients with a postoperative diagnosis of Crohn disease, data for increased incidence of pouchitis in patients with indeterminate colitis are less consistent.[67] Hahnloser and colleagues[33] conducted a long-term follow-up study and found no difference in the incidence of chronic pouchitis in patients with a postoperative diagnosis of UC (48%) and those with indeterminate colitis (49%). Patients diagnosed with Crohn disease de novo yielded a reported incidence of 56% at 10 years.

Pathogenesis

In light of its predominance as a major morbidity after IPAA, multiple risk factors for pouchitis have been suggested (**Box 2**) but its etiology remains ambiguous. Its predominance in patients with inflammatory bowel disease (IBD) and relatively infrequent occurrence in patients with FAP suggests that the underlying immune

Box 2
Reported risk factors for pouchitis
Postoperative complication (sepsis)[118]
Severe UC[2,157,158]
Extraintestinal manifestations with UC[81,118,159,160]
Age[161]
Primary sclerosing cholangitis[118,162]
Number of operations performed for IPAA[a][118]
Peripheral antineutrophil cytoplasmic antibodies[81,163]
Duration of diversion with ileostomy[a][118]
Nonsmokers[13,81,157,164]
Backwash ileitis[158,161]
Postoperative use of nonsteroidal anti-inflammatory drugs[13,157]
[a] Not found to be significant.

dysregulation in IBD plays an instrumental role in the development of pouchitis.[68,69] Conversely, the response to antibiotics with anaerobic activity, increased bacterial counts in the ileal pouch, and the predominance of neutrophils on histology suggest a bacterial etiology. For this reason, the most well-known and initial hypothesis regarding the pathogenesis of pouchitis is thought to be related to fecal stasis and bacterial overgrowth. However, O'Connell and colleagues[70] challenged the role of fecal stasis and found no correlation between incomplete emptying of the pouch and pouchitis; until recently, studies have failed to demonstrate a difference in stools to explain the divergence in incidence seen in patients with UC and FAP. Several studies have shown an increase in anaerobic bacteria, sulfate-reducing bacteria (SRB), which release hydrogen sulfide, which has been shown to be directly toxic to colonocytes and may play a role in the development of pouchitis. In a small study by Duffy and colleagues,[71] SRB were isolated from 80% (n = 8) of UC pouches, but were absent from FAP pouches. Ohge and colleagues[72] also demonstrated a similar finding in which SRB counts were significantly higher in patients who reported a history of pouchitis compared with those who never experienced pouchitis. Additionally, pouch contents from patients with FAP produced significantly less hydrogen sulfide than did any group of non–antibiotic-treated patients with UC.[72] Realistically, the pathogenesis of pouchitis is multifactorial and involves the interaction between epithelial metaplasia changes in luminal bacteria and altered mucosal immunity.[73]

Diagnosis

The diagnosis of pouchitis is often subjective and empirically based on clinical symptoms alone. A more accurate diagnosis should be acquired by considering clinical symptoms in addition to endoscopic appearance and histologic examination. Presenting symptoms can be classified as acute (<4 weeks) or chronic (>4 weeks) and often include increased stool frequency and urgency, liquid consistency of stool, anal bleeding, malaise, anorexia, lower abdominal cramps, and a low-grade fever. Additionally, endoscopic features of pouchitis typically include friable, erythematous ileal mucosa with occasional ulcerations, loss of vascular patterns, and hemorrhage, whereas histologic examination reveals villous atrophy, increased crypt depth, polymorphonuclear leukocyte infiltration, and ulcerations.

Objective assessments have been developed to diagnose pouchitis in patients with IPAA such as the Pouchitis Disease Activity Index (PDAI).[74] The PDAI is a diagnostic instrument that consists of three 6-point scales that are related to clinical symptoms, endoscopy, and histology. An index of 7 or higher is used to diagnose pouchitis. To increase the use of the PDAI as a clinical tool, Shen and colleagues[75] proposed a modified PDAI that omits histologic features from the index. Based only on clinical symptoms and endoscopic scores, the modified PDAI simplifies the diagnostic criteria but offers the same sensitivity and specificity as does the original PDAI.

Treatment

Most patients with acute pouchitis will respond to antibiotics. Patients with pouchitis are initially treated with a 14-day course of metronidazole (15–20 mg/kg/day) or ciprofloxacin (1000 mg/day).[76,77] Both treatments seem efficacious as first-line therapy, although a recent report from the Cochrane database suggests ciprofloxacin is more effective at inducing remission than is metronidazole.[78] Several randomized control trials have examined other medications in the treatment of acute pouchitis, including budesonide,[79] rifaximin,[80] lactobacillus GC,[81] and probiotics (VSL#3).[82] The Cochrane database, which included 11 randomized control trials, concluded that only budesonide enemas and VSL#3 were more effective than a placebo. Evidence did not support the use of lactobacillus GC, bismuth enemas, or butyrate and glutamine suppositories.[78]

Patients with recurrent or chronic pouchitis may require long-term maintenance therapy. Prompt recurrence of pouchitis after initial therapy should be treated initially with a second course of treatment. Combination antibiotic therapy has been recommended in patients who continue to recur and who can tolerate the medication. A combination of rifaximin (1 g twice daily), and ciprofloxacin (500 mg twice daily) for 15 days improved symptoms in 88% of patients with a complete response rate of 33%.[83] Additionally, the combination of metronidazole (500 mg twice daily) and ciprofloxacin (500 mg twice daily) for 28 days resulted in a remission rate of 82%.[84] Rotation of 3 or more antibiotics (ciprofloxacin, metronidazole, amoxicillin/clavulanic acid, and erythromycin) at weekly intervals has also been suggested for patients with chronic pouchitis; however, supporting data are limited.[85] The use of probiotics in patients with chronic pouchitis is promising and several studies have demonstrated them to be effective in inducing and maintaining remission.[78,82]

If pouchitis fails to respond to antimicrobial therapy, it is imperative to investigate other etiologies, such as Clostridium difficile, or cytomegalovirus (CMV) infection. C difficile may be treated with oral metronidazole or, more likely, oral vancomycin if the patient has already been on long-term metronidazole. CMV infection typically responds to antiviral therapy, such as ganciclovir. NSAID use, other autoimmune disorders, and ischemic pouchitis are additional etiologies that should be explored.[86] The risk of chronic refractory pouchitis ranges from 10% to 12% and is a leading cause of pouch failure. Refractory pouchitis may respond to immunosuppressive therapy, including azathioprine, 6-mercatpopurine, or infliximab.[87,88] In a recent retrospective study of patients with chronic refractory pouchitis, infliximab induced a complete response in 21% of patients and 63% patients experienced a partial clinical response.[89] Results are promising; however, one might suspect that response to immunosuppression may indicate an alternative underlying diagnosis, such as Crohn disease.

Pouchitislike symptoms are common and may be related to other etiologies, such as sphincter dysfunction, anastomotic stricture, pouch-outlet obstruction, rectal cuff inflammation, or irritable bowel syndromelike conditions.

Cuffitis

The adoption of the double-stapled technique in the construction of the IPAA has been associated with improved functional results,[90–92] shorter operative times, and reduced pelvic sepsis.[93] However, to accommodate the stapled anastomosis, several centimeters of rectal columnar mucosa within and above the anal transition zone is retained. The length of the retained rectal cuff varies and extends from 1 to 4 cm above the dentate line. This mucosa is at risk for disease recurrence or chronic inflammation, otherwise known as cuffitis. The incidence of cuffitis has been reported as high as 15%.[94,95] Clinical symptoms of cuffitis are similar to those experienced with pouchitis or irritable pouch syndrome, although cuffitis is often associated with small bloody bowel movements.[52,94,96] Patients with endoscopic inflammation of the rectal cuff, in the absence of endoscopic and histologic inflammation of the ileal pouch, are considered to have cuffitis. Endoscopic and histologic features of the mucosal inflammation are similar to that of pouchitis with ulceration, erythema, and neutrophil infiltration.[96]

Cuffitis often responds to topical steroids or suppositories or 5-aminosalicylic preparations. Shen and colleagues[52] recommend the use of mesalamine enemas and demonstrated a significant reduction in symptoms; endoscopy and histology scores were also associated with a Cuffitis Activity Index. At least 92% of patients with symptoms, including bloody bowel movements, improved with topical therapy. Systemic agents are rarely needed. If cuffitis fails to respond, other etiologies should be explored, including chronic pelvic sepsis. Additionally, inflammation of the rectal cuff may be indicative of a delayed diagnosis of Crohn disease. Chronic cuffitis may result in stricturing of pouch anastomosis, which could result in pouch dysfunction and, ultimately, pouch failure. If nonresponsive to medical therapy and in the absence of Crohn disease, operative intervention may be used. The residual mucosa can be resected off the rectal wall via a perineal approach; this technique is technically challenging and should be undertaken with vigilance.

Irritable Pouch Syndrome

First described in 2002 by Shen and colleagues,[96] irritable pouch syndrome (IPS) was described as a functional disorder in patients with IPAA. Except for rectal bleeding in patients with cuffitis, symptoms associated with IPS, pouchitis, and cuffitis widely overlap, which makes diagnosis of IPS rather difficult and one of exclusion. In the study by Shen and colleagues,[96,97] IPS was defined as clinical symptoms but with no evidence of cuffitis or endoscopic and histologic inflammation. Using the PDAI, previously mentioned in this text, patients with IPS have a PDAI index of less than 7 and no rectal cuff inflammation. Recent studies have suggested that IPS may be related to visceral hypersentivity[97] and enterochromaffin cell hyperplasia of the pouch mucosa,[98] as well as other factors, including depression.[99] Patients may be treated empirically with good response. For example, almost 50% of patients responded to a therapeutic approach similar to that used in patients with IBS, which included reassurance; dietary modification; dietary fiber supplementation; and antidiarrheal, antispasmodic, and antidepressant therapy.[96] In essence, the diagnosis of IPS largely relies on the exclusion of structural disorders of the ileal pouch. Clinical overlap with pouchitis and cuffitis underlines the importance of carefully evaluating clinical, endoscopic, and histologic data. The recognition of IPS as a distinct clinical entity, rather than a step in the progression to pouchitis, requires further investigation into the pathophysiology of the disease process.

Pouch Neoplasia

The development of dysplasia and cancer has been reported after restorative proctocolectomy, occurring in the residual rectal cuff (anal transition zone) or in the pouch itself. Data regarding the incidence and natural history of pouch neoplasia are limited, with few studies reporting follow-up periods of more than 10 years. Even so, current evidence suggests that for both the anal transition zone and the pouch itself, the incidence of invasive cancer remains low. In a meta-analysis by Chambers and McC Mortensen,[95] 25 published reports were identified that described adenocarcinoma of the pouch or the anal-transitional zone (ATZ), including the previously cited study. Of those patients, 11 developed cancer in the pouch, 4 at the anastomotic site, 4 in the residual rectal cuff, 3 in the anal canal, and 1 in the afferent limb remnant of an excised pouch.

The rectal cuff

The double-stapled technique is currently used in patients with UC or FAP. The retained rectal mucosa within and above the anal transition zone is at risk for the development of dysplasia and cancer. In patients with antecedent diagnosis of UC, reported potential risk factors for the development of dysplasia and cancer in the rectal cuff are similar to those for patients with UC-related colon cancer. Specifically, risk factors include duration and severity of disease,[100] family history of colonic cancer, and primary sclerosing cholangitis (PSC).[100] A finding of dysplasia or cancer on final pathology of the resected bowel also increases the odds of subsequent dysplasia.[101,102] Remzi and colleagues[102] examined dysplasia of the anal transition zone after construction of IPAA in patients with UC. A total of 289 patients with a minimum follow-up of 10 years were included in the study. Eight patients developed ATZ dysplasia, but no ATZ cancer was identified. Although the results of the study did not demonstrate an association between the risk of ATZ cancer with disease duration or extent of colitis, it did identify an association with the presence of cancer or dysplasia on the preoperative or postoperative histology.

Concerning patients with FAP, mucosectomy clearly reduces, but does not eliminate, the risk of developing polyps. In the meta-analysis by Chambers and McC Mortensen,[95] cancers were identified in the anastomosis in all patients who underwent IPAA for FAP. Of those 4 cases, 2 were mucosectomy. A similar finding was demonstrated by Remzi and colleagues,[103] who examined neoplasia surveillance in patients with FAP who underwent pouch surgery. One hundred eighteen patients were included in the study, 42 of whom had a mucosectomy and 76 a stapled anastomosis. Six (14%) of the mucosectomy group developed adenomas compared with 21 (28%) of the stapled group. Both groups were managed with local procedures and there was no difference between the 2 groups.[103]

The pouch

The occurrence of cancer within the pouch itself is infrequent and has been reported in patients who underwent IPAA for UC and FAP. Reported risk factors for intrapouch dysplasia or cancer include preoperative or postoperative diagnosis of cancer from underlying UC,[100,104] the presence of backwash ileitis,[105,106] villous atrophy of the pouch mucosa,[100,107] chronic pouchitis,[100,108] and PSC.[100] The average time to diagnosis of cancer from time of surgery ranged from 8 to 10 years.[95,100] In the meta-analysis by Chambers and McC Mortensen,[95] only 11 pouch cancers were reported by 2007; 9 of these patients underwent IPAA for UC and 2 patients for FAP. Eight of the 11 patients had a history of dysplasia or cancer in the resected specimen, which supports the idea that previous history of dysplasia and cancer is a significant risk factor for developing pouch neoplasia. In the most recent study to evaluate the rate of pouch neoplasia, the cumulative incidence for pouch neoplasia among 3203 patients, with a preoperative diagnosis of IBD who underwent restorative proctocolectomy with IPAA at the Cleveland Clinic, was estimated to be 0.9%, 1.3%, 1.9%, 4.2%, and 5.1% at 5, 10, 15, 20, and 25 years, respectively. Thirty-eight patients (1.19%) had pouch neoplasia, including 11 (0.36%) with adenocarcinoma of the pouch or ATZ. Not surprisingly, most patients with pouch neoplasia were found to arise from the ATZ with only 1 patient with cancer in the proximal pouch. In addition, 23 patients were identified with either high-grade or low-grade dysplasia (0.72%). Mucosectomy did not appear to prevent the development of cancer or dysplasia at the ATZ.[104]

Surveillance
Although the cumulative risk for pouch cancer is relatively low, the risk of developing dysplasia and cancer within the pouch or anal transition zone is not negligible and warrants further monitoring. Even though the data are limited, it is clear that mucosectomy does not eliminate the risk for cancer, and surveillance by endoscopy is less than perfect. In fact, dysplasia on surveillance endoscopy was not identified in any patient who underwent pouch excision for various reasons in the study by the Cleveland Clinic.[104]

Despite limitations, the current recommendation for surveillance of pouch dysplasia and ATZ in patients with an antecedent diagnosis of UC remains annual endoscopy with random biopsies of the pouch and anal transition zone. Based on the evidence, it may be reasonable to limit annual surveillance to the subgroup of patients with identified dysplasia or cancer on the resected colon, as this risk factor is consistent throughout the literature. Based on an algorithm proposed by Remzi and colleagues,[102] patients with high-grade dysplasia on 2 consecutive biopsies, 3 months apart, should undergo mucosectomy with pouch advancement. Additionally patients with low-grade dysplasia, identified on 3 consecutive biopsies, should undergo surgical intervention. Given the functional and technical advantages with the stapled IPAA, mucosectomy is reserved for patients with dysplasia or cancer with in the lower two-thirds of the rectum; however, careful surveillance should be discussed with all patients preoperatively.

In patients with FAP, surveillance of the pouch seems logical given that the prevalence of polyps in the pouch range from 8% to 62% with a risk of developing one or more adenomas at 10 years estimated to be between 35% and 75% at 15 years.[109,110] According to Church and Simmang,[111] the true prevalence of ileal polyps after IPAA for FAP is unknown and will likely remain for, at least, 20 years warranting close follow-up of these patients. The current recommendation includes annual endoscopic monitoring of the pouch and the anastomosis, biopsy of all suspicious lesions, destruction or removal of all small polyps, and transanal excision of large polyps.[111,112]

Crohn Disease and IPAA

In general, a preoperative diagnosis of Crohn disease is considered a contraindication to IPAA construction and as has been associated with increased disease recurrence, need for long-term medical therapy, increased morbidity with the development of chronic pouchitis, strictures, fistulas, pelvic sepsis, and pouch failure—all potentially leading to excision.[12,113–116] Differentiation between Crohn colitis and UC can often be difficult; therefore, it is no surprise that a certain percentage of patients will eventually be diagnosed with Crohn disease after construction of IPAA. The incidence of Crohn disease after IPAA ranges from 2.7% to 13.0%.[2,12,31–33,35,67,116,117] Additionally, the diagnosis of Crohn disease in the pouch may occur at any time after pouch construction, even before ileostomy reversal.[118] Even so, the diagnosis is often delayed, with manifestations of the disease occurring months to years after IPAA.

The pathogenesis of delayed-onset Crohn disease, or "de novo" Crohn disease, in patients with previously diagnosed UC is unclear. It has been hypothesized that the construction of the pouch created a "Crohn disease–friendly" environment by changing the bowel anatomy, which, in turn, leads to changes in the pouch environment and composition of commensal bacteria.[119] Several risk factors for the development of Crohn disease have been reported, and include a family history of Crohn disease,[120] being an active smoker,[12] a preoperative diagnosis of indeterminate colitis,[12,13] and seropositive anti-*Saccharomyces cerevisiae* immunoglobulin (Ig)A (ASCA). In a large retrospective study by Delaney and colleagues[12] in 2002, a diagnosis of indeterminate colitis was found to be associated with a higher risk of developing perineal fistula, pelvic abscess, and Crohn disease; however, pouch failure rate was equivalent to those patients diagnosed with UC. The role of histopathologic features in predicting the development of Crohn disease has also been evaluated. A large retrospective study by Nasseri and colleagues[121] suggested that neural hypertrophy in patients with UC may predict the development of delayed-onset Crohn disease. In a univariate analysis, de novo Crohn disease developed in 3 (30%) of 10 patients with neural hypertrophy compared with only 10 (7%) of the 143 patients without neural hypertrophy ($P = .01$). This finding was not significant in a multivariate regression.

Crohn disease of the ileal pouch is associated with a broad array of clinical presentations, and endoscopic and histologic features, which makes the diagnosis of de novo Crohn disease within the pouch complicated. Clinical symptoms of Crohn disease often overlap with other inflammatory disorders such as pouchitis, irritable pouch syndrome, NSAID ileitis, and cuffitis. This overlap underlies the importance of a detailed clinical history and endoscopic evaluation with subsequent histopathologic assessment. Clinical presentation often includes symptoms such as abdominal pain, nausea, anemia, weight loss, fevers, and frequent stools.[119] Patients may present with perianal disease, including fistulas and abscesses. Although Crohn disease should be considered with the early development of strictures and pelvic sepsis, including fistulas, abscesses, and sinuses, these complications can develop simply from postsurgical complications.

Endoscopic evaluation of the pouch may reveal mucosal ulcers, loss of vascular patterns, hemorrhage, or pseudopolyps, which are similar findings in pouchitis and cuffitis (**Fig. 9**). Location may help in the diagnosis, especially if the inflammation is limited to the rectal cuff, which suggests cuffitis, or located in the afferent limb of the pouch, which is more commonly seen in Crohn disease. In a small prospective study of 87 patients who underwent IPAA for inflammatory bowel disease, afferent limb ulcers were identified on endoscopy in 12 (45%) of 27 patients with Crohn disease and 4 of 28 patients with UC (14%) ($P = .019$). After adjusting for potential NSAID ileitis, afferent limb ulcers were found in 7 (39%) of 18 patients with Crohn disease and 0 of 17 patients with UC ($P = .010$).[122]

Histologic assessment is also beneficial, particularly if the presence of granulomas is identified, which suggests a diagnosis of Crohn disease. Foreign body granulomas can also be found along the staple line of the pouch and should not be considered indicative of Crohn disease.[123] Serologic markers have been useful in the

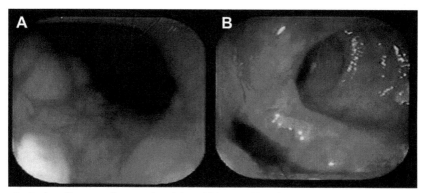

Fig. 9. Crohn disease of J-pouch with cobblestonelike features (A) and ulcerations at afferent limb outlet (B).

determination between Crohn colitis and UC; however, their utility in identifying Crohn disease of the pouch is yet to be determined. A small number of studies have shown that the preoperative presence of ASCA IgA antibodies in patients with UC or indeterminate colitis are associated with a higher risk of developing postoperative fistulae and may be more likely to develop de novo Crohn disease.[124,125] Other studies have not yielded such results, including a recent study by Tang and colleagues[126] who failed to show an association between serum ASCA antibodies and the development of Crohn disease–like complications after IPAA.

More recently, the stance concerning Crohn disease as a contraindication to restorative proctocolectomy with IPAA has been challenged. In 1996, Panis and colleagues[127] reported favorable functional results and low rates of pouch failure in select patients with Crohn disease confined to the large intestine in the absence of perianal disease. Nevertheless, the debate continues, mainly in part to the variation in the criteria for diagnosing Crohn disease. Variations in diagnostic criteria also increase the potential for misclassification and overestimating favorable outcomes in this population.

A number of studies have reported similar favorable results in patients with a known preoperative diagnosis of Crohn disease.[114,117,128–130] Regimbeau and colleagues[129] evaluated 41 patients with a preoperative diagnosis of Crohn disease who underwent IPAA. In patients in whom long-term follow-up was available (n = 20), the rates of Crohn disease–related complications (35%) and pouch excision (10%) were acceptable. A recent study by Melton and colleagues,[130] with a median follow-up of 7.4 years, reported an overall pouch retention rate of 55% with 71% of patients with Crohn disease keeping their pouch at 10 years. Specifically, the study population was divided into 3 groups: (1) those with Crohn disease before surgery (intentional), (2) those diagnosed immediately after IPAA construction on histology (incidental), and (3) those diagnosed later (delayed). Patients with known Crohn disease had favorable results with respect to pouch retention (85%) and manifestations of Crohn disease, including rates of pouchitis, fistula disease, and strictures compared with patients with a delayed diagnosis. Even functional results for patients with intentional or incidental pouches were more favorable, with 72% of patients with near-perfect to perfect continence. These patients were also less likely to have daytime and nighttime seepage or wear pads. Its unclear why patients with intentional or incidental Crohn yielded favorable results compared with those patients with a delayed diagnosis; however, it remains comprehensible, with proper counseling and set expectations, that IPAA may ultimately be accepted as an alternative for select patients with Crohn disease whose disease is confined to the colon and in the absence of perianal disease.

The previous data demonstrate that a fair amount of patients with Crohn disease may retain their pouch and avoid pouch failure with the assistance of medical therapy. Patients with inflammatory Crohn disease may be treated with topical and oral 5-aminoslaicylate agents, oral or topical steroids, antibiotics, immunomodulators or biologics, such as infliximab[131] or adalimumab.[132] Strictures may respond to endoscopic dilation in combination with medial therapy.[133] Endoscopic dilation appears to be more effective with shorter strictures. Refractory or complex strictures nonamenable to dilatation may be treated with surgical strictuloplasty, resection, and anastomosis, or proximal diversion. Management of fistulizing Crohn disease can be quite enduring and exhaust multiple medical therapies or combinations over time. Medical therapy can include those listed previously, although biologics offer the most promising results. In a small case series by Colombel and colleagues,[131] 62% of patients with fistulizing Crohn (n = 26) had a complete, short-term, response to infliximab with an additional 23% experiencing a partial response. Sixty-seven patients retained their pouch, whereas the remainder underwent pouch resection. Although favorable outcomes have been reported in patients with Crohn disease with IPAA, most of these patients will require lifelong medical therapy to avoid removal of their pouch and permanent ileostomy.

Pouch Failure

The definition of pouch failure varies throughout the literature; however, it is generally accepted that failure implies the need for indefinite defunctioning or excision of a pouch because of unmanageable pouch-specific complications.[9] When considered in failure, a patient may undergo construction of a permanent proximal diversion with loop ileostomy or pouch excision with creation of end ileostomy or continent stoma. Various articles in the literature report the rate of pouch failure to be between 3% and 30%,[2,6,18,31,33,34,134] with potential long-term rates as high as 48%.[33] The literature has also identified several factors as predictors of pouch failure (**Box 3**). The pouch failure rate for patients after septic complications in the Heuschen cohort was 29%.[15] Major causes of failure were persistent pouch fistula (36%), poor function secondary to a compromised anal sphincter (18%), outlet obstruction (13%), pelvic fibrosis (10%), pouchitis (10%), and unwillingness on patients' parts to undergo

---

Box 3
Risk factors associated with pouch failure

Pelvic sepsis[2,9,43,135,136]

Pouch-related fistulas[136,137]

Outlet obstruction[11]

Increased BMI (higher than 30)[136]

Chronic pouchitis[2,134]

Hand-sewn anastomosis[11]

Need for transanal drainage[11]

Need for laparotomy[11]

History of colectomy before IPAA[136]

Final diagnosis of Crohn disease[9,136,137]

ileostomy closure (13%). In the most recent Cleveland Clinic series for pelvic sepsis after IPAA, the pouch was saved in 75.8% of patients. They found that factors predictive of failure were hypertension, hand-sewn anastomosis, associated fistula, need for transanal drainage, need for laparotomy, delayed ileostomy closure, and the need for a new diverting ileostomy.[11]

Despite the lack of a standard definition for pouch failure, the 2 most consistent predictors of failure are pelvic sepsis and Crohn disease. Pelvic sepsis is typically never an isolated complication and is usually associated with other problems, such as stricture, fistulae, or anastomotic leak. The infection can lead to the development of pelvic fibrosis and scarring of the pouch within the pelvis, which could lead to decreased compliance of the pouch and deteriorated function of the pouch.[135] Research also suggests that the development of pouch-related fistulas has an adverse influence on long-term pouch function, including a failure rate as high as 29%.[9,136,137] Pouch fistulas may appear at any time after creation of IPAA and are associated with pouch failure rates as high as 29%.[136] Failure rates are particularly increased in patients with Crohn disease; however, the differentiation between Crohn-related complications and surgery-related complications or technical failure can be difficult. As discussed previously, there is significant overlap of the clinical symptoms associated with Crohn disease of the pouch, inflammation of the pouch (pouchitis, IPS, cuffitis), and septic complications (leak, fistula, and stricture). The difficulty in diagnosis, once again, underscores the importance of an appropriate evaluation, including endoscopic, histopathologic, and radiographic investigations.

Salvage Surgery

The inability of an IPAA to function correctly and provide an acceptable QoL may not necessarily lead to pouch failure. Conservative techniques, including transanal approaches for pouch revision, have been discussed and their use has been based on individual complications of the pouch being addressed. When these conservative approaches are not feasible, an abdominal approach to pouch salvage may be possible before the final diagnosis of pouch failure is given. Favorable results have been reported in patients who have undergone salvage surgery.[138–141] Several studies have suggested that outcomes may vary with the cause of pouch failure. Reconstruction of ileoanal pouches, related mechanical pouch outlet obstruction, and lack of reservoir capacity have resulted in good long-term results with a success or retention rate as high as 97%.[142,143] As one might expect, the factors that commonly lead to pouch failure also influence the results after salvage surgery.

Sepsis

Results for pouch salvage in the setting of septic complications are considered less favorable, although the data conflict. Early studies have suggested that sepsis results in scarring of the pouch into the pelvis and requires a technically difficult and unsafe dissection. In addition, patients who underwent pouch salvage for sepsis experienced poor results that ultimately led to pouch excision.[144,145] Ogunbiyi and colleagues[144] identified pelvic sepsis as a major predictor of pouch failure in 27 patients who underwent IPAA salvage surgery, which accounted for 58% (7 of 12) of pouch excisions.

Recent studies suggest that salvage surgery can be safely performed if the acute sepsis is well controlled.[138–140,146] Fazio and colleagues[138] reported an 86% success rate for patients who underwent reoperation for septic complications after IPAA. Repeat IPAA was performed in most patients, whereas complete excision and creation of a new IPAA occurred in 2 patients. With a median follow-up of 18 months, 30 patients retained their pouch, with 57% reporting good to excellent function. A more recent study by Baixauli and colleagues[146] similarly reported encouraging long-term function in patients who underwent salvage surgery for IPAA and sepsis. From 1985 to 2001, 101 patients underwent laparotomy, disconnection of the ileoanal anastomosis by either abdominal or combined abdominoperineal approach, pouch repair or re-fashioning, and repeat ileoanal anastomosis with sepsis as the indication in 64 cases. Five-year pouch survival was reported at 74%, with no difference between patients who underwent repeat IPAA for septic indications and those who underwent for non-septic indications.[146] In fact, the study demonstrated better functional results and higher satisfaction in patients who underwent repeat IPAA for septic complications.

Crohn disease

Not surprisingly, Crohn disease has also been associated with worse outcomes and increased pouch failure after salvage surgery. Studies by Fazio and colleagues[138] and Baixauli and colleagues[146] reported a pouch failure rate of 40% and 39% in patients diagnosed with Crohn disease, respectively. In the study by Fazio and colleagues,[138] all patients (n = 4) requiring excision or rediversion were diagnosed with Crohn disease after their salvage surgery. Even so, 60% of patients with Crohn disease retained their pouch after a median follow-up of 18 months. Similarly, Baixauli and colleagues[146] reported a 52.9% pouch retention rate at 5 years for patients with Crohn disease, with no difference in functional outcomes or QoL scores compared with those with UC. A recent study by Garret and colleagues[139] evaluated pouch salvage surgery in 33 patients with pouch failure and preoperative diagnosis of Crohn disease. Despite a referral diagnosis of Crohn disease, only 7 patients were diagnosed with Crohn disease after repeat IPAA. Of those 7 patients, only 2 developed pouch failure and the remaining required long-term immunosuppressive therapy. It is impor-tant to note that patients who were diagnosed with Crohn disease based on further evaluation at the Cleveland Clinic, were not offered salvage surgery and were excluded from the study.

Local versus laparotomy

The literature recommends local repair before abdominal revisions when possible. Local repair is ideal when (1) gross sepsis and edema are absent, (2) the granulation tissue associated with abscess cavities is minimal and can be completely eradicated, (3) the fistula is close to the anal verge and can be approached via a transanal approach, or (4) the stricture is short. If these conditions are not met, then laparotomy and complete pouch mobilization is suggested, which allows for excision of scar, debridement of infection, and repair of the pouch under direct vision.[138] Findings by Garret and colleagues[139] suggest that most patients diagnosed with Crohn disease after IPAA often do not have the disease. This is not surprising, as most patients are diagnosed based on empiric findings. An 84% pouch retention rate in patients thought to have Crohn disease highlights the importance of proper, detailed evaluation and potentially the avoidance of a permanent stoma and unnecessary treatment with immunosuppressant agents.

Pouch excision versus loop ileostomy

For patients who are not candidates for salvage surgery and restoration of intestinal continuity cannot be achieved, pouch excision with end ileostomy is generally per-formed. Similar to pouch salvage surgery, pouch excision is a major undertaking that is associated with significant perioperative morbidity.[147] Although few data exist regarding the outcomes after pouch excision, a small retrospective study by Karoui and colleagues[147] reported outcomes for 68 patients who underwent pouch excision and creation of either an end ileostomy (n = 61) or continent Kock ileostomy (n = 7).

The study reported a high rate of early and late morbidity of 62.3% and a low, but significant, mortality of 1.5%. Pelvic sepsis was the most frequent early complication and occurred in 6% of patients who all required drainage but not laparotomy. Most complications were considered late with a median follow-up period of 30.5 months. The most common late complications included those related to the perineal wound (40.3%) and SBO (14.9%). Other complications included perineal pain and sexual dysfunction (7%).

Given the associated risk with pouch excision, some investigators advocate the use of an alternative procedure (eg, diverting loop ileostomy). In performing an alternative procedure, one would avoid the technically more challenging dissection in the pelvis and its associated potential for damage to pelvic organs and risk for septic complications. Potential drawbacks include persistent drainage from the pouch and the risk of dysplasia or cancer in the pouch or anal transition zone.[100] Few studies evaluate the 2 options. In a recent study at the Cleveland Clinic, Kiran and colleagues[148] reported on 136 patients with pouch failure who underwent pouch excision (n = 105) or loop ileostomy with the pouch left in situ (n = 31). There was no difference between groups concerning baseline characteristics and preoperative details. Pelvic sepsis was the predominant indication for pouch failure in both the loop ileostomy (48.4%) and pouch excision (37.1%) groups. Thirty-day complication rates were similar between groups including pelvic sepsis and bowel obstruction. There was no difference between sexual and urinary dysfunction, although the proportion of patients who provided this information in follow-up was quite small. The median follow-up of the study was 9.8 years, of which QoL parameters were significantly better in those patients who underwent pouch excision compared with those with loop ileostomy. Further, patients with loop ileostomy reported persistent seepage with pad use and anal pain, and were associated with patients who underwent pouch excision for incontinence or outlet obstruction.[148] The findings were consistent with previous literature, including Das and colleagues,[149] who reported better QoL after pouch excision compared with loop ileostomy. Although limited, the current data suggest that, when feasible and associated with appropriate risk, pouch excision is the procedure of choice. Patients who undergo pouch excision may have better QoL compared with those who are permanently dysfunctioned with a loop ileostomy.

Long-Term Outcomes

The question remains whether IPAA function can withstand the test of time. When one asks this question, one must consider both function and QoL, which seem to be stable in most patients who keep their pouch (**Table 1**).

Bowel movements

Across multiple studies, time seemed to have little impact on the mean number of daily bowel movements, which typically range between 6 and 7 bowel movements (bms) or nightly bms, which range between 1 and 3.[31,33,34,150] The prospective study by Michelassi and colleagues[35] examined 391 patients who underwent IPAA and demonstrated a constant median bowel movement frequency of 6 bms per 24 hours over a median follow-up period of 5 years. Results also yielded an increase in bowel movements by 0.3 bm per decade of life ($P<.001$). Nighttime bms were also stable with a median of 1 bm per night.

Continence

Overall, the literature suggests a slight deterioration in continence over time; however, this decline was not a significant change in all but one study. In the retrospective study

Table 1
Summary of long-term function after restorative proctocolectomy with ileal anal pouch anastomosis

Author	Year	n	Median F/U, y	UC	ID	FAP	Conversion to CD (%)	BM Frequency	Good Daytime Continence	Good Nighttime Continence	Antidiarrheal	Pad Usage	Pouch Failure (%)	Satisfaction
McIntyre et al[34]	1994	61	10	75	nr	—	3 (4.0)	7	93%	49%	nr	nr	8 (11)	nr
Fazio et al[32]	1999	977	5	775	123	37	34 (3.5)		82.4%	nr	(↑)	20%	9 (0.9)	98%
Farouk et al[1]	2000	1386	8	1386	—	—	16 (1.2)	6–7	73%	43%	41.7% (↓)	28%	92 (6.6)	nr
Ko et al[165]	2001	25	11[a]	0	0	25	0	7.6	nr	nr	12%	16%	nr	nr
Bullard et al[31,b]	2002	154	12	146	—	2 (1)	6 (4.0)	7.1	83%	53%	19% (↓)	nr	11 (7)	91%
Michelassi et al[35]	2003	391	2	378	13	—	3 (0.7)	6	72.3%	72.3%	13% (±)	13.7%	12 (3)	96.3%
Hahnloser et al[33]	2007	1885	10.8	1885	76	0	47 (2.5)	6.1	89%	79%	59% (↑)	46%	(48)	nr

Abbreviations: BM, bowel movement; CD, Crohn disease; FAP, familial adenomatous polyposis; F/U, follow-up; ID, Indeterminate Colitis; nr, not reported; UC, ulcerative colitis; ↑, increased over study period; ↓, decreased over study period; ±, no change over study period.
[a] Mean follow-up.
[b] Most patients with S-pouch.

by Hahnloser and colleagues,[33] which studied long-term function of 1885 patients who underwent IPAA for chronic UC (median follow-up of 10.8 years), the number of patients with perfect continence during the day and night declined but remained relatively stable from 10 to 20 years. The number of patients with perfect incontinence decreased from 71% at 1 year after IPAA to 60% at 10 years and remained steady at 15 and 20 years. Similarly, in the study by Michelassi and colleagues,[35] 72.3% of patients were fully continent during the daytime and nighttime and results yielded an insignificant decrease from 74.4% of patients at 1 year after IPAA creation. Additionally, Bullard and colleagues[31] studied 154 patients who underwent restorative proctocolectomy with either J-pouches or S-pouches from 1992 to 2000. With a median follow-up of 12 years, most patients reported better or no change in major daytime (81%) or nighttime function (78%). Using a multivariate analysis, the results demonstrated that increased length of time from surgery (>12 years) was a predictor of poor function; however, all but 1 patient were reconstructed with an S-pouch. No comment could be made regarding J-pouches for longer than 12 years, given that the median follow-up for patients was 9 years.

Medication and pad usage

Despite the reported deterioration in function, the literature suggests that most patients require fewer antidiarrheal medications.[31,33,35] Bullard and colleagues[31] showed a decrease in the use of antidiarrheal medications from 34% to 19% over the course of 8 years with more than one-half of patients discontinuing the medications after initially requiring them when they first received their pouch. Michelassi and colleagues[35] also demonstrated that fewer than 25% of patients at 5 years required antimotility drugs to alter their stool frequency; this is a significant decrease from the 32% who required them at 1 year. Likewise, Hahnloser and colleagues[33] demonstrated no change in the use of antimotility agents or the use of protective pads over a median of 10.8 years.

Quality of life

In an era of increasing interest concerning QoL and patient satisfaction, one must consider that, despite the associated morbidity and mortality associated with the ileoanal pouch procedure, patients are satisfied with the results and overall QoL. Despite the heterogeneous use of metrics to assess QoL, the literature does demonstrate an overall high degree of patient satisfaction. In a large long-term study of patients with IPAA, Hahnloser and colleagues[33] demonstrated that all patients reported excellent QoL after IPAA, with good health performance scores in social activities, work, family relationships, recreation and sports, and sexual life. At 5 years after IPAA, Michelassi and colleagues[35] demonstrated that 81.1% of patients judged their QoL as "much better" or "better" with an overall satisfaction and adjustment as excellent or good in 96.3% and 97.5% of patients, respectively. Despite the decrease in function that was demonstrated in patients with S-pouches, Bullard and colleagues[31] also reported that patients were "satisfied" or "very satisfied" with their ileoanal pouch, and 97% said they would choose the pouch over a permanent ileostomy if given the option again.

Fazio and colleagues[32] prospectively evaluated long-term QoL and functional outcome after restorative proctocolectomy with ileal pouch anal anastomosis using the Cleveland Global Quality of Life instrument. With a median follow-up of 5 years, results revealed an increase in QoL 2 years after surgery. This change may be related in part to the increased prevalence of perfect continence from 75.5% before surgery to 82.4% after surgery. Although there was some deterioration over time, this finding was not significant and remained improved from preoperative incontinence with 75.1% of patients reporting prefect continence between 5 and 8 years after surgery. Based on the study, there was no deterioration in patient-reported function, QoL, or satisfaction over time in 98% of patients who continued to recommend surgery to others at 5 years.[32]

SUMMARY

Restorative proctocolectomy with ileal pouch anal anastomosis remains the standard operative approach for patients with UC and for most patients with FAP. Despite the many situations discussed in this review, most of the literature suggests an acceptable complication rate with good-to-excellent functional and acceptable QoL. Pouch-related problems can develop after several years of good function. Pelvic sepsis and delayed onset of Crohn disease remain critical obstacles in understanding the long-term outcomes in patients who undergo IPAA. Proper evaluation for underlying pathology, in addition to preoperative counseling and optimization of the patient's condition, adherence to meticulous surgical technique, and diligent postoperative care, contribute to improving surgical outcomes that result in the preservation of pouch function over time.

REFERENCES

1. Farouk R, Pemberton JH, Wolff BG, et al. Functional outcomes after ileal pouch-anal anastomosis for chronic ulcerative colitis. Ann Surg 2000;231(6):919–26.
2. Fazio VW, Ziv Y, Church JM, et al. Ileal pouch-anal anastomoses complications and function in 1005 patients. Ann Surg 1995;222(2):120–7.
3. Lian L, Serclova Z, Fazio VW, et al. Clinical features and management of post-operative pouch bleeding after ileal pouch-anal anastomosis (IPAA). J Gastrointest Surg 2008;12(11):1991–4.
4. Bach SP, Mortensen NJ. Revolution and evolution: 30 years of ileoanal pouch surgery. Inflamm Bowel Dis 2006;12(2):131–45.
5. Heuschen UA, Hinz U, Allemeyer EH, et al. Risk factors for ileoanal J pouch-related septic complications in ulcerative colitis and familial adenomatous polyposis. Ann Surg 2002;235(2):207–16.
6. Meagher AP, Farouk R, Dozois RR, et al. J ileal pouch-anal anastomosis for chronic ulcerative colitis: complications and long-term outcome in 1310 patients. Br J Surg 1998;85(6):800–3.
7. Belliveau P, Trudel J, Vasilevsky CA, et al. Ileoanal anastomosis with reservoirs: complications and long-term results. Can J Surg 1999;42(5):345–52.
8. Farouk R, Dozois RR, Pemberton JH, et al. Incidence and subsequent impact of pelvic abscess after ileal pouch-anal anastomosis for chronic ulcerative colitis. Dis Colon Rectum 1998;41(10):1239–43.
9. Fazio VW, Tekkis PP, Remzi F, et al. Quantification of risk for pouch failure after ileal pouch anal anastomosis surgery. Ann Surg 2003;238(4):605–14 [discussion: 614–7].
10. Cohen Z, McLeod RS, Stephen W, et al. Continuing evolution of the pelvic pouch procedure. Ann Surg 1992;216(4):506–11 [discussion: 511–2].
11. Sagap I, Remzi FH, Hammel JP, et al. Factors associated with failure in managing pelvic sepsis after ileal pouch-anal anastomosis (IPAA)–a multivariate analysis. Surgery 2006;140(4):691–703 [discussion: 703–4].
12. Delaney CP, Remzi FH, Gramlich T, et al. Equivalent function, quality of life and pouch survival rates after ileal pouch-anal anastomosis for indeterminate and ulcerative colitis. Ann Surg 2002;236(1):43–8.

13. Shen B, Fazio VW, Remzi FH, et al. Risk factors for diseases of ileal pouch-anal anastomosis after restorative proctocolectomy for ulcerative colitis. Clin Gastroenterol Hepatol 2006;4(1):81–9 [quiz: 2–3].

14. Heuschen UA, Allemeyer EH, Hinz U, et al. Outcome after septic complications in J pouch procedures. Br J Surg 2002;89(2):194–200.

15. Thoeni RF, Fell SC, Engelstad B, et al. Ileoanal pouches: comparison of CT, scintigraphy, and contrast enemas for diagnosing postsurgical complications. AJR Am J Roentgenol 1990;154(1):73–8.

16. Broder JC, Tkacz JN, Anderson SW, et al. Ileal pouch-anal anastomosis surgery: imaging and intervention for post-operative complications. Radiographics 2010; 30:221–33.

17. Kirat HT, Kiran RP, Remzi FH, et al. Diagnosis and management of afferent limb syndrome in patients with ileal pouch-anal anastomosis. Inflamm Bowel Dis 2011;17(6):1287–90.

18. MacLean AR, Cohen Z, MacRae HM, et al. Risk of small bowel obstruction after the ileal pouch-anal anastomosis. Ann Surg 2002;235(2):200–6.

19. Fichera A, Silvestri MT, Hurst RD, et al. Laparoscopic restorative proctocolectomy with ileal pouch anal anastomosis: a comparative observational study on long-term functional results. J Gastrointest Surg 2009;13(3):526–32.

20. Marcello PW, Roberts PL, Schoetz DJ Jr, et al. Obstruction after ileal pouch-anal anastomosis: a preventable complication? Dis Colon Rectum 1993;36(12): 1105–11.

21. Francois Y, Dozois RR, Kelly KA, et al. Small intestinal obstruction complicating ileal pouch-anal anastomosis. Ann Surg 1989;209(1):46–50.

22. Sagar PM, Pemberton JH. Intraoperative, postoperative and reoperative problems with ileoanal pouches. Br J Surg 2012;99(4):454–68.

23. Scott NA, Dozois RR, Beart RW Jr, et al. Postoperative intra-abdominal and pelvic sepsis complicating ileal pouch-anal anastomosis. Int J Colorectal Dis 1988;3(3):149–52.

24. Smith L, Friend WG, Medwell SJ. The superior mesenteric artery. The critical factor in the pouch pull-through procedure. Dis Colon Rectum 1984;27(11):741–4.

25. Utsunomiya J, Iwama T, Imajo M, et al. Total colectomy, mucosal proctectomy, and ileoanal anastomosis. Dis Colon Rectum 1980;23(7):459–66.

26. Thirlby RC. Optimizing results and techniques of mesenteric lengthening in ileal pouch-anal anastomosis. Am J Surg 1995;169(5):499–502.

27. Nicholls RJ, Pezim ME. Restorative proctocolectomy with ileal reservoir for ulcerative colitis and familial adenomatous polyposis: a comparison of three reservoir designs. Br J Surg 1985;72(6):470–4.

28. Cherqui D, Valleur P, Perniceni T, et al. Inferior reach of ileal reservoir in ileoanal anastomosis. Experimental anatomic and angiographic study. Dis Colon Rectum 1987;30(5):365–71.

29. Michels NA, Siddharth P, Kornblith PL, et al. The variant blood supply to the descending colon, rectosigmoid and rectum based on 400 dissections. Its importance in regional resections: a review of medical literature. Dis Colon Rectum 1965;8:251–78.

30. Martel P, Majery N, Savigny B, et al. Mesenteric lengthening in ileoanal pouch anastomosis for ulcerative colitis: is high division of the superior mesenteric pedicle a safe procedure? Dis Colon Rectum 1998;41(7):862–6 [discussion: 866–7].

31. Bullard KM, Madoff RD, Gemlo BT. Is ileoanal pouch function stable with time? Results of a prospective audit. Dis Colon Rectum 2002;45(3):299–304.

32. Fazio VW, O'Riordain MG, Lavery IC, et al. Long-term functional outcome and quality of life after stapled restorative proctocolectomy. Ann Surg 1999;230(4): 575–84 [discussion: 584–6].

33. Hahnloser D, Pemberton JH, Wolff BG, et al. Results at up to 20 years after ileal pouch-anal anastomosis for chronic ulcerative colitis. Br J Surg 2007;94(3): 333–40.

34. McIntyre PB, Pemberton JH, Wolff BG, et al. Comparing functional results one year and ten years after ileal pouch-anal anastomosis for chronic ulcerative colitis. Dis Colon Rectum 1994;37(4):303–7.

35. Michelassi F, Lee J, Rubin M, et al. Long-term functional results after ileal pouch anal restorative proctocolectomy for ulcerative colitis: a prospective observational study. Ann Surg 2003;238(3):433–41 [discussion: 442–5].

36. Kiely JM, Fazio VW, Remzi FH, et al. Pelvic sepsis after IPAA adversely affects function of the pouch and quality of life. Dis Colon Rectum 2012;55(4):387–92.

37. Heriot AG, Tekkis PP, Smith JJ, et al. Management and outcome of pouch-vaginal fistulas following restorative proctocolectomy. Dis Colon Rectum 2005; 48(3):451–8.

38. Johnson PM, O'Connor BI, Cohen Z, et al. Pouch-vaginal fistula after ileal pouch-anal anastomosis: treatment and outcomes. Dis Colon Rectum 2005; 48(6):1249–53.

39. Shah NS, Remzi F, Massmann A, et al. Management and treatment outcome of pouch-vaginal fistulas following restorative proctocolectomy. Dis Colon Rectum 2003;46(7):911–7.

40. Paye F, Penna C, Chiche L, et al. Pouch-related fistula following restorative proctocolectomy. Br J Surg 1996;83(11):1574–7.

41. Groom JS, Nicholls RJ, Hawley PR, et al. Pouch-vaginal fistula. Br J Surg 1993; 80(7):936–40.

42. Breen EM, Schoetz DJ Jr, Marcello PW, et al. Functional results after perineal complications of ileal pouch-anal anastomosis. Dis Colon Rectum 1998;41(6):691–5.

43. MacRae HM, McLeod RS, Cohen Z, et al. Risk factors for pelvic pouch failure. Dis Colon Rectum 1997;40(3):257–62.

44. Tsujinaka S, Ruiz D, Wexner SD, et al. Surgical management of pouch-vaginal fistula after restorative proctocolectomy. J Am Coll Surg 2006;202(6):912–8.

45. Gajsek U, McArthur DR, Sagar PM. Long-term efficacy of the button fistula plug in the treatment of ileal pouch-vaginal and Crohn's-related rectovaginal fistulas. Dis Colon Rectum 2011;54(8):999–1002.

46. Gonsalves S, Sagar P, Lengyel J, et al. Assessment of the efficacy of the rectovaginal button fistula plug for the treatment of ileal pouch-vaginal and rectovaginal fistulas. Dis Colon Rectum 2009;52(11):1877–81.

47. Shen B, Lian L, Kiran RP, et al. Efficacy and safety of endoscopic treatment of ileal pouch strictures. Inflamm Bowel Dis 2011;17(12):2527–35.

48. Lewis WG, Kuzu A, Sagar PM, et al. Stricture at the pouch-anal anastomosis after restorative proctocolectomy. Dis Colon Rectum 1994;37(2):120–5.

49. Fleshman JW, Cohen Z, McLeod RS, et al. The ileal reservoir and ileoanal anastomosis procedure. Factors affecting technical and functional outcome. Dis Colon Rectum 1988;31(1):10–6.

50. Prudhomme M, Dozois RR, Godlewski G, et al. Anal canal strictures after ileal pouch-anal anastomosis. Dis Colon Rectum 2003;46(1):20–3.

51. Kirat HT, Kiran RP, Lian L, et al. Influence of stapler size used at ileal pouch-anal anastomosis on anastomotic leak, stricture, long-term functional outcomes, and quality of life. Am J Surg 2010;200(1):68–72.

52. Shen B, Lashner BA, Bennett AE, et al. Treatment of rectal cuff inflammation (cuffitis) in patients with ulcerative colitis following restorative proctocolectomy and ileal pouch-anal anastomosis. Am J Gastroenterol 2004;99(8):1527–31.
53. Shen B, Fazio VW, Remzi FH, et al. Endoscopic balloon dilation of ileal pouch strictures. Am J Gastroenterol 2004;99(12):2340–7.
54. Fazio VW, Tjandra JJ. Pouch advancement and neoileoanal anastomosis for anastomotic stricture and anovaginal fistula complicating restorative proctocolectomy. Br J Surg 1992;79(7):694–6.
55. Cornish JA, Tan E, Teare J, et al. The effect of restorative proctocolectomy on sexual function, urinary function, fertility, pregnancy and delivery: a systematic review. Dis Colon Rectum 2007;50(8):1128–38.
56. Olsen KO, Joelsson M, Laurberg S, et al. Fertility after ileal pouch-anal anastomosis in women with ulcerative colitis. Br J Surg 1999;86(4):493–5.
57. Olsen KO, Juul S, Bulow S, et al. Female fecundity before and after operation for familial adenomatous polyposis. Br J Surg 2003;90(2):227–31.
58. Rajaratnam SG, Eglinton TW, Hider P, et al. Impact of ileal pouch-anal anastomosis on female fertility: meta-analysis and systematic review. Int J Colorectal Dis 2011;26(11):1365–74.
59. Gorgun E, Remzi FH, Goldberg JM, et al. Fertility is reduced after restorative proctocolectomy with ileal pouch anal anastomosis: a study of 300 patients. Surgery 2004;136(4):795–803.
60. Fazio VW, Cohen Z, Fleshman JW, et al. Reduction in adhesive small-bowel obstruction by Seprafilm adhesion barrier after intestinal resection. Dis Colon Rectum 2006;49(1):1–11.
61. Hahnloser D, Pemberton JH, Wolff BG, et al. Pregnancy and delivery before and after ileal pouch-anal anastomosis for inflammatory bowel disease: immediate and long-term consequences and outcomes. Dis Colon Rectum 2004;47(7):1127–35.
62. Graham ID, Carroli G, Davies C, et al. Episiotomy rates around the world: an update. Birth 2005;32(3):219–23.
63. Ramalingam T, Box B, Mortensen NM. Pregnancy delivery and pouch function after ileal pouch-anal anastomosis for ulcerative colitis. Dis Colon Rectum 2003;46(9):1292.
64. Remzi FH, Gorgun E, Bast J, et al. Vaginal delivery after ileal pouch-anal anastomosis: a word of caution. Dis Colon Rectum 2005;48(9):1691–9.
65. Lovegrove RE, Tilney HS, Heriot AG, et al. A comparison of adverse events and functional outcomes after restorative proctocolectomy for familial adenomatous polyposis and ulcerative colitis. Dis Colon Rectum 2006;49(9):1293–306.
66. Penna C, Dozois R, Tremaine W, et al. Pouchitis after ileal pouch-anal anastomosis for ulcerative colitis occurs with increased frequency in patients with associated primary sclerosing cholangitis. Gut 1996;38(2):234–9.
67. Murrell ZA, Melmed GY, Ippoliti A, et al. A prospective evaluation of the long-term outcome of ileal pouch-anal anastomosis in patients with inflammatory bowel disease-unclassified and indeterminate colitis. Dis Colon Rectum 2009; 52(5):872–8.
68. Sandborn WJ. Pouchitis following ileal pouch-anal anastomosis: definition, pathogenesis, and treatment. Gastroenterology 1994;107(6):1856–60.
69. Rubinstein MC, Fisher RL. Pouchitis: pathogenesis, diagnosis, and management. Gastroenterologist 1996;4(2):129–33.
70. O'Connell PR, Pemberton JH, Kelly KA. Motor function of the ileal J pouch and its relation to clinical outcome after ileal pouch-anal anastomosis. World J Surg 1987;11(6):735–41.

71. Duffy M, O'Mahony L, Coffey JC, et al. Sulfate-reducing bacteria colonize pouches formed for ulcerative colitis but not for familial adenomatous polyposis. Dis Colon Rectum 2002;45(3):384–8.

72. Ohge H, Furne JK, Springfield J, et al. Association between fecal hydrogen sulfide production and pouchitis. Dis Colon Rectum 2005;48(3):469–75.

73. Coffey JC, Rowan F, Burke J, et al. Pathogenesis of and unifying hypothesis for idiopathic pouchitis. Am J Gastroenterol 2009;104(4):1013–23.

74. Sandborn WJ, Tremaine WJ, Batts KP, et al. Pouchitis after ileal pouch-anal anastomosis: a Pouchitis Disease Activity Index. Mayo Clin Proc 1994;69(5): 409–15.

75. Shen B, Achkar JP, Connor JT, et al. Modified pouchitis disease activity index: a simplified approach to the diagnosis of pouchitis. Dis Colon Rectum 2003; 46(6):748–53.

76. Madden MV, McIntyre AS, Nicholls RJ. Double-blind crossover trial of metronidazole versus placebo in chronic unremitting pouchitis. Dig Dis Sci 1994; 39(6):1193–6.

77. Shen B, Achkar JP, Lashner BA, et al. A randomized clinical trial of ciprofloxacin and metronidazole to treat acute pouchitis. Inflamm Bowel Dis 2001;7(4):301–5.

78. Holubar SD, Cima RR, Sandborn WJ, et al. Treatment and prevention of pouchitis after ileal pouch-anal anastomosis for chronic ulcerative colitis. Cochrane Database Syst Rev 2010;(6):CD001176.

79. Sambuelli A, Boerr L, Negreira S, et al. Budesonide enema in pouchitis—a double-blind, double-dummy, controlled trial. Aliment Pharmacol Ther 2002; 16(1):27–34.

80. Isaacs KL, Sandler RS, Abreu M, et al. Rifaximin for the treatment of active pouchitis: a randomized, double-blind, placebo-controlled pilot study. Inflamm Bowel Dis 2007;13(10):1250–5.

81. Kuisma J, Jarvinen H, Kahri A, et al. Factors associated with disease activity of pouchitis after surgery for ulcerative colitis. Scand J Gastroenterol 2004;39(6): 544–8.

82. Mimura T, Rizzello F, Helwig U, et al. Once daily high dose probiotic therapy (VSL#3) for maintaining remission in recurrent or refractory pouchitis. Gut 2004;53(1):108–14.

83. Gionchetti P, Rizzello F, Venturi A, et al. Antibiotic combination therapy in patients with chronic, treatment-resistant pouchitis. Aliment Pharmacol Ther 1999;13(6):713–8.

84. Mimura T, Rizzello F, Helwig U, et al. Four-week open-label trial of metronidazole and ciprofloxacin for the treatment of recurrent or refractory pouchitis. Aliment Pharmacol Ther 2002;16(5):909–17.

85. Mahadevan U, Sandborn WJ. Diagnosis and management of pouchitis. Gastroenterology 2003;124(6):1636–50.

86. Shen B, Plesec TP, Remer E, et al. Asymmetric endoscopic inflammation of the ileal pouch: a sign of ischemic pouchitis? Inflamm Bowel Dis 2010;16(5):836–46.

87. Viscido A, Kohn A, Papi C, et al. Management of refractory fistulizing pouchitis with infliximab. Eur Rev Med Pharmacol Sci 2004;8(5):239–46.

88. Ferrante M, D'Haens G, Dewit O, et al. Efficacy of infliximab in refractory pouchitis and Crohn's disease-related complications of the pouch: a Belgian case series. Inflamm Bowel Dis 2010;16(2):243–9.

89. Acosta MB, Garcia-Bosch O, Souto R, et al. Efficacy of infliximab rescue therapy in patients with chronic refractory pouchitis: a multicenter study. Inflamm Bowel Dis 2012;18(5):812–7.

90. Deen KI, Williams JG, Grant EA, et al. Randomized trial to determine the optimum level of pouch-anal anastomosis in stapled restorative proctocolectomy. Dis Colon Rectum 1995;38(2):133–8.

91. Lovegrove RE, Constantinides VA, Heriot AG, et al. A comparison of hand-sewn versus stapled ileal pouch anal anastomosis (IPAA) following proctocolectomy: a meta-analysis of 4183 patients. Ann Surg 2006;244(1):18–26.

92. Hallgren TA, Fasth SB, Oresland TO, et al. Ileal pouch anal function after endoanal mucosectomy and handsewn ileoanal anastomosis compared with stapled anastomosis without mucosectomy. Eur J Surg 1995;161(12): 915–21.

93. Lian L, Kiran RP, Remzi FH, et al. Outcomes for patients developing anastomotic leak after ileal pouch-anal anastomosis: does a handsewn vs. stapled anastomosis matter? Dis Colon Rectum 2009;52(3):387–93.

94. Thompson-Fawcett MW, Mortensen NJ, Warren BF. "Cuffitis" and inflammatory changes in the columnar cuff, anal transitional zone, and ileal reservoir after stapled pouch-anal anastomosis. Dis Colon Rectum 1999;42(3):348–55.

95. Chambers WM, McC Mortensen NJ. Should ileal pouch-anal anastomosis include mucosectomy? Colorectal Dis 2007;9(5):384–92.

96. Shen B, Achkar JP, Lashner BA, et al. Irritable pouch syndrome: a new category of diagnosis for symptomatic patients with ileal pouch-anal anastomosis. Am J Gastroenterol 2002;97(4):972–7.

97. Shen B, Sanmiguel C, Bennett AE, et al. Irritable pouch syndrome is characterized by visceral hypersensitivity. Inflamm Bowel Dis 2011;17(4):994–1002.

98. Shen B, Liu W, Remzi FH, et al. Enterochromaffin cell hyperplasia in irritable pouch syndrome. Am J Gastroenterol 2008;103(9):2293–300.

99. Schmidt C, Hauser W, Giese T, et al. Irritable pouch syndrome is associated with depressiveness and can be differentiated from pouchitis by quantification of mucosal levels of proinflammatory gene transcripts. Inflamm Bowel Dis 2007; 13(12):1502–8.

100. Das P, Johnson MW, Tekkis PP, et al. Risk of dysplasia and adenocarcinoma following restorative proctocolectomy for ulcerative colitis. Colorectal Dis 2007;9(1):15–27.

101. O'Riordain MG, Fazio VW, Lavery IC, et al. Incidence and natural history of dysplasia of the anal transitional zone after ileal pouch-anal anastomosis: results of a five-year to ten-year follow-up. Dis Colon Rectum 2000;43(12): 1660–5.

102. Remzi FH, Fazio VW, Delaney CP, et al. Dysplasia of the anal transitional zone after ileal pouch-anal anastomosis: results of prospective evaluation after a minimum of ten years. Dis Colon Rectum 2003;46(1):6–13.

103. Remzi FH, Church JM, Bast J, et al. Mucosectomy vs. stapled ileal pouch-anal anastomosis in patients with familial adenomatous polyposis: functional outcome and neoplasia control. Dis Colon Rectum 2001;44(11):1590–6.

104. Kariv R, Remzi FH, Lian L, et al. Preoperative colorectal neoplasia increases risk for pouch neoplasia in patients with restorative proctocolectomy. Gastroenterology 2010;139(3):806–12, 812.e1–2.

105. Heuschen UA, Hinz U, Allemeyer EH, et al. Backwash ileitis is strongly associated with colorectal carcinoma in ulcerative colitis. Gastroenterology 2001; 120(4):841–7.

106. Veress B, Reinholt FP, Lindquist K, et al. Long-term histomorphological surveillance of the pelvic ileal pouch: dysplasia develops in a subgroup of patients. Gastroenterology 1995;109(4):1090–7.

107. Gullberg K, Stahlberg D, Liljeqvist L, et al. Neoplastic transformation of the pelvic pouch mucosa in patients with ulcerative colitis. Gastroenterology 1997;112(5):1487–92.
108. Gullberg K, Lindforss U, Zetterquist H, et al. Cancer risk assessment in long-standing pouchitis. DNA aberrations are rare in transformed neoplastic pelvic pouch mucosa. Int J Colorectal Dis 2002;17(2):92–7.
109. Parc YR, Olschwang S, Desaint B, et al. Familial adenomatous polyposis: prevalence of adenomas in the ileal pouch after restorative proctocolectomy. Ann Surg 2001;233(3):360–4.
110. Groves CJ, Beveridge G, Swain DJ, et al. Prevalence and morphology of pouch and ileal adenomas in familial adenomatous polyposis. Dis Colon Rectum 2005; 48(4):816–23.
111. Church J, Simmang C. Practice parameters for the treatment of patients with dominantly inherited colorectal cancer (familial adenomatous polyposis and hereditary nonpolyposis colorectal cancer). Dis Colon Rectum 2003;46(8):1001–12.
112. Kartheuser A, Stangherlin P, Brandt D, et al. Restorative proctocolectomy and ileal pouch-anal anastomosis for familial adenomatous polyposis revisited. Fam Cancer 2006;5(3):241–60 [discussion: 261–2].
113. Gemlo BT, Wong WD, Rothenberger DA, et al. Ileal pouch-anal anastomosis. Patterns of failure. Arch Surg 1992;127(7):784–6 [discussion: 787].
114. Reese GE, Lovegrove RE, Tilney HS, et al. The effect of Crohn's disease on outcomes after restorative proctocolectomy. Dis Colon Rectum 2007;50(2): 239–50.
115. Brown CJ, Maclean AR, Cohen Z, et al. Crohn's disease and indeterminate colitis and the ileal pouch-anal anastomosis: outcomes and patterns of failure. Dis Colon Rectum 2005;48(8):1542–9.
116. Yu CS, Pemberton JH, Larson D. Ileal pouch-anal anastomosis in patients with indeterminate colitis: long-term results. Dis Colon Rectum 2000;43(11):1487–96.
117. Hartley JE, Fazio VW, Remzi FH, et al. Analysis of the outcome of ileal pouch-anal anastomosis in patients with Crohn's disease. Dis Colon Rectum 2004; 47(11):1808–15.
118. Hoda KM, Collins JF, Knigge KL, et al. Predictors of pouchitis after ileal pouch-anal anastomosis: a retrospective review. Dis Colon Rectum 2008;51(5):554–60.
119. Shen B. Crohn's disease of the ileal pouch: reality, diagnosis, and management. Inflamm Bowel Dis 2009;15(2):284–94.
120. Shen B, Remzi FH, Hammel JP, et al. Family history of Crohn's disease is associated with an increased risk for Crohn's disease of the pouch. Inflamm Bowel Dis 2009;15(2):163–70.
121. Nasseri Y, Melmed G, Wang HL, et al. Rigorous histopathological assessment of the colectomy specimen in patients with inflammatory bowel disease unclassified does not predict outcome after ileal pouch-anal anastomosis. Am J Gastroenterol 2010;105(1):155–61.
122. Wolf JM, Achkar JP, Lashner BA, et al. Afferent limb ulcers predict Crohn's disease in patients with ileal pouch-anal anastomosis. Gastroenterology 2004; 126(7):1686–91.
123. Kariv R, Plesec TP, Gaffney K, et al. Pyloric gland metaplasia and pouchitis in patients with ileal pouch-anal anastomoses. Aliment Pharmacol Ther 2010; 31(8):862–73.
124. Dendrinos KG, Becker JM, Stucchi AF, et al. Anti-*Saccharomyces cerevisiae* antibodies are associated with the development of postoperative fistulas following ileal pouch-anal anastomosis. J Gastrointest Surg 2006;10(7):1060–4.

125. Melmed GY, Fleshner PR, Bardakcioglu O, et al. Family history and serology predict Crohn's disease after ileal pouch-anal anastomosis for ulcerative colitis. Dis Colon Rectum 2008;51(1):100–8.

126. Tang LY, Cai H, Navaneethan U, et al. Utility of fecal and serum anti-*Saccharomyces cerevisiae* antibodies in the diagnosis of Crohn's disease-like condition of the pouch. Int J Colorectal Dis 2012;27(11):1455–63.

127. Panis Y, Poupard B, Nemeth J, et al. Ileal pouch/anal anastomosis for Crohn's disease. Lancet 1996;347(9005):854–7.

128. Le Q, Melmed G, Dubinsky M, et al. Surgical outcome of ileal pouch-anal anastomosis when used intentionally for well-defined Crohn's disease. Inflamm Bowel Dis 2012. [Epub ahead of print].

129. Regimbeau JM, Panis Y, Pocard M, et al. Long-term results of ileal pouch-anal anastomosis for colorectal Crohn's disease. Dis Colon Rectum 2001;44(6):769–78.

130. Melton GB, Fazio VW, Kiran RP, et al. Long-term outcomes with ileal pouch-anal anastomosis and Crohn's disease: pouch retention and implications of delayed diagnosis. Ann Surg 2008;248(4):608–16.

131. Colombel JF, Ricart E, Loftus EV Jr, et al. Management of Crohn's disease of the ileoanal pouch with infliximab. Am J Gastroenterol 2003;98(10):2239–44.

132. Shen B, Remzi FH, Lavery IC, et al. Administration of adalimumab in the treatment of Crohn's disease of the ileal pouch. Aliment Pharmacol Ther 2009;29(5):519–26.

133. Matzke GM, Kang AS, Dozois EJ, et al. Mid pouch strictureplasty for Crohn's disease after ileal pouch-anal anastomosis: an alternative to pouch excision. Dis Colon Rectum 2004;47(5):782–6.

134. Korsgen S, Keighley MR. Causes of failure and life expectancy of the ileoanal pouch. Int J Colorectal Dis 1997;12(1):4–8.

135. Forbes SS, O'Connor BI, Victor JC, et al. Sepsis is a major predictor of failure after ileal pouch-anal anastomosis. Dis Colon Rectum 2009;52(12):1975–81.

136. Nisar PJ, Kiran RP, Shen B, et al. Factors associated with ileoanal pouch failure in patients developing early or late pouch-related fistula. Dis Colon Rectum 2011;54(4):446–53.

137. Foley EF, Schoetz DJ Jr, Roberts PL, et al. Rediversion after ileal pouch-anal anastomosis. Causes of failures and predictors of subsequent pouch salvage. Dis Colon Rectum 1995;38(8):793–8.

138. Fazio VW, Wu JS, Lavery IC. Repeat ileal pouch-anal anastomosis to salvage septic complications of pelvic pouches: clinical outcome and quality of life assessment. Ann Surg 1998;228(4):588–97.

139. Garrett KA, Remzi FH, Kirat HT, et al. Outcome of salvage surgery for ileal pouches referred with a diagnosis of Crohn's disease. Dis Colon Rectum 2009;52(12):1967–74.

140. Shawki S, Belizon A, Person B, et al. What are the outcomes of reoperative restorative proctocolectomy and ileal pouch-anal anastomosis surgery? Dis Colon Rectum 2009;52(5):884–90.

141. Cohen Z, Smith D, McLeod R. Reconstructive surgery for pelvic pouches. World J Surg 1998;22(4):342–6.

142. Herbst F, Sielezneff I, Nicholls RJ. Salvage surgery for ileal pouch outlet obstruction. Br J Surg 1996;83(3):368–71.

143. Fonkalsrud EW, Phillips JD. Reconstruction of malfunctioning ileoanal pouch procedures as an alternative to permanent ileostomy. Am J Surg 1990;160(3):245–51.

144. Ogunbiyi OA, Korsgen S, Keighley MR. Pouch salvage. Long-term outcome. Dis Colon Rectum 1997;40(5):548–52.
145. Sagar PM, Dozois RR, Wolff BG, et al. Disconnection, pouch revision and reconnection of the ileal pouch-anal anastomosis. Br J Surg 1996;83(10):1401–5.
146. Baixauli J, Delaney CP, Wu JS, et al. Functional outcome and quality of life after repeat ileal pouch-anal anastomosis for complications of ileoanal surgery. Dis Colon Rectum 2004;47(1):2–11.
147. Karoui M, Cohen R, Nicholls J. Results of surgical removal of the pouch after failed restorative proctocolectomy. Dis Colon Rectum 2004;47(6):869–75.
148. Kiran RP, Kirat HT, Rottoli M, et al. Permanent ostomy after ileoanal pouch failure: pouch in situ or pouch excision? Dis Colon Rectum 2012;55(1):4–9.
149. Das P, Smith JJ, Tekkis PP, et al. Quality of life after indefinite diversion/pouch excision in ileal pouch failure patients. Colorectal Dis 2007;9(8):718–24.
150. Michelassi F, Hurst R. Restorative proctocolectomy with J-pouch ileoanal anastomosis. Arch Surg 2000;135(3):347–53.
151. Kiran RP, da Luz Moreira A, Remzi FH, et al. Factors associated with septic complications after restorative proctocolectomy. Ann Surg 2010;251(3):436–40.
152. Efron JE, Uriburu JP, Wexner SD, et al. Restorative proctocolectomy with ileal pouch anal anastomosis in obese patients. Obes Surg 2001;11(3):246–51.
153. Ferrante M, D'Hoore A, Vermeire S, et al. Corticosteroids but not infliximab increase short-term postoperative infectious complications in patients with ulcerative colitis. Inflamm Bowel Dis 2009;15(7):1062–70.
154. Mor IJ, Vogel JD, da Luz Moreira A, et al. Infliximab in ulcerative colitis is associated with an increased risk of postoperative complications after restorative proctocolectomy. Dis Colon Rectum 2008;51(8):1202–7 [discussion: 1207–10].
155. Selvasekar CR, Cima RR, Larson DW, et al. Effect of infliximab on short-term complications in patients undergoing operation for chronic ulcerative colitis. J Am Coll Surg 2007;204(5):956–62 [discussion: 962–3].
156. Madbouly KM, Senagore AJ, Remzi FH, et al. Perioperative blood transfusions increase infectious complications after ileoanal pouch procedures (IPAA). Int J Colorectal Dis 2006;21(8):807–13.
157. Achkar JP, Al-Haddad M, Lashner B, et al. Differentiating risk factors for acute and chronic pouchitis. Clin Gastroenterol Hepatol 2005;3(1):60–6.
158. Schmidt CM, Lazenby AJ, Hendrickson RJ, et al. Preoperative terminal ileal and colonic resection histopathology predicts risk of pouchitis in patients after ileoanal pull-through procedure. Ann Surg 1998;227(5):654–62 [discussion: 663–5].
159. Hata K, Watanabe T, Shinozaki M, et al. Patients with extraintestinal manifestations have a higher risk of developing pouchitis in ulcerative colitis: multivariate analysis. Scand J Gastroenterol 2003;38(10):1055–8.
160. Lohmuller JL, Pemberton JH, Dozois RR, et al. Pouchitis and extraintestinal manifestations of inflammatory bowel disease after ileal pouch-anal anastomosis. Ann Surg 1990;211(5):622–7 [discussion: 627–9].
161. Ferrante M, Declerck S, De Hertogh G, et al. Outcome after proctocolectomy with ileal pouch-anal anastomosis for ulcerative colitis. Inflamm Bowel Dis 2008;14(1):20–8.
162. Rahman M, Desmond P, Mortensen N, et al. The clinical impact of primary sclerosing cholangitis in patients with an ileal pouch-anal anastomosis for ulcerative colitis. Int J Colorectal Dis 2011;26(5):553–9.
163. Fleshner PR, Vasiliauskas EA, Kam LY, et al. High level perinuclear antineutrophil cytoplasmic antibody (pANCA) in ulcerative colitis patients before colectomy

predicts the development of chronic pouchitis after ileal pouch-anal anastomosis. Gut 2001;49(5):671–7.

164. Merrett MN, Mortensen N, Kettlewell M, et al. Smoking may prevent pouchitis in patients with restorative proctocolectomy for ulcerative colitis. Gut 1996;38(3): 362–4.

165. Ko CY, Rusin LC, Schoetz DJ Jr, et al. Long-term outcomes of the ileal pouch anal anastomosis: the association of bowel function and quality of life 5 years after surgery. J Surg Res 2001;98(2):102–7.

Management and Complications of Stomas

Andrea C. Bafford, MD[a], Jennifer L. Irani, MD[b],*

KEYWORDS

- Stoma • Complications • Hernia • Prolapse • Retraction • Skin

KEY POINTS

- Parastomal hernias are a common complication of ostomy creation. Mesh repairs either via a laparoscopic or via an open approach are superior to both stoma relocation and primary suture repair with respect to hernia recurrence. Prophylactic mesh placement seems to decrease subsequent parastomal herniation without increasing morbidity.
- Stoma prolapse can lead to difficulty with appliance fitting, bowel obstruction, and ischemia. Multiple surgical options for repair are available, most of which can be accomplished locally.
- High stoma output losses can lead to dehydration, electrolyte abnormalities, vitamin deficiencies, and malnutrition. Patients with high ostomy output are managed with a combination of oral and intravenous fluid and electrolyte replacement, vitamin supplementation, hypotonic fluid intake restriction, and antidiarrheal and antisecretory medications.
- Peristomal skin irritation is a common complication that is often managed with local skin care and stoma nursing support.
- While loop ileostomy is a better choice than loop colostomy for temporary fecal diversion, end stomas function better than loop stomas.
- Stoma stricture is a rare complication of stoma formation, usually resulting from ischemia. Local dilation can be attempted; however, definitive treatment often requires stoma revision.
- Stoma retraction is often an early complication that occurs when insufficient bowel length is procured when creating a stoma.

BACKGROUND

Ostomy creation is associated with an overall complication rate between 21% and 70%.[1,2] Many patients feel liberated after creation of an ostomy, whereas others feel imprisoned. This paradox highlights the importance and tremendous impact of

Financial disclosures: The authors have nothing to disclose.
[a] Section of Colon and Rectal Surgery, Division of General and Oncologic Surgery, Department of Surgery, University of Maryland Medical Center, University of Maryland School of Medicine, 22 South Greene Street, S4B10, Baltimore, MD 21230, USA; [b] Department of Surgery, Harvard Medical School, Brigham and Women's Hospital, 75 Francis Street, Boston, MA 02115, USA
* Corresponding author.
E-mail address: jirani@partners.org

Surg Clin N Am 93 (2013) 145–166
http://dx.doi.org/10.1016/j.suc.2012.09.015
0039-6109/13/$ – see front matter © 2013 Elsevier Inc. All rights reserved.

the surgeon's role in dealing with ostomies. The surgeon must be proficient at not only creating the stoma but also handling postoperative complications. This article discusses the more common stoma complications.

PARASTOMAL HERNIAS
Introduction

Parastomal hernias are incisional hernias occurring at the site of or directly adjacent to a stoma (**Figs. 1** and **2**). Although Goligher[3] originally declared that the occurrence of a parastomal hernia is an inevitable consequence of having a stoma, the reported incidence of parastomal hernias is highly variable. One comprehensive review demonstrated an incidence between 0 and 48.1%, depending on the type of stoma.[4] Although frequently asymptomatic, parastomal hernias can lead to pain, bulging, poor stoma appliance fitting, obstructive symptoms, and changes in stool quantity or caliber. While common indications for surgery include these symptoms, incarceration, complete obstruction, and strangulation are absolute indications for surgical repair.

Risk Factors

Technical factors

The incidence of parastomal herniation depends on the type of ostomy, with higher rates seen for end as opposed to loop stomas and for colostomies as opposed to ileostomies.[4-7] This difference has been explained by the direct relationship between the tangential forces on any opening in the abdominal wall and the radius of the opening itself.[8] One study demonstrated a 10% increase in risk of parastomal herniation for each 1-mm increase in fascial aperture size.[7] The appropriate stoma fascial aperture size is classically described as the width of 2 fingerbreadths. A better guideline, however, is the smallest possible opening that will accommodate the stoma without causing ischemia from constriction.[4] Although stoma placement through, rather than lateral, to the rectus muscle is frequently believed to be associated with lower rates of subsequent hernia formation, there is minimal data to support this practice.[4,9-16] Transrectus stoma placement at the time of parastomal hernia repair with mesh does, however, seem to decrease future hernia recurrence.[17] Although previously advocated, fixation of the ostomy mesentery to the fascia does not seem to decrease the risk of parastomal herniation.[18]

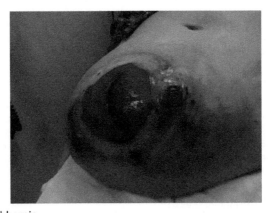

Fig. 1. Parastomal hernia.

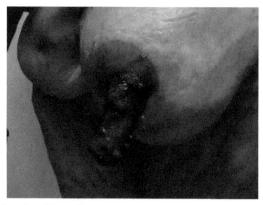

Fig. 2. Parastomal hernia with prolapse.

Patient factors

Despite multiple studies attempting to determine the patient-related risk factors for parastomal herniation, little scientific evidence exists. Patient factors that have been suggested to increase hernia formation include conditions that lead to increases in abdominal pressure, such as obesity and chronic obstructive pulmonary disease; increased patient age; weight gain after ostomy creation; poor nutritional status; underlying malignancy; emergent rather than elective stoma creation; and immuno-suppressive medications such as steroids.[7,19–24] Patients with stomas for longer lengths of time also seem to have a higher risk of parastomal hernia formation.[25]

Diagnosis

Parastomal hernias are typically diagnosed clinically by physical examination. An appropriate examination should include assessment of the patient in upright and supine positions with the ostomy appliance removed, such that the stoma fascial aperture can be palpated. The Valsalva maneuver increases the detection of parasto-mal hernias.[26] Computed tomography can also be used to diagnose parastomal hernias and is especially useful in obese patients.

Treatment

Nonoperative management of parastomal hernias with patient reassurance, abdom-inal support belts, and patient education regarding the avoidance of heavy work and heavy lifting is frequently successful.[3,5,27] Pouching difficulties can be rectified with the use of flexible ostomy appliances with appropriate-sized apertures and with the application of skin protectants. Approximately 20% to 30% of patients with parastomal hernias require surgical repair.[28,29] More emergent operations for absolute indications account for half of parastomal hernia repairs.[25] The remaining elective indi-cations include pain, poor appliance fitting, difficulty with evacuation, and cosmesis.[5] Before deciding upon a parastomal hernia repair, stoma closure should always be considered. Also critical is determining whether the current stoma location is appro-priate, as stoma relocation may be the best surgical option.

Primary fascial repair without mesh

Primary fascial repair is an attractive surgical option because it avoids the morbidity associated with a laparotomy and preserves the integrity of the abdominal wall in case future stoma relocation is necessary. In this technique, a skin incision is made well away from the stoma and dissection is performed within the subcutaneous tissues to isolate and reduce the hernia sac and its contents. In a mesh-free local repair, the fascial defect is suture-repaired primarily. This type of parastomal hernia repair has been largely abandoned because associated recurrence rates have been reported to be between 46% and 100%.[25,30–33]

Stoma relocation

Stoma resiting involves stoma takedown followed by re-creation of the stoma at a new, planned premarked location. The hernia and old stoma defect are closed, with or without mesh reinforcement. Although stoma relocation is associated with lower rates of recurrent parastomal herniation compared with primary fascial repair,[25,30–33] reherniation rates are still significant. Furthermore, laparotomy is often necessary for stoma relocation and suitable sites for resiting may be limited. Stomas relocated to the contralateral abdomen seem to have a lower risk of subsequent herniation than those relocated to the ipsilateral abdomen.[30,32]

Mesh repairs

In 1977, Rosin and Bonardi[34] first described the repair of parastomal hernias via a local approach using mesh reinforcement. Although synthetic prosthetic reinforcement decreases parastomal hernia recurrence, mesh-related complications, including adhesions, possibly leading to bowel obstruction, infection, erosion, and fistulization, are not uncommon.[1,30,35–37] Newer prosthetics with lower polypropylene content, larger pore sizes, and absorbable material coverings may decrease the incidence of these complications.[38] Parastomal hernia repairs with mesh are typically classified according to the mesh position into onlay, sublay, and underlay repairs. For incisional hernias, sublay and underlay grafts are associated with a lower rate of hernia recurrence compared with onlay grafts, being less than 10% versus 20% to 40%.[28,39] Furthermore, dissection close to the stoma opening is avoided with both these techniques, possibly leading to lower infection rates.[40] Many investigators therefore believe that sublay and underlay mesh repairs are preferable.[13,14,41,42] Mesh repairs can be accomplished via local and transabdominal approaches, using both open and laparoscopic techniques. In addition, stomas can be placed directly through an opening in the mesh (keyhole technique) or lateral to the mesh (Sugarbaker technique).[40]

Onlay mesh repair

In an onlay mesh repair, a skin incision is made away from the stoma; dissection is performed within the subcutaneous tissues to isolate and reduce the hernia sac and its contents. The fascial opening is then narrowed with sutures, and the mesh is placed over the anterior rectus aponeurosis and around the stoma, either by cutting a keyhole in the mesh or by mobilizing and passing the bowel through a preexisting opening in the mesh. In general, the prosthetic should overlap the hernia defect by 3 to 4 cm. Recurrence rates have been reported to be between 0% and 26%, significantly lower than those seen after direct suture repair.[28,35,43–47] Mesh-related complications, including obstruction, infection, and mesh erosion, however, occur at a rate of up to 13%.[28,44,48]

Sublay mesh

In sublay mesh repair, the prosthetic is placed between the rectus sheath and posterior fascia. Sublay mesh repairs may lead to lower rates of mesh infection, although the exact reasons are debatable.[41,49,50] Dissection within these abdominal wall layers, however, may be difficult because of postoperative scarring and adhesions.

Intraperitoneal mesh

Parastomal hernia repairs with intraperitoneal mesh are performed using either the keyhole or the modified Sugarbaker technique. In the Sugarbaker repair, a mesh underlay is placed over the ostomy opening. The bowel exits at the lateral border of the mesh before traveling intraperitoneally.[40] The keyhole technique involves stoma passage through a mesh opening positioned directly in line with the fascial opening. There is minimal data comparing these 2 techniques performed in the open manner. Studies have shown a gradual widening of the keyhole aperture over time with associated hernia recurrence.[14,37,40,47] Furthermore, in a recently published systematic review of the literature regarding parastomal hernia repair, a significantly higher recurrence rate was found for laparoscopic repairs using the keyhole technique compared with those using the Sugarbaker technique (odds ratio, 2.3; 95% confidence interval, 1.2–4.6).[47] Mesh erosion and mesh infection have been described at similar rates after both techniques.[35,37,51]

Parastomal hernia repair with biologic mesh

Concerns over mesh infection and mesh erosion have led to the use of biologic rather than synthetic grafts for parastomal hernia repairs. One study of 22 open bioprosthetic mesh repairs using the Sugarbaker technique resulted in no mesh infections and a hernia recurrence rate of 9% after a median follow-up of 18 months.[12] A subsequent meta-analysis also demonstrated a graft infection rate of 0%.[52] In this study, however, recurrences occurred in 15.7% of patients and wound complications in 26.2%, rates being similar to those seen after synthetic mesh repairs.

Laparoscopic parastomal hernia repair

Laparoscopic parastomal hernia repair has been shown to be both feasible and safe.[47,53–55] Evidence demonstrating acceptable long-term recurrence rates or significant benefits over open repair, however, is lacking. Laparoscopic repairs involve intraperitoneal mesh placement, principally using either the keyhole or the Sugarbaker techniques. Ports are placed contralateral to the stoma, adhesions surrounding the stoma and to the abdominal wall are taken down, the hernia contents are reduced, and the mesh is placed. When the keyhole technique is used, the mesh should overlap the fascial defect by 4 to 5 cm.[13,56] Hansson and colleagues[47] analyzed the results of 363 laparoscopic parastomal hernia repairs reported in 11 studies. The overall morbidity rate was 17.2%, including a 3.3% rate of wound infection, a 2.7% rate of mesh infection, and a 4.1% rate of intraoperative iatrogenic bowel injury. Laparoscopic mesh repairs using the Sugarbaker technique resulted in a pooled hernia recurrence rate of 11.6%, compared with a recurrence rate of 20.8% after laparoscopic keyhole-type repairs. The results after laparoscopic and open repairs were comparable.

Prevention

In some studies, limiting the size of the ostomy fascial opening, stoma creation through rather than lateral to the rectus muscle, fixation of the ostomy limb to the abdominal fascia, extraperitoneal stoma placement, preoperative stoma marking, and training by an enterostomal therapist have all been shown to decrease the incidence of parastomal herniation.[4,7,12–15,17,57] Of these, only limiting the size of the fascial aperture has demonstrated a consistent benefit.[4,7,13,14] Recently, the hypothesis that parastomal herniation can be prevented through the use of mesh reinforcement at the time of ostomy creation has also been studied. Janes and colleagues[58] compared the results of permanent colostomy creation with and without prophylactic synthetic mesh in a randomized controlled trial of 54 patients. The mesh was placed in the sublay position using the keyhole technique. There was no difference between the groups regarding the rate of infection, fistula, or postoperative pain. At 12 months of follow-up, only 1 of 21 patients in whom mesh was used developed a parastomal hernia versus 13 of 26 patients without mesh. In a meta-analysis of 3 randomized controlled trials, which included 129 patients receiving ostomies, preperitoneal or sublay mesh reinforcement was associated with a significant reduction in parastomal herniation without a difference in stoma-related morbidity.[42] A second systematic review of prophylactic mesh placement reported a hernia rate of 12.5% with mesh compared with 53% without mesh, again with no difference in operative morbidity.[59] Figel and colleagues[60] demonstrated the safety and efficacy of bioprosthetic mesh placement at the time of ostomy creation and calculated that a parastomal hernia rate of 39% or greater without mesh or a bioprosthetic cost of less than $2267 to $4312 would be needed for prophylactic mesh placement to be cost effective.

Conclusions

The current literature regarding parastomal hernia repair consists primarily of small retrospective studies that examine variable stoma types in heterogeneous patient populations. The definitions of recurrence and infection vary, as do the durations of follow-up. Therefore, a clear consensus regarding the optimal type and approach to parastomal hernia repair is yet to be reached. Suture repair has been shown to be inferior to mesh repair or stoma relocation with respect to hernia recurrence. Laparoscopic parastomal hernia repair is safe and feasible; however, studies have yet to demonstrate a decrease in morbidity after laparoscopic repair compared with open repair and data on long-term recurrence rates are not yet available. Biologic grafts are associated with lower rates of infection, but at a much higher cost than synthetics. Finally, prophylactic mesh placement at the time of ostomy creation seems to decrease subsequent parastomal herniation without increasing perioperative morbidity.

STOMA PROLAPSE
Introduction

Stoma prolapse refers to the condition in which a full thickness of bowel protrudes through an ostomy (**Fig. 3**). Prolapse results largely from intestinal redundancy and lack of fixation, whereas parastomal herniation occurs when the size of the fascial opening is excessive. The incidence of stoma prolapse has been reported to be 3% for ileostomies, 2% for colostomies, and 1% for urostomies, based on a large review from the United Ostomy Association Registry.[61] Other studies, however, have shown a prolapse rate as high as 42% for loop colostomies.[62]

Risk Factors

Advanced patient age, patient obesity, bowel obstruction at the time of stoma creation, and lack of preoperative enterostomal nurse ostomy site marking have all been shown to be associated with a higher incidence of stoma prolapse.[62–64] Loop colostomies seem to prolapse more often than end colostomies.[65–67] Furthermore, the distal limb of loop colostomies prolapses more frequently than the proximal limb, possibly because of bowel atrophy and shrinkage due to a defunctionalized state. Stoma prolapse frequently coexists with parastomal herniation.[30,67] Other factors that may lead to increased prolapse include intraperitoneal versus extraperitoneal

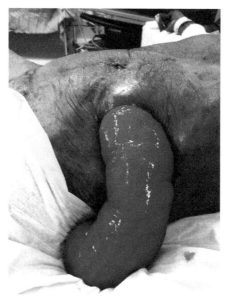

Fig. 3. Stoma prolapse.

stoma creation,[68] failure to fix the mesentery of the stoma to the abdominal wall,[69] and failure to limit the size of the stoma fascial aperture.[70]

Classification

Stoma prolapse can be classified into 2 types: fixed and sliding. Fixed stoma prolapse refers to permanent eversion of an excessive length of bowel. Sliding prolapse is characterized by intermittent protrusion of bowel through the stoma orifice, usually because of an increase in intra-abdominal pressure, such as with Valsalva maneuver.[71]

Symptoms

Stoma prolapse can lead to pain, bulging, poor appliance fitting (possibly with local skin irritation), obstruction, incarceration, and strangulation. The last 3 complications are absolute indications for repair.

Treatment

Surgical treatment options for stoma prolapse include resection of the prolapsed segment, conversion of a prolapsed loop ostomy to an end ostomy, restoration of gastrointestinal continuity in the case of temporary stomas, and ostomy resiting. An acutely prolapsed and incarcerated stoma can sometimes be reduced with the aid of topical sugar, allowing for elective rather than urgent repair. Sugar leads to desiccation of the prolapsed tissue with a subsequent reduction in edema. Although the use of sugar was originally described by veterinarians, it has been described successfully in humans as well.[72]

Resection

Resection is most commonly used for end ostomies and involves disconnection of the ostomy at the mucocutaneous junction, eversion of the prolapsed segment, resection of the redundant bowel, and rematuration of the stoma. A mucosal rather than full-thickness resection, similar to the Delorme procedure for rectal prolapse, has also been described.[73]

Revision

A prolapsed loop stoma can also be repaired by conversion to an end stoma or end loop stoma. In the case of a prolapsed distal limb, a peristomal skin incision is made, after which the distal limb is dissected free, closed, and either returned to the abdominal cavity as a Hartmann's pouch or sutured to the peritoneal surface or within the subcutaneous tissues. Alternatively, the distal limb can be matured into a mucous fistula. A prolapsed proximal limb can be resected in an identical manner to that described above and rematured as an end stoma. The distal limb is either converted to a mucous fistula or Hartmann's pouch or secured to the abdominal wall. Various techniques of stoma prolapse repair using stapling devices have been described.[74–77]

Relocation

Finally, stoma prolapse can be surgically corrected by resiting the stoma. This option should be considered when there is an associated parastomal hernia or if the stoma is in a poor location.

Conclusions

Stoma prolapse is not uncommon after colostomy or ileostomy creation, with rates up to 42% reported for loop colostomies. Although typically asymptomatic, obstruction, difficulty with appliance fitting, and ischemia can occur. Multiple surgical options for repair are available, most of which can be accomplished locally. Stoma closure should always be considered.

HIGH-OUTPUT STOMAS
Introduction

The definition of a high-output stoma is variable, with some describing it as a daily output greater than 2 L and others defining it as the amount that leads to dehydration.[78] Small bowel lengths less than 200 cm are typically associated with fluid and nutrient imbalance.[79] Correspondingly, high stoma output is primarily seen after ileostomy or jejunostomy creation. The typical ileostomy output is between 200 and 700 mL/d, with a median output of approximately 500 mL/d. This varies based on patient body mass and the quantity and type of oral intake.[80] Fasting, for example, is associated with daily ileostomy outputs of only 50 to 100 mL. Elemental diets have been found to decrease ileostomy output, whereas diets high in fat increase the output.[81]

Causes

High stoma output most commonly results from extensive small bowel resection, intrinsic bowel diseases such as Crohn disease, and postoperative states. Other causes include radiation enteritis; partial small bowel obstruction; infectious enteritis; abrupt withdrawal of medications, such as steroids and opioids; bacterial overgrowth; and enteroenteral fistulae.[78]

Postoperative high stoma output

After ileostomy creation, 3 distinct periods of adaptation occur. Output initially increases daily up until the third or fourth day postoperatively. Postoperative days 4 through 6 are characterized by stabilizing output. Finally, a 7-week period of steady decrease in volume and thickening of output ensues.[82,83] Accordingly, dehydration and electrolyte derangements most frequently occur in the early postoperative period.

In a recent study, dehydration was found to be the most frequent indication for hospital readmission after diverting ileostomy creation.[84]

Metabolic effects of high stoma output

High stoma output can lead to electrolyte abnormalities, including hyponatremia, hypokalemia, and hypomagnesemia, all of which can have their own secondary and tertiary effects. The usual amount of sodium lost via ileostomy effluent is 60 mEq/d, which is 2 to 3 times the amount normally lost in stool.[85] Enhanced renal conservation of salt and water lead to a compensatory decrease in urine output and sodium excretion.[86] Excess ostomy output, however, results in salt depletion and hyponatremia. Salt depletion may lead to secondary hyperaldosteronism, causing increased urinary potassium and magnesium loss and subsequent hypokalemia and hypomagnesemia.[87,88] Hypomagnesemia can also occur because of magnesium chelation with unabsorbed fatty acids, resulting in reduced absorption.[89] Malabsorption of fat and vitamin B_{12} occur when more than 60 to 100 cm of the terminal ileum is resected.[79] Deficiency of vitamin B_{12}, necessary for normal hemoglobin synthesis, results in macrocytic anemia.[90] Fat malabsorption can in turn lead to deficiency of the fat-soluble vitamins A, D, E, and K. Because of chronic dehydration and acidic urine, patients who undergo ileostomy are predisposed to kidney stone formation. Increased fluid intake and sodium bicarbonate supplementation may decrease this incidence.[91,92]

Treatment

The management of patients with high stoma output starts with identifying and treating any underlying cause of elevated output, such as Crohn disease, partial obstruction, and infectious enteritis. As with other stoma complications, stoma reversal should always be sought out as a possible treatment of high output. In the long-term, a combination of oral and intravenous fluid and electrolyte replacement, hypotonic fluid intake restriction, and antidiarrheal and antisecretory medications are used in the care of these complicated patients. Long-term total parenteral nutrition is often needed in patients with less than 150 cm of small bowel length remaining.

Intravenous support

Profound dehydration is initially addressed with bowel rest and intravenous fluid and electrolyte replacement with normal saline.[79] Further supplementation with intravenous magnesium and potassium may be necessary, although serum potassium levels typically normalize with the correction of salt depletion and hypomagnesemia alone. Similar to other states, care must be taken to avoid too rapid electrolyte correction to avoid resultant morbidity. Once electrolyte derangements are corrected and the urine output improves, more durable treatment strategies are commenced.

Oral fluid restriction and replacement

Consumption of hypotonic fluids results in net sodium efflux into the intestinal lumen with subsequent hyponatremia.[78] Hypertonic fluids, high in glucose or sorbitol content, can also lead to stoma water and sodium loss. Substituting the intake of both hypotonic and hypertonic fluids with that of balanced glucose–saline replacement solutions is therefore important in the management of high-output stomas. For patients with marginally high stoma outputs, oral fluid restriction to 1 L/d as well as dietary salt supplementation can prevent dehydration.[79]

Antidiarrheal and antisecretory agents

Antidiarrheal agents, including loperamide, codeine phosphate, diphenoxylate–atropine, and tincture of opium have all been shown to decrease ileostomy output.[93–96]

Loperamide seems to be more effective than codeine phosphate in decreasing stoma sodium and potassium losses with the added benefit of causing fewer side effects, such as sedation and fat malabsorption.[93] H2 antagonists and proton pump inhibitors significantly reduce ostomy output and electrolyte losses.[96–100] The somatostatin analog, octreotide, has also been shown to reduce ileostomy output and sodium and chloride losses and to prolong small bowel transit time. Plasma levels of glucagon, C peptide, insulin, renin, and aldosterone, and absorption of potassium, calcium, magnesium, phosphate, zinc, nitrogen, and fat, seem to be unaffected by octreotide administration.[101–103]

Conclusions

High output is commonly encountered after jejunostomy or ileostomy creation and can be either transient, such as in the early postoperative period, or chronic. Excessive stoma losses can lead to dehydration, electrolyte abnormalities, vitamin deficiencies, and malnutrition. The management of patients with high ostomy output depends on a combination of oral and intravenous fluid and electrolyte replacement, vitamin supplementation, and hypotonic fluid intake restriction, along with antidiarrheal and antisecretory medications.

PERISTOMAL SKIN IRRITATION

Peristomal skin irritation is a common complication of stomas. The incidence of peristomal skin irritation ranges from 3% to 42%,[18,19,57,62] and the degree of irritation ranges from mild dermatitis to full-thickness skin necrosis and ulceration. Highlighting the significance of this problem, in a study of 1616 patients with stomas compiled by Cook County Hospital[62] the most common early (<1 month postoperative) complication was skin irritation (12%). Likewise, Pearl and colleagues[104] found that in 610 patients who underwent stoma creation, the most commonly seen early complication was peristomal skin irritation (42.1%). Of 358 end ileostomies constructed, Carlsen and Bergan[105] noted peristomal dermatitis in 8%. Patients with Crohn disease had significantly more problems than patients with ulcerative colitis. This difference may be related to increased appliance leakage seen in patients with Crohn disease.[105]

Causes and Treatment

It is usually an ill-fitting appliance that results in leakage and ultimately a chemical dermatitis. In addition, desquamation of peristomal skin can occur because of frequent appliance changes.[57] In a prospective audit of 97 patients in whom stomas were created, multivariate analysis confirmed an independent association of higher body mass index with early skin excoriation. Diabetes was also found to have an independent correlation with late skin excoriation.[24] Ideally, an appliance should be changed no more often than once every 3 to 7 days to avoid skin breakdown. Owing to the more liquid caustic nature of the bilious small bowel contents, peristomal skin irritation is more frequently seen with ileostomies than with colostomies.[57] Colostomy output contains less bile acid and is more formed, resulting in less skin contact and therefore less irritation.[106]

Candida albicans

The most common peristomal skin infection is from *Candida albicans*. Breakdown of the peristomal skin secondary to mechanical trauma in combination with the warm moist environment makes this location suitable for fungal infection. The appearance is often of a raised rash, and the edges demonstrate well-circumscribed papules and pustules or satellite lesions.[106] Application of miconazole nitrate 2% powder is often sufficient treatment.

Contact dermatitis

Contact dermatitis secondary to an allergic reaction from any of the stoma management products is not uncommon. Symptoms may range from mild erythema and itching to full skin breakdown, blistering, burning, and pain. The hallmark of allergic dermatitis is of the presence of an outline of irritation, which perfectly matches the shape and size of the skin appliance (**Fig. 4**). Given the multitude of products that an ostomite uses, there must be a systematic method of removal to try to identify the allergen. Once the allergen is identified, it is avoided and the patient can enjoy relief. Topical steroid creams and oral antihistamines are often helpful.[106]

Pyoderma gangrenosum

Cutaneous ulceration in patients with Crohn disease was first described in 1970.[107] In 1984, pyoderma gangrenosum was described at the parastomal site in patients with Crohn disease.[108] Pyoderma gangrenosum is a rare, idiopathic, inflammatory ulcerative condition that begins as small erythematous pustules or papules and rapidly coalesces, resulting in superficial ulceration, surrounding induration, and undermining at the edges. The characteristic lesion is a painful ulcer with sharply demarcated violaceous edges (**Fig. 5**).[106,108–110] In more than 80% of cases, the diagnosis is based on physical appearance alone.[111] Furthermore, it is often a diagnosis of exclusion because cultures fail to reveal a pathogen and biopsy results show a nonspecific inflammatory reaction.[109] The onset of pyoderma gangrenosum from the time of stoma creation is variable, with periods ranging from 2 weeks to 25 years reported.[109–111] It is often associated with inflammatory bowel disease, and its appearance is largely believed to parallel intestinal disease activity.[106,109] However, some studies dispute this association with disease activity.[110,112] Definitive treatment of pyoderma gangrenosum is lacking. Local treatment, systemic treatment, and surgery have all been used

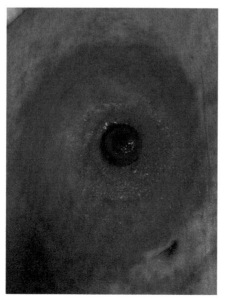

Fig. 4. Contact dermatitis.

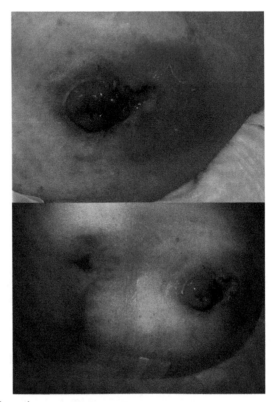

Fig. 5. Peristomal pyoderma gangrenosum.

with variable results. In a series[110] reviewing 16 patients with pyoderma gangrenosum, 6 patients had a complete response to local debridement and intralesional injection of corticosteroids and 14 patients required systemic therapy in the form of corticosteroids, pentoxifylline, 6-mercaptopurine, dapsone, antibiotics, cyclosporine, infliximab, or azathioprine. Of the 7 patients who underwent stoma relocation, only 1 had lasting resolution of pyoderma gangrenosum. The investigators concluded that initial treatment consists of local debridement and wound care with intralesional steroid injection, that systemic therapy may also be required in those who fail local therapy, and that relocation of the stoma should be avoided unless other options have been exhausted.[110] There are conflicting reports regarding healing after stoma relocation. Some investigators have shown that patients develop ulceration at the new stoma site,[109,111] and others suggest that relocation may result in healing.[108] Still others promote stoma closure as the best therapy, if possible.[112]

Prevention

Skin issues secondary to leakage have been reduced by modern stoma equipment and improved stoma nursing. Preoperative stoma site marking and a visit to an enterostomal therapist is the best way to prevent stoma complications.[64,113,114] The site should be centered on a flat area, away from scars, skin creases, and bony prominences, and the surrounding skin should be healthy.[57] The patient should be evaluated sitting and standing, and a note should be made of the belt line. Ideally, the stoma is below the belt line, however, still in a convenient place for the patient to reach. In the obese patient, higher location is often better for visualization.

Ileostomies should always be everted, and the spout should be at least 1 cm above skin level,[57] and ideally 2 cm to 3 cm,[115] to allow the effluent to flow into the pouch rather than on the skin. In general, the opening in the appliance should exactly match the outer diameter of the stoma to protect the skin. There are several pouching accessories, including belts, specially shaped appliances, adhesive seals, and caulking paste that can help with pouch fitting. Patient education and technique is important in avoiding and treating peristomal dermatitis.[57,106]

Conclusion

Peristomal skin irritation is a common complication of stoma creation, more so with ileostomies than colostomies. Precise stoma construction and meticulous stoma and skin care are key to prevention and treatment of this troublesome problem. Local treatment is often successful.

COLOSTOMY VERSUS ILEOSTOMY

There are conflicting data as to what type of stoma has the highest complication rate. Many groups have shown equivalent overall complication rates with colostomies and ileostomies,[1,24,64,114,116] whereas others have shown higher complications with ileostomies.[62,104] There may be differences in individual complications even when overall complication rates are equivalent.

Duchesne and colleagues[114] evaluated 164 patients with intestinal stomas and did not find a statistically significant difference in complication rates between ileostomy and colostomy. Robertson and colleagues[116] showed that the overall complication rates between ileostomies and colostomies did not differ among 408 patients prospectively studied. However, they did note that colostomy patients complained of odor more frequently and ileostomy patients complained of leakage and nighttime emptying more frequently.[116] Of 266 patients with 345 stomas of the small and large bowel, Leenen and Kuypers[64] found that ileostomies were not associated with a higher overall rate of complications than colostomies and that localization in the colon had no influence on the outcome of stoma surgery. When individual complications are analyzed, patients who underwent transverse colostomy had the greatest hernia rate (19%) and those who underwent ileostomy had the greatest incidence of high output and local irritation.[64] Arumugam and colleagues[24] prospectively studied 97 patients who underwent end colostomy, end ileostomy, loop colostomy and loop ileostomy. They analyzed the type of stoma against each complication (necrosis, ischemia, retraction, skin excoriation, detachment, sepsis, parastomal hernia, prolapse, overflow, and other complications) and found no associations.

In contrast, in a study of 1616 patients with stomas compiled by Cook County Hospital,[62] the enteric stoma with the most complications was loop ileostomy (75%), whereas the enteric stoma with the least complications was end transverse colostomy (6%). Although Makela and Niskasaari[117] found ileostomies to have a lower overall complication rate, leakage was seen more frequently with ileostomies than colostomies.

Loop Colostomy Versus Loop Ileostomy for Fecal Diversion

When comparing loop colostomy with loop ileostomy for fecal diversion after low colorectal or coloanal anastomoses, many studies favor loop ileostomy[2,118–122] because of fewer and/or less-severe associated complications. Some studies, however, show equivalence.[122–124] Two meta-analyses consisting of 5 randomized controlled trials comparing loop ileostomy with loop colostomy demonstrated comparable overall morbidity and mortality rates.[123,124] A Cochrane review did find a higher prolapse rate with loop colostomy compared with loop ileostomy.[123]

Rullier and colleagues[125] evaluated 462 rectal resections for cancer and found that the overall morbidity rate was significantly higher after loop colostomy than after loop ileostomy. The higher morbidity rate in the colostomy group was primarily due to the higher rate of parastomal abscess, prolapse, retraction, and hernia compared with the ileostomy group. Also, the colostomy group had a significantly higher complication rate after stoma closure. This high complication rate was primarily due to higher wound infection and hernia rates after colostomy closure compared with ileostomy closure. Both groups were similar with regard to age, gender, obesity, tumor stage, and duration before closure. Tilney and colleagues[122] performed a meta-analysis of 3 randomized controlled trials and 4 cohort studies, including 1204 patients who underwent loop ileostomy or loop colostomy after distal colorectal resection. The investigators found that, in a subgroup of high-quality studies, overall complications were less frequent for patients who underwent ileostomy compared with those who underwent colostomy. Ileostomy patients did have higher stoma outputs but fewer wound infections and incisional hernias after reversal.

In a recent large meta-analysis including 12 comparative studies and 1529 patients, Rondelli and colleagues[121] found that patients with a loop ileostomy had a lower risk of prolapse and sepsis but an increased risk of occlusion after stoma closure and dehydration. These factors were the only ones found to be significant after looking at the following outcome measures: general outcome measures (wound infection, dehydrations), stoma construction outcome measures (necrosis, prolapse, retraction, parastomal hernia, stenosis, sepsis, hemorrhage), stoma closure outcome measures (occlusion, wound infection, anastomotic leak or fistula, hernia), and functioning of the stoma outcome measures (skin irritations, occlusion).[121] Finally, in a prospective randomized clinical trial, Edwards and colleagues[118] compared 36 patients who underwent loop transverse colostomy to 34 patients who underwent loop ileostomy for diversion after rectal resection. Although they found no difference in the difficulty of formation or closure or in postoperative recovery between the groups, they did find 10 complications in the loop colostomy group (1 fecal fistula, 2 prolapse, 2 parastomal hernia, 5 incisional hernias) and no complication in the loop ileostomy group. Based on the frequency of herniation before or after colostomy closure, the investigators supported loop ileostomy for defunctioning a low anastomosis.

End Versus Loop Stoma

There are few studies comparing loop to end stomas. In a small study, Caricato and colleagues[126] compared 44 patients with loop ileostomy, 77 patients with loop colostomy, and 11 patients with end colostomy. The stoma with the lowest complication rate was end colostomy. Although not evaluated in their study, the investigators pointed out that end colostomy reversal is associated with a higher complication rate than loop colostomy or ileostomy closure because it requires laparotomy. Other investigators dispute this claim, and concede that although it may take longer to close an end colostomy, closure of end and loop colostomies have similar complication rates.[126–129]

Harris and colleagues[119] retrospectively studied 345 stomas created in 320 patients and found that loop colostomy had the highest complication rate and end ileostomy had the lowest. Prolapse occurred in 13% of loop colostomies, which increased to 17% in the transverse loop colostomy group. Retraction was the most frequent end ileostomy complication (7%). Notably, they did not include skin excoriation or dehydration as potential complications.

Conclusion

Many investigators declare that for temporary fecal diversion, loop ileostomy is a better choice than loop colostomy.[1,2,118,121,122,125] End stomas tend to function better than loop stomas for permanent stoma formation.[1,119,126] Ileostomies tend to have a higher leakage rate, whereas colostomies have a higher hernia rate.

STRICTURE/STENOSIS

Stoma stricture can occur at the level of the skin or the fascia. It is a relatively rare complication, being found in only 1% to 10% of stomas.[18,64,105,115,116,130,131] Strictures can act as a mechanical obstruction, leading to noisy bowel function, especially with flatus, and also periods of low stoma output followed by large-volume output. There are varying reports on whether colostomies or ileostomies have a higher rate of stenosis.[117,132,133]

Causes

Stenosis usually results from ischemia or infection; however, it can also result from a technical error if either the skin or the fascia is left too tight at the time of operation. The latter scenario presents in the early postoperative period and is rare. Ischemia, the most common underlying factor in stenosis, usually renders stenosis a late complication.[106,132] Stoma stenosis is more often seen in patients with Crohn disease, because of the difficulty in length with the thickened foreshortened mesentery.[120] Although uncommon, it should be kept in mind that stenosis could be a sign of an underlying carcinoma causing mass effect; this has been described in patients with inflammatory bowel disease and familial polyposis syndromes who have a long-standing permanent stoma.[120,134–137]

Management

First, one must rule out recurrent disease (Crohn disease, malignancy, and so forth), usually by inspection and biopsy. Initial treatment is usually in the form of dilation, either digitally or with the use of Hegar dilators, and usually requiring multiple sessions. Unfortunately, tissue trauma during mechanical dilation often promotes further fibrosis and stricturing. Definitive treatment often requires stoma revision, either locally, if stenosis is at the skin-level, or via laparotomy, if it is deeper.[30,106,132]

Conclusion

Stoma stricture is a rare complication of stoma formation, usually resulting from ischemia. Once recurrent disease is ruled out, local dilation can be attempted; however, definitive treatment often requires stoma revision.

STOMA RETRACTION

Stoma retraction is usually an immediate postsurgical problem resulting from tension on the bowel, although it is possible to occur later.[57] Patients who are malnourished, immunosuppressed, or obese may experience retraction because of poor wound healing and difficult anatomy. Patients with stoma ischemia who are managed expectantly may later experience retraction.[57] Many series have shown stoma retraction to occur in 1% to 6% of all colostomies[64,115,130] and 3% to 17% of all ileostomies.[18,64,105,138] In a study of 358 end ileostomies, Carlsen and Bergan[105] noted retraction in 2.7% after primary stoma construction and in 6.7% after reconstruction. Fixation of the stoma to the rectus fascia or closing the lateral gutter did not prevent retraction of the ileostomy. Disease indication also did not influence retraction rate. High body mass index has been shown to be associated with retraction.[24] One of the main problems with retraction involves difficulty in pouching and leakage.

Prevention

Sufficient length of the bowel is needed to prevent tension and retraction. This problem is rarely encountered for ileostomies but often encountered when creating colostomies, especially in the setting of abdominal sepsis. For example, when constructing an end left colostomy, it is often necessary to mobilize the splenic flexure and also ligate the inferior mesenteric artery at or near its takeoff, thus relying on the marginal artery to ensure sufficient length for a well-constructed colostomy. If bowel length is still a problem, end loop ostomy is an option because one can obviate more mesenteric length, as the mesenteric vessels are often what are tethering the bowel. By pulling up the antimesenteric side of the bowel, and leaving the stapled end intra-abdominal, the surgeon can often gain some length.[115,138] It may be helpful to mature the bowel over a stoma bar.

Treatment

The use of a convex stoma appliance may result in decreased leakage; however, definitive treatment usually requires stoma revision. An attempt at local revision is acceptable and is usually more successful with ileostomies, but in most cases, laparotomy is required.[106,115] Stoma revision techniques are the same as for the initial creation, ensuring adequate length and excellent blood supply. If the skin at the original stoma location is not compromised, the same site can be used for the new stoma.[106,115] In the instance of complete mucocutaneous separation with the stoma retracting below the fascia, intra-abdominal contamination and peritonitis may ensue, necessitating emergent laparotomy.[57]

Conclusion

Stoma retraction is often an early complication that occurs when insufficient bowel length is procured when creating a stoma and/or the patient is unable to heal a well-constructed stoma. Mobilization of the bowel and creation of an end loop stoma may allow greater length for stoma creation. Local revision may be attempted; however, laparotomy is often required for repair.

SUMMARY

Beyond simply exteriorizing a piece of bowel to the skin surface, there are a wide variety of issues that a surgeon needs to consider when creating a stoma. Having a thorough understanding of the technical details and potential complications from ostomy placement is an essential tool for all providers caring for these patients.

REFERENCES

1. Shabbir J, Britton DC. Stoma complications: a literature overview. Colorectal Dis 2010;12(10):958–64.
2. Parmar KL, Zammit M, Smith A, et al. A prospective audit of early stoma complications in colorectal cancer treatment throughout the greater Manchester and Cheshire colorectal cancer network. Colorectal Dis 2011;13(8):935–8.

3. Goligher JC. Surgery of the anus, rectum and colon. 5th edition. London: Bailliere Tindall; 1984.
4. Carne PW, Robertson GM, Frizelle FA. Parastomal hernia. Br J Surg 2003;90(7): 784–93.
5. Martin L, Foster G. Parastomal hernia. Ann R Coll Surg Engl 1996;78(2):81–4.
6. Hiranyakas A, Ho YH. Laparoscopic parastomal hernia repair. Dis Colon Rectum 2010;53(9):1334–6.
7. Pilgrim CH, McIntyre R, Bailey M. Prospective audit of parastomal hernia: prevalence and associated comorbidities. Dis Colon Rectum 2010;53(1):71–6.
8. de Ruiter P, Bijnen AB. Successful local repair of paracolostomy hernia with a newly developed prosthetic device. Int J Colorectal Dis 1992;7(3):132–4.
9. Birnbaum W, Ferrier P. Complication of abdominal colostomy. Am J Surg 1952; 83:64–7.
10. Grier WR, Postel AH, Syarse A, et al. An evaluation of colonic stoma management without irrigations. Surg Gynecol Obstet 1964;118:1234–42.
11. Sjodahl R, Anderberg B, Bolin T. Parastomal hernia in relation to site of the abdominal stoma. Br J Surg 1988;75(4):339–41.
12. Ellis CN. Short-term outcomes with the use of bioprosthetics for the management of parastomal hernias. Dis Colon Rectum 2010;53(3):279–83.
13. Israelsson LA. Parastomal hernias. Surg Clin North Am 2008;88(1):113–25, ix.
14. Lo Menzo E, Martinez JM, Spector SA, et al. Use of biologic mesh for a complicated paracolostomy hernia. Am J Surg 2008;196(5):715–9.
15. Janes A, Cengiz Y, Israelsson LA. Experiences with a prophylactic mesh in 93 consecutive ostomies. World J Surg 2010;34(7):1637–40.
16. Williams JG, Etherington R, Hayward MW, et al. Paraileostomy hernia: a clinical and radiological study. Br J Surg 1990;77(12):1355–7.
17. Smart NJ, Velineni R, Khan D, et al. Parastomal hernia repair outcomes in relation to stoma site with diisocyanate cross-linked acellular porcine dermal collagen mesh. Hernia 2011;15(4):433–7.
18. Leong AP, Londono-Schimmer EE, Phillips RK. Life-table analysis of stomal complications following ileostomy. Br J Surg 1994;81(5):727–9.
19. Pearl RK. Parastomal hernias. World J Surg 1989;13(5):569–72.
20. McGrath A, Porrett T, Heyman B. Parastomal hernia: an exploration of the risk factors and the implications. Br J Nurs 2006;15(6):317–21.
21. Leslie D. The parastomal hernia. Surg Clin North Am 1984;64(2):407–15.
22. De Raet JDG, Haentjens P, Van Nieuwenhove Y. Waist circumference is an independent risk factor for the development of parastomal hernia after permanent colostomy. Dis Colon Rectum 2008;51(12):1806–9.
23. Nastro P, Knowles CH, McGrath A, et al. Complications of intestinal stomas. Br J Surg 2010;97(12):1885–9.
24. Arumugam PJ, Bevan L, Macdonald L, et al. A prospective audit of stomas–analysis of risk factors and complications and their management. Colorectal Dis 2003;5(1):49–52.
25. Rubin MS, Schoetz DJ Jr, Matthews JB. Parastomal hernia. Is stoma relocation superior to fascial repair? Arch Surg 1994;129(4):413–8 [discussion: 418–9].
26. Gurmu A, Matthiessen P, Nilsson S, et al. The inter-observer reliability is very low at clinical examination of parastomal hernia. Int J Colorectal Dis 2011;26(1):89–95.
27. Thompson MJ. Parastomal hernia: incidence, prevention and treatment strategies. Br J Nurs 2008;17(2):S16, S18–20.
28. Luning TH, Spillenaar-Bilgen EJ. Parastomal hernia: complications of extraperitoneal onlay mesh placement. Hernia 2009;13(5):487–90.

29. Horgan K, Hughes LE. Para-ileostomy hernia: failure of a local repair technique. Br J Surg 1986;73(6):439–40.
30. Allen-Mersh TG, Thomson JP. Surgical treatment of colostomy complications. Br J Surg 1988;75(5):416–8.
31. Rieger N, Moore J, Hewett P, et al. Parastomal hernia repair. Colorectal Dis 2004; 6(3):203–5.
32. Riansuwan W, Hull TL, Millan MM, et al. Surgery of recurrent parastomal hernia: direct repair or relocation? Colorectal Dis 2010;12(7):681–6.
33. Cheung MT, Chia NH, Chiu WY. Surgical treatment of parastomal hernia complicating sigmoid colostomies. Dis Colon Rectum 2001;44(2):266–70.
34. Rosin JD, Bonardi RA. Paracolostomy hernia repair with Marlex mesh: a new technique. Dis Colon Rectum 1977;20(4):299–302.
35. Steele SR, Lee P, Martin MJ, et al. Is parastomal hernia repair with polypropylene mesh safe? Am J Surg 2003;185(5):436–40.
36. Morris-Stiff G, Hughes LE. The continuing challenge of parastomal hernia: failure of a novel polypropylene mesh repair. Ann R Coll Surg Engl 1998;80(3):184–7.
37. Aldridge AJ, Simson JN. Erosion and perforation of colon by synthetic mesh in a recurrent paracolostomy hernia. Hernia 2001;5(2):110–2.
38. Simmermacher RK, Schakenraad JM, Bleichrodt RP. Reherniation after repair of the abdominal wall with expanded polytetrafluoroethylene. J Am Coll Surg 1994; 178(6):613–6.
39. Shell DH 4th, de la Torre J, Andrades P, et al. Open repair of ventral incisional hernias. Surg Clin North Am 2008;88(1):61–83, viii.
40. Sugarbaker PH. Peritoneal approach to prosthetic mesh repair of paraostomy hernias. Ann Surg 1985;201(3):344–6.
41. Kasperk R, Klinge U, Schumpelick V. The repair of large parastomal hernias using a midline approach and a prosthetic mesh in the sublay position. Am J Surg 2000;179(3):186–8.
42. Wijeyekoon SP, Gurusamy K, El-Gendy K, et al. Prevention of parastomal herniation with biologic/composite prosthetic mesh: a systematic review and meta-analysis of randomized controlled trials. J Am Coll Surg 2010;211(5):637–45.
43. Ho KM, Fawcett DP. Parastomal hernia repair using the lateral approach. BJU Int 2004;94:598–602.
44. De Ruiter P, Bijnen AB. Ring-reinforced prosthesis for paracolostomy hernia. Dig Surg 2005;22:152–6.
45. Venditti D, Gargiani M, Milito G. Parastomal hernia surgery: personal experience with use of polypropylene mesh. Tech Coloproctol 2001;5(2):85–8.
46. Amin SN, Armitage NC, Abercrombie JF, et al. Lateral repair of parastomal hernia. Ann R Coll Surg Engl 2001;83(3):206–8.
47. Hansson BM, Slater NJ, van der Velden AS, et al. Surgical techniques for parastomal hernia repair: a systematic review of the literature. Ann Surg 2012;255(4): 685–95.
48. Geisler DJ, Reilly JC, Vaughan SG, et al. Safety and outcome of use of nonabsorbable mesh for repair of fascial defects in the presence of open bowel. Dis Colon Rectum 2003;46(8):1118–23.
49. Longman RJ, Thomson WH. Mesh repair of parastomal hernia – a safety modification. Colorectal Dis 2005;7:292–4.
50. Guzman-Valdivia G, Guerrero TS, Laurrabaquio HV. Parastomal hernia repair using mesh and an open technique. World J Surg 2008;32:465–70.
51. Mancini GJ, McClusky DA 3rd, Khaitan L, et al. Laparoscopic parastomal hernia repair using a nonslit mesh technique. Surg Endosc 2007;21(9):1487–91.

52. Slater NJ, Hansson BM, Buyne OR, et al. Repair of parastomal hernias with biologic grafts: a systematic review. J Gastrointest Surg 2011;15(7): 1252–8.
53. Mizrahi H, Bhattacharya P, Parker MC. Laparoscopic slit mesh repair of parastomal hernia using a designated mesh: long-term results. Surg Endosc 2012; 26(1):267–70.
54. Safadi B. Laparoscopic repair of parastomal hernias: early results. Surg Endosc 2004;18(4):676–80.
55. Hansson BM, de Hingh IH, Bleichrodt RP. Laparoscopic parastomal hernia repair is feasible and safe: early results of a prospective clinical study including 55 consecutive patients. Surg Endosc 2007;21(6):989–93.
56. Saber AA, Rao AJ, Rao CA, et al. Simplified laparoscopic parastomal hernia repair: the scroll technique. Am J Surg 2008;196(3):e16–8.
57. Kann BR. Early stomal complications. Clin Colon Rectal Surg 2008;21(1):23–30.
58. Janes A, Cengiz Y, Israelsson LA. Preventing parastomal hernia with a prosthetic mesh. Arch Surg 2004;139(12):1356–8.
59. Shabbir J, Chaudhary BN, Dawson R. A systematic review on the use of prophylactic mesh during primary stoma formation to prevent parastomal hernia formation. Colorectal Dis 2011;14(8):931–6.
60. Figel NA, Rostas JW, Ellis CN. Outcomes using a bioprosthetic mesh at the time of permanent stoma creation in preventing a parastomal hernia: a value analysis. Am J Surg 2012;203(3):323–6 [discussion: 326].
61. Fleshman JW, Lewis MG. Complications and quality of life after stoma surgery: a review of 16,470 patients in the UOA data registry. Semin Colon Rectal Surg 1991;2:66–72.
62. Park JJ, Del Pino A, Orsay CP, et al. Stoma complications: the Cook County Hospital experience. Dis Colon Rectum 1999;42(12):1575–80.
63. Black P. Managing physical postoperative stoma complications. Br J Nurs 2009; 18(17):S4–10.
64. Leenen LP, Kuypers JH. Some factors influencing the outcome of stoma surgery. Dis Colon Rectum 1989;32(6):500–4.
65. Chandler JG, Evans BP. Colostomy prolapse. Surgery 1978;84(5):577–82.
66. Cheung MT. Complications of an abdominal stoma: an analysis of 322 stomas. Aust N Z J Surg 1995;65(11):808–11.
67. Gooszen AW, Geelkerken RH, Hermans J, et al. Temporary decompression after colorectal surgery: randomized comparison of loop ileostomy and loop colostomy. Br J Surg 1998;85(1):76–9.
68. Whittaker M, Goligher JC. A comparison of the results of extraperitoneal and intraperitoneal techniques for construction of terminal iliac colostomies. Dis Colon Rectum 1976;19(4):342–4.
69. Ng WT, Book KS, Wong MK, et al. Prevention of colostomy prolapse by peritoneal tethering. J Am Coll Surg 1997;184(3):313–5.
70. Law WL, Chu KW, Choi HK. Randomized clinical trial comparing loop ileostomy and loop transverse colostomy for faecal diversion following total mesorectal excision. Br J Surg 2002;89(6):704–8.
71. Gordon PH, Nivatvongs S. Principles and practice of surgery for the colon, rectum and anus. 3rd edition. New York: Informa Healthcase; 2006.
72. Myers JO, Rothenberger DA. Sugar in the reduction of incarcerated prolapsed bowel. Report of two cases. Dis Colon Rectum 1991;34(5):416–8.
73. Abulafi AM, Sherman IW, Fiddian RV. Delorme operation for prolapsed colostomy. Br J Surg 1989;76(12):1321–2.

74. Masumori K, Maeda K, Koide Y, et al. Simple excision and closure of a distal limb of loop colostomy prolapse by stapler device. Tech Coloproctol 2012;16(2):143–5.
75. Hata F, Kitagawa S, Nishimori H, et al. A novel, easy, and safe technique to repair a stoma prolapse using a surgical stapling device. Dig Surg 2005; 22(5):306–9 [discussion: 310].
76. Maeda K, Maruta M, Utsumi T, et al. Local correction of a transverse loop colostomy prolapse by means of a stapler device. Tech Coloproctol 2004;8(1):45–6.
77. Tepetes K, Spyridakis M, Hatzitheofilou C. Local treatment of a loop colostomy prolapse with a linear stapler. Tech Coloproctol 2005;9(2):156–8.
78. Baker ML, Williams RN, Nightingale JM. Causes and management of a high-output stoma. Colorectal Dis 2011;13(2):191–7.
79. Nightingale J, Woodward JM. Guidelines for management of patients with a short bowel. Gut 2006;55(Suppl 4):iv1–12.
80. Hill GL, Millward SF, King RF, et al. Normal ileostomy output: close relation to body size. Br Med J 1979;2(6194):831–2.
81. Ladas SD, Isaacs PE, Murphy GM, et al. Fasting and postprandial ileal function in adapted ileostomates and normal subjects. Gut 1986;27(8):906–12.
82. Tang CL, Yunos A, Leong AP, et al. Ileostomy output in the early postoperative period. Br J Surg 1995;82(5):607.
83. Soybel DI. Adaptation to ileal diversion. Surgery 2001;129(2):123–7.
84. Messaris E, Sehgal R, Deiling S, et al. Dehydration is the most common indication for readmission after diverting ileostomy creation. Dis Colon Rectum 2012; 55(2):175–80.
85. Dozois RR. Alternatives to conventional ileostomy. Chicago: Year Book Medical Publishers; 1985.
86. Gallagher ND, Harrison DD, Skyring AP. Fluid and electrolyte disturbances in patients with long-established ileostomies. Gut 1962;3:219–23.
87. Hanna S, Mac II. The influence of aldosterone on magnesium metabolism. Lancet 1960;2(7146):348–50.
88. Ladefoged K, Olgaard K. Fluid and electrolyte absorption and renin-angiotensin-aldosterone axis in patients with severe short-bowel syndrome. Scand J Gastroenterol 1979;14(6):729–35.
89. Hessov I, Andersson H, Isaksson B. Effects of a low-fat diet on mineral absorption in small-bowel disease. Scand J Gastroenterol 1983;18(4):551–4.
90. Booth CC. The metabolic effects of intestinal resection in man. Postgrad Med J 1961;37:725–39.
91. Modlin M. Urinary calculi and ulcerative colitis. Br Med J 1972;3(5821):292.
92. Fukushima T, Sugita A, Masuzawa S, et al. Prevention of uric acid stone formation by sodium bicarbonate in an ileostomy patient–a case report. Jpn J Surg 1988;18(4):465–8.
93. King RF, Norton T, Hill GL. A double-blind crossover study of the effect of loperamide hydrochloride and codeine phosphate on ileostomy output. Aust N Z J Surg 1982;52:121–4.
94. Tytgat GN, Huibregtse K. Loperamide and ileostomy output–placebo-controled double-blind crossover study. Br Med J 1975;2(5972):667.
95. Kramer P. Effect of antidiarrheal and antimotility drugs on ileal excreta. Am J Dig Dis 1977;22(4):327–32.
96. Newton CR. Effect of codeine phosphate, Lomotil, and Isogel on iileostomy function. Gut 1978;19(5):377–83.
97. Nightingale JM, Walker ER, Farthing MJ, et al. Effect of omeprazole on intestinal output in the short bowel syndrome. Aliment Pharmacol Ther 1991;5(4):405–12.

98. Jeppesen PB, Staun M, Tjellesen L, et al. Effect of intravenous ranitidine and omeprazole on intestinal absorption of water, sodium, and macronutrients in patients with intestinal resection. Gut 1998;43(6):763–9.

99. Jacobsen O, Ladefoged K, Stage JG, et al. Effects of cimetidine on jejunostomy effluents in patients with severe short-bowel syndrome. Scand J Gastroenterol 1986;21(7):824–8.

100. Aly A, Barany F, Kollberg B, et al. Effect of an H2-receptor blocking agent on diarrhoeas after extensive small bowel resection in Crohn's disease. Acta Med Scand 1980;207(1–2):119–22.

101. Ladefoged K, Christensen KC, Hegnhoj J, et al. Effect of a long acting somatostatin analogue SMS 201-995 on jejunostomy effluents in patients with severe short bowel syndrome. Gut 1989;30(7):943–9.

102. Cooper JC, Williams NS, King RF, et al. Effects of a long-acting somatostatin analogue in patients with severe ileostomy diarrhoea. Br J Surg 1986;73(2):128–31.

103. Kusuhara K, Kusunoki M, Okamoto T, et al. Reduction of the effluent volume in high-output ileostomy patients by a somatostatin analogue, SMS 201-995. Int J Colorectal Dis 1992;7(4):202–5.

104. Pearl RK, Prasad ML, Orsay CP, et al. Early local complications from intestinal stomas. Arch Surg 1985;120(10):1145–7.

105. Carlsen E, Bergan A. Technical aspects and complications of end-ileostomies. World J Surg 1995;19(4):632–6.

106. Husain SG, Cataldo TE. Late stomal complications. Clin Colon Rectal Surg 2008;21(1):31–40.

107. Mountain JC. Cutaneous ulceration in Crohn's disease. Gut 1970;11(1):18–26.

108. McGarity WC, Robertson DB, McKeown PP, et al. Pyoderma gangrenosum at the parastomal site in patients with Crohn's disease. Arch Surg 1984;119(10):1186–8.

109. Hughes AP, Jackson JM, Callen JP. Clinical features and treatment of peristomal pyoderma gangrenosum. JAMA 2000;284(12):1546–8.

110. Kiran RP, O'Brien-Ermlich B, Achkar JP, et al. Management of peristomal pyoderma gangrenosum. Dis Colon Rectum 2005;48(7):1397–403.

111. Cairns BA, Herbst CA, Sartor BR, et al. Peristomal pyoderma gangrenosum and inflammatory bowel disease. Arch Surg 1994;129(7):769–72.

112. Poritz LS, Lebo MA, Bobb AD, et al. Management of peristomal pyoderma gangrenosum. J Am Coll Surg 2008;206(2):311–5.

113. Bass EM, Del Pino A, Tan A, et al. Does preoperative stoma marking and education by the enterostomal therapist affect outcome? Dis Colon Rectum 1997;40(4):440–2.

114. Duchesne JC, Wang YZ, Weintraub SL, et al. Stoma complications: a multivariate analysis. Am Surg 2002;68(11):961–6 [discussion: 966].

115. Shellito PC. Complications of abdominal stoma surgery. Dis Colon Rectum 1998;41(12):1562–72.

116. Robertson I, Leung E, Hughes D, et al. Prospective analysis of stoma-related complications. Colorectal Dis 2005;7(3):279–85.

117. Makela JT, Niskasaari M. Stoma care problems after stoma surgery in northern Finland. Scand J Surg 2006;95(1):23–7.

118. Edwards DP, Leppington-Clarke A, Sexton R, et al. Stoma-related complications are more frequent after transverse colostomy than loop ileostomy: a prospective randomized clinical trial. Br J Surg 2001;88(3):360–3.

119. Harris DA, Egbeare D, Jones S, et al. Complications and mortality following stoma formation. Ann R Coll Surg Engl 2005;87(6):427–31.

120. Kaidar-Person O, Person B, Wexner SD. Complications of construction and closure of temporary loop ileostomy. J Am Coll Surg 2005;201(5):759–73.
121. Rondelli F, Reboldi P, Rulli A, et al. Loop ileostomy versus loop colostomy for fecal diversion after colorectal or coloanal anastomosis: a meta-analysis. Int J Colorectal Dis 2009;24(5):479–88.
122. Tilney HS, Sains PS, Lovegrove RE, et al. Comparison of outcomes following ileostomy versus colostomy for defunctioning colorectal anastomoses. World J Surg 2007;31(5):1142–51.
123. Guenaga KF, Lustosa SA, Saad SS, et al. Ileostomy or colostomy for temporary decompression of colorectal anastomosis. Cochrane Database Syst Rev 2007;(1):CD004647.
124. Lertsithichai P, Rattanapichart P. Temporary ileostomy versus temporary colostomy: a meta-analysis of complications. Asian J Surg 2004;27(3):202–10 [discussion: 211–2].
125. Rullier E, Le Toux N, Laurent C, et al. Loop ileostomy versus loop colostomy for defunctioning low anastomoses during rectal cancer surgery. World J Surg 2001;25(3):274–7 [discussion: 277–8].
126. Caricato M, Ausania F, Ripetti V, et al. Retrospective analysis of long-term defunctioning stoma complications after colorectal surgery. Colorectal Dis 2007;9(6):559–61.
127. Mileski WJ, Rege RV, Joehl RJ, et al. Rates of morbidity and mortality after closure of loop and end colostomy. Surg Gynecol Obstet 1990;171(1):17–21.
128. Mosdell DM, Doberneck RC. Morbidity and mortality of ostomy closure. Am J Surg 1991;162(6):633–6 [discussion: 636–7].
129. Segreti EM, Levenback C, Morris M, et al. A comparison of end and loop colostomy for fecal diversion in gynecologic patients with colonic fistulas. Gynecol Oncol 1996;60(1):49–53.
130. Mealy K, O'Broin E, Donohue J, et al. Reversible colostomy–what is the outcome? Dis Colon Rectum 1996;39(11):1227–31.
131. Porter JA, Salvati EP, Rubin RJ, et al. Complications of colostomies. Dis Colon Rectum 1989;32(4):299–303.
132. Nunoo R, Asgeirsson T. Stomal strictures. Semin Colon Rectal Surg 2012;23(1):10–2.
133. Takahashi K, Funayama Y, Fukushima K, et al. Stoma-related complications in inflammatory bowel disease. Dig Surg 2008;25(1):16–20.
134. Gadacz TR, McFadden DW, Gabrielson EW, et al. Adenocarcinoma of the ileostomy: the latent risk of cancer after colectomy for ulcerative colitis and familial polyposis. Surgery 1990;107(6):698–703.
135. Johnson WR, McDermott FT, Pihl E, et al. Adenocarcinoma of an ileostomy in a patient with ulcerative colitis. Dis Colon Rectum 1980;23(5):351–2.
136. Smart PJ, Sastry S, Wells S. Primary mucinous adenocarcinoma developing in an ileostomy stoma. Gut 1988;29(11):1607–12.
137. Vasilevsky CA, Gordon PH. Adenocarcinoma arising at the ileocutaneous junction occurring after proctocolectomy for ulcerative colitis. Br J Surg 1986;73(5):378.
138. Hebert JC. A simple method for preventing retraction of an end colostomy. Dis Colon Rectum 1988;31(4):328–9.

Surgical Management of Crohn's Disease

Kim C. Lu, MD[a],*, Steven R. Hunt, MD[b]

KEYWORDS

- Crohn's disease • Anal abscess/fistula • Enteric fistula • Enteric stricture • Short gut
- Extraintestinal manifestations

KEY POINTS

- Crohn's disease can be classified by various methods, although the Vienna classification is most commonly used, and is based on 3 categories/phenotypes: penetrating (fistulizing), stricturing, and nonpenetrating, nonstricturing disease.
- Despite the relatively common incidence of Crohn's disease, its pathogenesis remains incompletely understood.
- Patients with Crohn's disease often require multiple intestinal surgeries. As such, it is important to recognize that future function must be considered when deciding on the extent and aggressiveness of the surgical intervention.
- Although medical management can control symptoms in a recurring, incurable disease, such as Crohn's disease, surgical management is reserved for disease complications or those problems refractory to medical management.

INTRODUCTION

Crohn's disease was originally described in 1932 by Drs Crohn, Ginzburg, and Oppenheimer, and has since carried the eponym based on the alphabetical order of the authors.[1] Although patients can develop inflammation in the gastrointestinal tract anywhere between the mouth and anus, 50% of patients have ileocolic disease, 30% have ileal disease only, and 20% have colonic disease only.[2] Felt to be a marker of more aggressive disease, 26.5% of patients also have perianal disease.[3] Overall, Crohn's disease can be classified by various methods, although the Vienna classification, published in 2000, is most commonly used. This created 3

Financial Disclosure: The author have no relevant financial disclosures.
[a] Division of Gastrointestinal and General Surgery, Department of Surgery, Oregon Health & Science University, 3181 Southwest Sam Jackson Park Road, Mailcode L223A, Portland, OR 97239, USA; [b] Section of Colon and Rectal Surgery, Department of Surgery, Washington University School of Medicine, Campus Box 8109, 660 South Euclid Avenue, Suite 14102 Queeny Tower, St Louis, MO 63110, USA
* Corresponding author.
E-mail address: luk@ohsu.edu

categories/phenotypes: penetrating (fistulizing), stricturing, and nonpenetrating, non-stricturing disease.[4] Despite its relatively common incidence, its pathogenesis remains incompletely understood. Increasingly, the genetic component is being explored, with the NOD2/CARD 15 gene among numerous mutations having been associated with Crohn's disease.[5,6] It is currently felt that this gene may play a role in the innate immunity recognition of peptidoglycans.[7] Because the pathogenesis of Crohn's disease has a presumed autoimmune component like ulcerative colitis, medical management is aimed at suppressing the immune system and includes mesalamine derivatives, azathioprine, 6-mercaptopurine, methotrexate, budesonide, corticosteroids, and antibodies targeting tumor necrosis factor alpha.[8,9] Yet, as Crohn's disease tends to recur and cannot be cured, surgery is reserved for patients with symptomatic disease refractory to medical management or in those with complications, including retardation of growth in children, hemorrhage, perforation, abscess, fistula, stricture, or malignancy.[10–13] In this article, we cover the various aspects involved in the surgical management of each of these processes, as well as the unique considerations by anatomic site.

ANORECTAL CROHN'S DISEASE

Granulomatous perianal disease without tuberculosis was first described in 1921.[14] This was later recognized as a presentation of Crohn's disease by Dr Bissel in 1934.[15] Crohn described similar findings in 1938.[16] Crohn's perianal disease includes large perianal skin tags, recurrent perirectal abscesses, complicated fistula-in-ano, and strictures.[13,17–19] A careful anorectal examination (under anesthesia if necessary), including anoscopy and flexible sigmoidoscopy, is critical for diagnosis.[13]

Large Perianal Tags

It is important to distinguish between the 2 major types of perianal tags that patients with Crohn's disease can develop. One type typically appears large, hard, and blue, and they become painful during flares. In general, these should not be excised, because of the risk of poor wound healing or possible anal stenosis, which may ultimately require proctectomy. The second type consists of large, flat, painless "elephant ear" anal skin tags that may be safely excised without as much of a risk of nonhealing complications.[17–19]

Anal Fissure

Patients with Crohn's disease with typical anterior or posterior midline anal fissure can be treated with standard medical treatments, including glyceryl trinitrate, calcium channel blockers, and botulinum toxin. Although it is prudent to err on side of caution, without proctitis, these patients can undergo lateral internal anal sphincterotomy with good results.[20] However, in the presence of proctitis, sphincterotomy should be avoided.[17]

Abscess/Fistula-in-Ano/Rectovaginal Fistula

Patients with acute anorectal abscesses should undergo a careful anorectal examination under anesthesia and have their abscesses drained in a timely fashion. The incision should be as close to the anal verge as possible to minimize the risk of a long fistula tract, should one ensue.[13] Simple fistulas involving minimal muscle may be treated with fistulotomy with marsupialization of wound edges in patients with otherwise normal continence. Repeat fistulotomy should be avoided, because of the risk of fecal incontinence.[21] Unfortunately, in Crohn's disease, fistula-in-ano may have an internal opening above the dentate line, multiple internal openings, and/or may involve a large amount (>50%) of the external anal sphincter. Pelvic magnetic resonance imaging or endorectal ultrasound with hydrogen peroxide injected into the fistula tract can elucidate the anatomy of more complex fistulae.[13] Setons should be placed to control every internal opening. Flexible sigmoidoscopy should be done to rule out proctitis.[21,22] Although endorectal mucosal advancement flap remains the gold standard, severe proctitis is associated with worse results.[23] There is weaker evidence for the anal fistula plug or the ligation of the intersphincteric fistula tract.[21,24] In the presence of proctitis, one should just leave setons and continue with aggressive medical therapy aimed at controlling the rectal disease. Severe perianal disease refractory to setons may require temporary or permanent fecal diversion (ileostomy vs colostomy).[21]

Rectovaginal fistula requires special mention. Patients with Crohn's disease with rectovaginal fistula can be successfully treated with an endorectal advancement flap, but with a lower success rate than patients without Crohn's, especially in the presence of proctitis.[23,25]

Anorectal Stricture

Because of the chronic inflammatory nature of Crohn's disease, anorectal strictures can be extremely symptomatic. Similar to other Crohn's anorectal disease, one of the important initial variables involved in decision making is to determine whether or not there is active proctitis present. Second, the exact location of the stricture will help dictate therapy. An anal stricture without anorectal inflammation can be dilated gently under anesthesia.[18] A rectal stricture without proctitis can be treated with a low anterior resection and coloanal anastomosis, although initial attempt at dilation is often warranted.[18,26] Anorectal Crohn's strictures associated with severe proctitis refractory to medical management will ultimately often require proctectomy and end colostomy.[18,27]

INTESTINAL FISTULA

Patients with Crohn's disease often require multiple intestinal surgeries. As such, it is important to recognize that function must be considered when deciding on the extent and aggressiveness of the surgical intervention. Adult population cohort studies found that 40% to 55% of patients require surgery within 10 years of diagnosis. Furthermore, 16%, 28%, and 35% of patients require a second surgery at 5, 10, and 15 years after the first surgery, respectively.[28,29] In a pediatric population cohort, 17% and 29% of patients require a second surgery at 5 and 10 years, respectively.[30]

Guiding Principles

In approaching intestinal fistulizing Crohn's disease, one can be guided by a few sound principles.

1. Nutrition should be optimized preoperatively, if possible.[31,32]
2. For preoperative workup, esophagogastroduodenoscopy and colonoscopy are helpful. CT enterography can identify both luminal and extraluminal intestinal disease.[33–35]
3. Laparoscopy is a reasonable approach for operating on complicated Crohn's disease.[36,37]
4. Only diseased bowel should be resected. See **Figs. 1** and **2**. The nondiseased target of the fistula can be repaired safely.[38,39] There is an important caveat: fistula targeting the mesenteric side of nondiseased bowel may compromise the blood supply of the nondiseased bowel and mandate resection.[40]

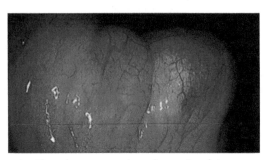

Fig. 1. Diseased bowel with corkscrew vessels and creeping fat.

5. Resection margins should be small (2 cm) and within grossly normal bowel.[41]
6. Although stapled side-to-side anastomoses might have a lower early complication rate,[42,43] it does not decrease the rate of recurrent Crohn's disease.[44]
7. Steroid use (>10 mg of prednisone a day for 4 weeks before surgery) and preoperative abscess significantly increase the risk of anastomotic leak.[45] Although use of anti–tumor necrosis factor biologics before surgery does not appear to increase the risk of a leak, this is still controversial, with data supporting each side.[46–49]

Enteroenteric or Enterocolic Fistula

Asymptomatic enteroenteric fistula should be left alone.[11] Large acute abscesses should be drained, percutaneously, if possible. For those fistula associated with diarrhea, the diseased bowel should be resected.[12]

Enterocutaneous Fistula

Acute sepsis should be treated with aggressive fluid resuscitation, intravenous antibiotics, and drainage of large intra-abdominal abscesses. The skin opening should be pouched. Nutrition should be optimized.[32] Either a fistulogram or CT enterography could be helpful to delineate fistula anatomy.[33] Finally, the diseased bowel and fistula tract should be resected.[50] For further information on the management of enterocutaneous fistulas, see the article by Drs Johnson and Davis elsewhere in this issue.

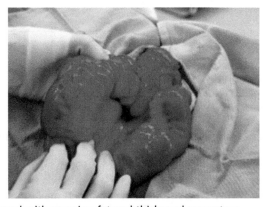

Fig. 2. Diseased bowel with creeping fat and thickened mesentery.

Duodenal Fistula

Duodenal fistula is rare. Typically, the duodenum is the target of a fistula arising from diseased ileum or colon. The diseased bowel is resected, and the duodenum can be repaired.[51]

Ureteral Fistula

The most common urologic complication from Crohn's disease is an ileovesical fistula. Preoperative temporary ureteral stents can be helpful during a difficult dissection. The fistula can be treated with an ileal resection and repair of the bladder, if necessary.[52]

An enteroureteral fistula is much less common. A preoperatively placed double J ureteral stent is helpful when dissecting out the associated ureter. The ureter can be repaired or reimplanted by a urologist.[52]

Musculoskeletal/Psoas Complications

CT scan can diagnose an abscess within the psoas. Acute sepsis should be treated with percutaneous drainage if possible. Depending on the result, oftentimes intravenous antibiotics can aid in clearing the rest of the infectious process. Diseased bowel should be resected. An omental flap can be mobilized to cover the psoas. An orthopedic surgeon can be helpful in avoid injuring nerves within the psoas.[53]

INFLAMMATORY AND FIBROTIC STRICTURES

Surgery for small bowel strictures in patients with Crohn's disease should be reserved only for complications. Timing of operative intervention should be such that the patient is not compromised from the standpoint of their systemic health and nutritional status.

Preoperative Planning

History and physical

The preoperative preparation of the patient with stricturing disease begins with a detailed history. The patient's symptoms are important in establishing the operative indications. The nature of any pain and its relationship to oral intake can help to delineate between active inflammatory disease and obstruction. Weight loss and solid food intolerance are important clues to the severity of obstructive disease. Significant weight loss is a sign of malnutrition.

Medication history, relative to Crohn's treatment, must be detailed. Although a surgeon should not be expected to medically manage a patient with complicated Crohn's disease, one must be able to recognize if a patient has had an appropriate trial of medical management. It is important to note the experience of the medical specialist who has been overseeing the patient's medical management. In elective cases, if there were any doubt that a patient has had less than adequate medical treatment, a referral should be made to a gastroenterologist with an expertise in inflammatory bowel disease. Often, appropriate treatment will obviate the need for operation.

If a patient has been on steroids in recent months, the dose and duration of the treatment is important. Consideration for perioperative stress dosing should be given to patients on relatively high doses for extended periods of time. Other immunomodulators or biologics should be noted.

The history of prior surgeries must be obtained from the patient, but the details of the procedure should be verified in the operative notes. Disease location, the type and location of any anastomoses or strictureplasties, length of resected bowel, and length of remaining bowel should be recorded. Often, the records for surgeries performed remotely are not available. In these cases, the surgeon must rely on patient history, preoperative imaging, and endoscopic findings for clues as to the nature of prior operations.

Routine preoperative laboratory evaluation should be performed. Pay special attention to the hemoglobin and albumin, because these values may be predictive of complications.

Imaging

Imaging plays an important role in the surgical evaluation of the patient with small bowel structuring disease. As patients with Crohn's disease may have disease flares and complications over the course of many decades, the exposure to ionizing radiation must be taken into consideration when considering an imaging examination. The risk of malignancy with repeated exposure is real and cumulative over a patient's lifetime.[54]

- In acute flares, a CT scan can help to make the initial diagnosis, define the extent and location of the disease, and rule out the possibility of perforation and abscess. CT enterography is valuable in preoperative planning, as it can provide precise anatomic delineation of disease.
- Magnetic resonance enterography (MRE), is often more difficult for the surgeon to interpret, but can provide valuable information to guide therapy. MRE gives an accurate anatomic location of diseased bowel and can help distinguish between active inflammatory disease and more chronic fibrotic disease. This differentiation assists in the decision making regarding escalation of medical therapy, or the decision to proceed with surgery. Additionally, MRE does not expose the patient to ionizing radiation and its potential risks.
- The small bowel follow through (SBFT) provides a clear picture of the extent and severity of stricturing disease. Although this study cannot differentiate between fibrosis and inflammation, it can be complementary to other imaging modalities in the preoperative evaluation. In patients who have had large or multiple prior resections, SBFT allows the surgeon to estimate the amount of remaining normal small bowel. Although this modality exposes the patient to less radiation than CT, the dose is not negligible.
- A distal obstruction can doom an anastomosis to failure. Before a strictureplasty or resection, any suspected colonic disease must be assessed by either a contrast enema or a colonoscopy.
- Although capsule endoscopy is an increasingly used diagnostic examination, it should have no role in the preoperative evaluation of patients with Crohn's disease, owing to the near certainty that the capsule will obstruct at the point of symptomatic disease. The use of this modality should be limited to the early detection of disease or recurrence.
- Enteroclysis has a limited utility in today's evaluation of patients with Crohn's disease, and it has largely been supplanted by CT enterography and MRE.
- Ultrasound, although a cost-effective screening and diagnostic examination, offers little information that is useful in operative planning.

Surgical Planning

In the later stages of obstructing Crohn's disease, the disease tends to respond less readily to medical therapy, and obstructive episodes tend to become more frequent and less responsive to conservative management. It is under these circumstances that elective surgery should be considered. Although there are no hard and fast rules for the timing of surgical intervention, operative indications for stricturing disease include persistent or recurrent obstruction in the face of adequate medical management, significant weight loss, inability to tolerate a solid diet, inability to tolerate medications, and inability to wean from steroids.

Patients with severe malnutrition should be considered for preoperative total parenteral nutrition (TPN). There is evidence that patients with moderate to severe Crohn's disease can improve their nutritional status and have significantly fewer postoperative complications and mortality if treated for several weeks with hyperalimentation.[55,56]

Once the decision to proceed with surgery has been reached, a frank discussion should take place regarding the risks and benefits of the procedure. Patients must understand that, although surgery will provide symptomatic relief, it is not always a curative endeavor. Reoperation rates for Crohn's disease approach 50% over the long term.[57]

Additionally, smoking confers a 2.5-fold increased risk of postoperative recurrence requiring surgery, and patients should be counseled extensively, both in the preoperative and postoperative setting, on smoking cessation techniques.[58]

The operative plan may be quite clear before surgery, as is the case with index surgeries (resection) for isolated ileocolic disease. Alternatively, the nature and the extent of the surgery may not be clear until the time of operation, as is often the case with recurrent disease or diffuse jejunoileal Crohn's disease. In addition to the standard discussion of surgical risks, the risks unique to these patients must be addressed. The possibility of short bowel syndrome (SBS) must be mentioned to these patients, not only as a risk of the impending surgery, but as a long-term risk should other procedures become necessary. Every patient with Crohn's disease who is undergoing surgery should understand that there is some lifelong risk of intestinal failure and that bowel conservation is the goal.

Operative Management

Surgical decision making in Crohn's disease should be influenced by the overarching concerns that are prevalent in this population: malnutrition, immunosuppression, and intestinal conservation. Bowel sparing should be the guiding principle to all elective surgery for Crohn's disease.

Preparation

- A mechanical bowel prep should be avoided in patients undergoing surgery for stricturing disease. Aside from the lack of evidence to support this undertaking for small bowel or ileocolic resection, it can be extremely uncomfortable for the patient. Moreover, in the case of more severe obstruction, it can lead to massive dilation of the bowel proximal to the diseased segments and enteric spillage during the procedure.
- If there is any chance an ostomy will be created during the surgery, the patient should be marked preoperatively (by an enterostomal therapist, if available). Improper site selection can lead to postoperative leakage, skin irritation and breakdown, inability to pouch the ostomy, stress, and costs. Pouching problems can have an enormous influence on quality of life and can be debilitating, yet most of such problems can be avoided by proper site selection.
- Antibiotic prophylaxis should be given before the incision and consist of a broad-spectrum antibiotic with anaerobic coverage. For cases that have the potential to last for several hours, consideration should be given to antibiotics with longer half-lives, as redosing during long procedures is often overlooked.
- Patients with inflammatory bowel disease (IBD) have a more than threefold risk of venous thromboembolic (VTE) events in the postoperative period.[59] Additionally, VTE is associated with a twofold increased risk of mortality. For this reason,

patients with Crohn's disease should have both mechanical and pharmacologic prophylaxis during the perioperative period. Mechanical prophylaxis has been shown to reduce the incidence of VTE's and includes graded compression stockings, sequential pneumatic compression devices, and early postoperative ambulation.[60] Patients should be given heparin immediately before, and for at least 1 week after surgery. No study has been able to demonstrate a difference in the VTE or bleeding risk between unfractionated and low-molecular-weight heparin.[61]

- Although supine positioning is adequate for extracolonic disease, lithotomy should be used if there is any chance that the colon could be involved as a bystander. Additionally, if the laparoscopic approach were considered, lithotomy positioning affords another place for the operator or assistant to stand.

Surgical Approach

The decision to proceed with an operation in the open or laparoscopic fashion is influenced by many factors. First and foremost is the surgeon's comfort and experience with a particular approach. Although it is more time consuming than open surgery, it is generally accepted that laparoscopy for ileocolic Crohn's disease allows for earlier return of bowel function, shorter length of stay, and decreased postoperative pain.[62–64] Other perceived benefits, such as decreased physiologic stress, decreased inflammatory response, fewer adhesions, and safer reoperative surgery, are not proven. Although these considerations are important in patients who are at risk for frequent reoperations, they should not be the only factors guiding the choice of approach. Risk factors for conversion from laparoscopic to open procedures include prior resection or strictureplasty, fistulizing disease, multifocal disease, large inflammatory masses, and acute disease.[65] Conversion is not a complication or failure, and dogged pursuit of laparoscopy under difficult circumstances may lead to serious complications forcing a reactive, rather than proactive, conversion. If multiple strictureplasties or resections were planned, laparoscopy should not be considered.

Technical Considerations

Resection

Resection is the treatment of choice in patients with isolated, initial ileocolic disease. The length of the resected segment should include only the grossly diseased bowel. There is no increased risk of recurrence with a 2-cm grossly normal margin, regardless of presence of histologic disease at the site of resection.[41]

A distal diseased segment may put a proximal anastomosis or strictureplasty at risk for dehiscence. In every operation for Crohn's disease, the entire bowel should be inspected if it is safe to do so. Nonetheless, rigorous adhesiolysis or mobilization should not be undertaken if there is no reason to suspect disease in a nonvisualized segment. In the interest of bowel conservation, asymptomatic disease should be left in situ.

One method of determining the need for intervention is to introduce a Foley catheter into the bowel at a point where a resection or strictureplasty is to be performed. The catheter can be introduced into the diseased segment in question, the balloon partially inflated, and the catheter withdrawn. Inability to pass the balloon through a diseased segment is an indication that surgical correction is needed.

The choice of anastomotic techniques is often a point of contention. The literature is clear that the risk of anastomotic leak after ileocolic resection is significantly lower with a stapled side-to-side, functional end-to-end anastomosis, when compared with a handsewn anastomosis.[43,66] Additionally, although early studies suggested the risk of anastomotic recurrence requiring resection was also lower with the stapled anastomosis,[67] this was disproven in a randomized trial.[44]

Patients with Crohn's disease are at increased risk for anastomotic complications after resection. Although this risk is not prohibitive, surgeons should consider forgoing an anastomosis in patients who have multiple risk factors. Patient factors that have been associated with anastomotic leaks include long-term steroids, impaired nutritional status, hypoalbuminemia (albumin <3.0 mg/dL), anemia (hemoglobin <10 g/mL), emergent surgery, and the presence of an abscess or fistula.[12] There is no clear evidence that immunomodulators (azathioprine, mercaptopurine, and methotrexate) or biologic agents (tumor necrosis factor antagonists) have any increased risk for anastomotic complications.

Bypass

Historically, intestinal bypass was an accepted procedure for obstructing or phlegmonous small bowel disease. In fact, on June 9, 1956, President Eisenhower underwent a bypass of 30 to 40 cm of distal terminal ileal disease affected by Crohn's disease. Unfortunately, early articles showed an increased rate of recurrent disease, with the risk of recurrence for terminal ileal Crohn's disease twice that of resection.[68] Today, bypass should be reserved for cases in which small bowel resection is not feasible. Generally, such situations occur in the acute setting with significant inflammation that would threaten an unacceptable length of small bowel, the superior mesenteric artery or vein, or surrounding organs. When bypass has been performed, the risk of recurrence, carcinoma, and blind loop syndrome necessitates a subsequent resection after an interval in which the inflammation has had sufficient time to subside.[12]

For gastroduodenal Crohn's disease, bypass is often the optimal treatment. In patients with obstructing duodenal disease, resection has a fourfold increased risk of major morbidity when compared with gastrojejunal bypass.[69] Some investigators advocate for strictureplasty in the case of duodenal disease. To accomplish this, the duodenum must be mobilized, which can be challenging in the setting of inflammatory changes. Gastroduodenal strictureplasty frequently fails, has a high rate of reoperation, and confers little advantage over gastrojejunal bypass.[70] Strictureplasty is best used for selected, proximal duodenal lesions near the pylorus.

Traditionally, a truncal vagotomy was considered mandatory when performing a gastrojejunal bypass to avoid the complication of marginal ulceration. This resulted in a high rate of diarrhea in patients already predisposed to this affliction. Because of the introduction of effective acid suppression medications, several groups have shown that the rate of marginal ulceration is negligible, with most investigators recommending lifelong proton pump inhibitors and foregoing vagotomy.[70–72]

Small Bowel Strictureplasty

More than 30 years ago, the technique of strictureplasty was described for the treatment of small bowel strictures from tuberculosis.[73] Shortly thereafter, Lee and Papaioannou published the first series using this technique for patients with Crohn's disease.[74] Since that time, strictureplasty has played a crucial role in the surgical treatment of patients with recurrent and/or diffuse disease.

Although most patients with Crohn's disease have terminal ileal disease, some patients have a more malignant phenotype with diffuse jejunoileal involvement. It is this group of patients who are least responsive to medical therapy and are most at risk for SBS. This patient population stands to benefit the most from the strictureplasty.

Originally, indications for strictureplasty included diffuse jejunoileal disease with single or multiple short fibrotic strictures, multiple or extensive prior resections, early recurrence (<1 year) after resection, and isolated ileocolic anastomotic stricture.[75]

More recently, other investigators have advocated for the use of strictureplasty techniques in the setting of active, mild inflammation, demonstrating that the technique is safe in this situation.[76]

Contraindications to strictureplasty are sepsis, perforation, fistulizing disease, malnutrition (albumin <2 g/dL), a stricture near a segment of bowel to be resected, and multiple strictures over a short segment of bowel.

Various strictureplasty techniques exist, with the choice depending on the length of the stricture. Although there are multiple variations, there are essentially 3 techniques for small bowel strictureplasty. For short (<10 cm) strictures, the Heineke-Mikulicz strictureplasty should be used. In this technique, the bowel is incised longitudinally on the antimesenteric border through the stricture and extending 2 cm onto normal bowel on each end of the stricture. The enterotomy is then sutured transversely.

Longer strictures (10–25 cm) can be treated using the Finney technique. The strictured bowel is folded in a U-configuration and opened across the stricture on the antimesenteric border, extending 1 to 2 cm onto normal bowel at each end of the stricture. The enterotomy is then sutured, opposing the posterior and anterior bowel walls together, much as one would fashion a side-to-side functional end-to-end anastomosis. Alternatively, a stapler can be used to achieve this, but one should be careful to take note of the bowel wall thickness before attempting a stapled Finney strictureplasty. There are no data comparing the stapled and handsewn strictureplasty; most of the reports on the safety and efficacy of this procedure, however, involve the handsewn technique.

Attempting to perform a Finney strictureplasty on a stricture longer than 20 to 25 cm would put the patient at risk for blind-loop syndrome. The apex of such a long strictureplasty forms a large diverticulum and creates stasis of enteric contents with resultant bacterial overgrowth. For this reason, in early reports, resection was the only option for longer strictures. In the mid-1990s, Michelassi[77] published the technique of side-to-side isoperistaltic strictureplasty, which can be used for strictures up to 90 cm in length. Additionally, this procedure can be used for multiple short strictures that are closely clustered over a segment of bowel.

In this technique, the bowel and mesentery are divided at the midpoint of the stricture, the 2 limbs of bowel are then placed side by side, antimesenteric enterotomies are created on each limb, and the 2 limbs are then sutured together to create a larger common channel.

In an analysis of isoperistaltic side-to-side strictureplasties, Michalassi and colleagues[78] evaluated the outcomes of 184 patients undergoing this technique at 6 international centers. Most of the patients in this series had other resections or strictureplasties performed simultaneously. The cumulative 5-year reoperation-free survival was 77% for this group and only 8% of patients had a surgical recurrence at the site of the previous isoperistaltic strictureplasty. The overall complication rate was 10%, with intraluminal bleeding (2%) and anastomotic dehiscence (1%) among the technical complications. This experience supports the use of this technique in skilled hands.

In one of the largest series reported, Dietz and colleagues[75] described more than 1000 strictureplasties performed in 314 patients. Twenty-two patients in this series had 10 or more strictureplasties performed during the same procedure, demonstrating the safety of multiple serial strictureplasties. Most (88%) of the strictures in this series were short and treated with a Heineke-Mikulicz technique, with the balance predominately Finney strictureplasties. Two-thirds of the patients also had a synchronous bowel resection performed.

In this series, 5% of the patients suffered septic complications related to the strictureplasty. Intraluminal bleeding was a common complication (occurring in 7% of patients), but it was almost always self-limited and responded to transfusion. There were no deaths. Older age and recent weight loss were significantly associated with morbidity. The surgical recurrence rate was 34%, with younger patients requiring surgery for recurrence at an earlier time point.

A more recent meta-analysis reports on 3259 strictureplasties in multiple series comprising 1112 patients.[57] The morbidity in this series was similar to that described by Dietz and colleagues,[75] with a 4% rate of anastomotic septic complications (leak, abscess, or fistula). Risk factors for complications in this meta-analysis are similar to the risks for anastomotic complications after resection in Crohn's disease and include hypoalbuminemia, anemia, preoperative weight loss, older age, emergent surgery, and intra-abdominal abscess. Steroids, synchronous resections, and the number or length of the strictureplasties were not associated with complications.

Although it is a much-feared consequence of strictureplasty, only 2 patients (0.2%) developed adenocarcinoma at the site of the strictureplasty in this report. Although this rate is low, one must be mindful of this risk and perform frozen-section biopsy of any suspicious ulcers or masses before performing strictureplasty.

One-half of patients who undergo an index ileocolic resection will have a preanastomotic recurrence requiring surgery. Strictureplasty for ileocolonic anastomotic recurrence is safe, but 48% of these patients have recurrent disease at the site of strictureplasty requiring another operation.[79] There is no difference in the rate of surgical recurrence between anastomotic strictureplasty or anastomotic resection with long-term follow-up.[80] The decision to perform strictureplasty or resection for ileocolic anastomotic recurrence should be based on the patient factors and the need for bowel conservation. Strictureplasty should be considered in patients who are young, have had an early recurrence, or who have a recurrence in the setting of other small bowel disease.

Endoscopic Dilation

Although resection and strictureplasty are relatively safe, they are not curative and still have considerable morbidity and costs. The practice of endoscopic dilation has proven to be a safe alternative to surgery for short (<4 cm) strictures, especially at site of a prior ileocolic anastomosis. In a review of 347 patients, Hassan and colleagues[81] showed that this procedure could provide a durable cure, and avoid surgery in two-thirds of patients. The perforation rate of 2%, although low, obliges that surgical support be available when endoscopic dilation is attempted.

Complications and Management

Although complications cannot be eliminated in this difficult patient population, they can be minimized by properly preparing these patients for surgery and using sound intraoperative judgment. Preoperative optimization with parenteral nutrition should be considered for the severely malnourished patients. Preoperative broad-spectrum antibiotics and perioperative prevention of thromboembolism must be routine. Anastomosis and strictureplasty should be avoided, when possible, in patients at risk for dehiscence. The general tenets regarding the avoidance of tension, good blood supply, and a technically sound anastomosis apply in the creation of a strictureplasty or an anastomosis after resection.

Bleeding

Although postoperative bleeding can complicate any intra-abdominal procedure, it is particularly common following strictureplasty procedures. In these instances, the bleeding is frequently intraluminal and occurs within the first week after surgery.[82] This complication can generally be managed with blood transfusions. In severe refractory bleeding, it may be necessary to perform angiography with catheter-directed vasopressin infusion. In the rare case that a patient requires operative intervention for bleeding after multiple strictureplasties or resections, preoperative localization should be performed and the catheter left in place to allow identification of the bleeding.

Anastomotic Complications

The management of anastomotic dehiscence is guided by the timing and the clinical manifestations of the complication. The abdominal examination in the early postoperative patient is often unreliable. The surgeon should have a high suspicion for leak in patients with fever, tachycardia, decreased urine output, rising white blood cell counts, or frank sepsis.

When a leak is suspected, a contrast-enhanced CT scan is the most useful diagnostic tool. Contained leaks and abscesses can frequently be treated with percutaneous drainage. Free intraperitoneal leaks in the early postoperative period should be treated with operative intervention. At exploration, the circumstances should dictate the treatment. In cases in which there is minimal inflammation and tissues are pliable, simple repair and drainage may suffice. In other situations in which there is profound edema or sepsis, resection and an end-ostomy should be performed.

Short bowel syndrome

A patient with SBS has less than 200 cm of small intestine with signs and symptoms of malabsorption, malnutrition, diarrhea, steatorrhea, and fluid/electrolyte disturbances.[83] The extreme manifestation is lifelong dependence on TPN.

Risk factors for the development of SBS in patients with Crohn's disease include a long duration of disease, diffuse jejunoileal disease, multiple resections, ostomy creation, loss of the ileocecal valve, and colectomy.[84]

Bowel conservation through the use of strictureplasty and limited resection of grossly involved symptomatic disease has decreased the incidence of SBS in patients with Crohn's disease. Nonetheless, Crohn's disease is the most common underlying condition leading to intestinal failure and accounts for 20% of patients with SBS.[85]

Small bowel length is a surrogate predictor for nutritional deficiency. Any patient who has had a significant amount of bowel resected should have the length of the remaining bowel measured and recorded at the time of surgery to allow for future surgical planning and the prediction of intestinal failure. Although dependence on TPN can be predicted in those with less than 100 cm of remaining bowel (60 cm in the presence of a completely functional colon and ileocecal valve), the degree of adaptation can be highly variable.[86]

SBS results from decreased absorptive area or decreased bowel transit time and can be a functional, as well as an anatomic problem. The management of this complex problem must be multidisciplinary, involving dieticians, pharmacists, surgeons, and gastroenterologists. The treatment of this problem can be divided into 2 phases: the immediate postoperative period (3–4 weeks), and the recovery and adaptation period.

The immediate postoperative period should be focused on the identification and supportive treatment of patients with SBS. Volume and electrolyte homeostasis should be achieved early and monitored closely during this time. Patients who have been identified by the surgeon to be at risk for SBS should have TPN initiated soon after surgery. Oral intake should be advanced as early as possible, but TPN should be continued as a supplement to enteral feedings.

Medical therapy should be aimed at decreasing fluid losses and increasing transit time. Proton pump inhibitors should be used routinely to suppress gastric secretion. Antidiarrheal medications (loperamide, diphenoxylate/atropine [Lomotil], and tincture of opium) help to decrease diarrhea, mitigate fluid losses, and increase time for absorption. The somatostatin analog octreotide is available in a long-lasting depo formulation and has been shown to decrease intestinal transit time and symptomatically reduce diarrhea.[87]

During the recovery and adaptation phase, the bowel continues to adapt and absorptive capacity increases through an increase in bowel diameter and villous height. Enteral nutrition is essential to promote adaptation. Diarrhea should be controlled medically during this period, as patients with severe diarrhea may learn to avoid oral intake.

Over time, an attempt should be made to wean patients with adequate intestinal length from TPN by reducing the caloric content of the parenteral nutrition and increasing their oral intake. During this period, the patient's weight, electrolytes, and volume status must be carefully monitored.

If a patient transitions to an oral diet, he or she still requires lifelong monitoring to ensure that symptoms are controlled and that vitamin deficiencies do not develop. Vitamin supplementation of the fat-soluble vitamins (A, D, E, and K) should be considered in those with steatorrhea, and serum levels should be monitored. If the terminal ileum has been resected, vitamin B-12 supplementation is essential.

Although reconstructive and transplant procedures exist for those with intestinal failure and lifelong TPN dependence, these techniques have shown variable clinical success and should be performed only at specialized centers of expertise.

EXTRAINTESTINAL MANIFESTATIONS OF CROHN'S DISEASE

Nearly one-quarter of patients with Crohn's disease have some extraintestinal manifestations (EIM) of their disease, and in some cases, the EIM causes more problems than the intestinal symptoms.[88] Musculoskeletal, ocular, and mucocutaneous problems are the most common EIMs in Crohn's disease.

Musculoskeletal

The most common site of EIMs in Crohn's disease is the musculoskeletal system.[89] Musculoskeletal involvement can be divided into peripheral joint and axial inflammatory conditions. Axial manifestations include psoriatic arthritis, and ankylosing spondylitis. Although the peripheral arthropathies tend to track intestinal disease and respond to medical or surgical treatment of the primary Crohn's, the axial inflammation flares independently from the bowel disease.[90]

Although nonsteroidal anti-inflammatory drugs are a mainstay in the treatment of musculoskeletal inflammation, these drugs may precipitate IBD flares and should be used with caution.[91]

In addition to the inflammatory conditions that can parallel IBD, longstanding disease and nutritional deficiencies can also lead to severe osteoporosis, which is more pronounced in Crohn's disease than ulcerative colitis.[92] These patients have a higher fracture risk that is independent of bone density.

Osteoporosis in the setting of IBD should be managed in the same manner as it is in the general population, with exercise, correction of hormone deficiencies, smoking cessation, supplementation of calcium and vitamin D, and bisphosphonates.[92] A specialist in bone diseases should manage this aspect of the patient's care.

Ocular Manifestations

Ocular disease can manifest with symptoms such as erythema, itching, burning, pain, visual disturbances, and photophobia. Ocular disease is generally independent of the intestinal flares. The most common ocular EIM is episcleritis, which presents with hyperemia and normal vision.[93]

Painful visual disturbances that occur in patients with IBD must be considered urgent and promptly referred to an ophthalmologist, as this may signify the onset of uveitis (inflammation of the iris, ciliary body, or choroid layer of the globe). Other symptoms of uveitis include photophobia, erythema, and floaters. Uveitis can be a serious condition that can result in blindness; hence, early recognition and treatment are crucial.

Mucocutaneous Manifestations

The 3 dermatologic manifestations of Crohn's disease are erythema nodosum (EN), pyoderma gangrenosum (PG), and aphthous ulcerations.[91]

The most common cutaneous lesion is EN, which is more common in women with IBD. It presents with small (1–5 cm) raised, red, warm, tender nodules distributed symmetrically on the legs, especially over the tibia. It is usually associated with intestinal flares, and is self-limited, with resolution within 1 to 2 months.

PG is a more virulent cutaneous process and causes painful ulcers that have a violaceous border and a necrotic, purulent center. It generally occurs over the lower extremities, but also can cause significant problems to the peristomal skin. Mild disease can be treated with local wound care and cleansing, whereas more severe disease may require systemic steroid or biologic agents. When PG occurs in the peristomal skin, stoma reversal should be considered if feasible, as this is generally curative of the local disease.

Aphthous ulcers generally reflect intestinal inflammation and should be treated symptomatically and with appropriate therapy directed at the underlying bowel disease.

Other EIMs

More recently, other, less classic, extraintestinal manifestations have been associated with Crohn's disease. Among these are an increase in the frequency of common pulmonary, biliary, and urinary collecting system diseases.

Pulmonary problems are prevalent in the IBD population, with bronchitis and bronchiectasis occurring in a significant number of these patients.[91] The pulmonary diseases can sometimes present in the postoperative period. More commonly, they occur subclinically with increased coughing and sputum production.

Lithiasis, both in the gallbladder and the urinary collecting system, is more common in patients with Crohn's disease than in the general population or in patients with ulcerative colitis. These stones should be treated similarly to those in the general population, with interventions reserved for symptomatic patients.

SUMMARY

In an incurable, recurring disease, medical management can often control symptoms. Yet surgical management is reserved for Crohn's disease refractory to medical management and complications resulting from the condition. In perianal disease, large painful blue skin tags should not be excised. Abscesses should be promptly drained. Anal fistula should be controlled with setons. Without proctitis, fistula can be treated definitively with endorectal advancement flaps. Anal stenosis associated with proctitis may require proctectomy.

Intestinal fistulae require resection of diseased bowel with grossly normal margins. Noninflamed strictures can be safely treated with strictureplasty, which can avoid SBS. Some extraintestinal manifestations (peripheral arthropathies, erythema nodosum, and aphthous ulcers) may respond to treatment of intestinal disease.

ACKNOWLEDGMENTS

The authors thank Mary Kwatkosky-Lawlor for her editorial assistance.

REFERENCES

1. Crohn BB, Ginzburg L, Oppenheimer GD. Regional ileitis; a pathologic and clinical entity. Am J Med 1952;13(5):583–90.
2. McClane SJ, Rombeau JL. Anorectal Crohn's disease. Surg Clin North Am 2001; 81(1):169–83, ix.
3. Eglinton TW, Roberts R, Pearson J, et al. Clinical and genetic risk factors for perianal Crohn's disease in a population-based cohort. Am J Gastroenterol 2012; 107(4):589–96.
4. Gasche C, Scholmerich J, Brynskov J, et al. A simple classification of Crohn's disease: report of the working party for the World Congresses of Gastroenterology, Vienna 1998. Inflamm Bowel Dis 2000;6(1):8–15.
5. Hugot JP, Chamaillard M, Zouali H, et al. Association of NOD2 leucine-rich repeat variants with susceptibility to Crohn's disease. Nature 2001;411(6837): 599–603.
6. Ogura Y, Bonen DK, Inohara N, et al. A frameshift mutation in NOD2 associated with susceptibility to Crohn's disease. Nature 2001;411(6837):603–6.
7. Hugot JP. CARD15/NOD2 mutations in Crohn's disease. Ann N Y Acad Sci 2006; 1072:9–18.
8. Sands BE. IBD: medical management. In: Beck DE, Roberts PL, Saclarides TJ, et al, editors. The ASCRS Textbook of Colon and Rectal Surgery. New York: Springer Sciences Business Media LLC; 2011. p. 463–70.
9. Cottone M, Renna S, Orlando A, et al. Medical management of Crohn's disease. Expert Opin Pharmacother 2011;12(16):2505–25.
10. Efron JE. Crohn's disease. 2011 Available at: http://www.fascrs.org/physicians/education/core_subjects/2011/Crohns/. Accessed June 8, 2012.
11. Strong SA. Crohn's disease: surgical management. In: Beck DE, Roberts PL, Saclarides TJ, et al, editors. The ASCRS Textbook of Colon and Rectal Surgery. New York: Springer Sciences Business Media LLC; 2011. p. 499–516.
12. Strong SA, Koltun WA, Hyman NH, et al. Practice parameters for the surgical management of Crohn's disease. Dis Colon Rectum 2007;50(11):1735–46.
13. Steele SR. Operative management of Crohn's disease of the colon including anorectal disease. Surg Clin North Am 2007;87(3):611–31.
14. Gabriel WB. Results of an experimental and histological investigation into seventy-five cases of rectal fistulae. Proc R Soc Med 1921;14(Surg Sect):156–61.
15. Bissell AD. Localized chronic ulcerative ileitis. Ann Surg 1934;99(6):957–66.
16. Penner A, Crohn BB. Perianal fistulae as a complication of regional ileitis. Ann Surg 1938;108(5):867–73.
17. Lewis RT, Maron DJ. Anorectal Crohn's disease. Surg Clin North Am 2010;90(1): 83–97.
18. Bouguen G, Siproudhis L, Bretagne JF, et al. Nonfistulizing perianal Crohn's disease: clinical features, epidemiology, and treatment. Inflamm Bowel Dis 2010;16(8):1431–42.

19. Sandborn WJ, Fazio VW, Feagan BG, et al. AGA technical review on perianal Crohn's disease. Gastroenterology 2003;125(5):1508–30.

20. Fleshner PR, Schoetz DJ Jr, Roberts PL, et al. Anal fissure in Crohn's disease: a plea for aggressive management. Dis Colon Rectum 1995;38(11): 1137–43.

21. Steele SR, Kumar R, Feingold DL, et al. Practice parameters for the management of perianal abscess and fistula-in-ano. Dis Colon Rectum 2011;54(12): 1465–74.

22. van Dongen LM, Lubbers EJ. Perianal fistulas in patients with Crohn's disease. Arch Surg 1986;121(10):1187–90.

23. Jarrar A, Church J. Advancement flap repair: a good option for complex anorectal fistulas. Dis Colon Rectum 2011;54(12):1537–41.

24. O'Riordan JM, Datta I, Johnston C, et al. A systematic review of the anal fistula plug for patients with Crohn's and non-Crohn's related fistula-in-ano. Dis Colon Rectum 2012;55(3):351–8.

25. Pinto RA, Peterson TV, Shawki S, et al. Are there predictors of outcome following rectovaginal fistula repair? Dis Colon Rectum 2010;53(9):1240–7.

26. Lawal TA, Frischer JS, Falcone RA, et al. The transanal approach with laparoscopy or laparotomy for the treatment of rectal strictures in Crohn's disease. J Laparoendosc Adv Surg Tech A 2010;20(9):791–5.

27. Michelassi F, Melis M, Rubin M, et al. Surgical treatment of anorectal complications in Crohn's disease. Surgery 2000;128(4):597–603.

28. Peyrin-Biroulet L, Loftus EV Jr, Harmsen WS, et al. Postoperative recurrence of Crohn's disease in a population-based cohort. Gastroenterology 2010;138(5 Suppl 1):S-198–9.

29. Dhillon SL, Loftus EV Jr, Colombel JF, et al. The national history of adult Crohn's disease in a population-based cohort from Olmstead County, Minnesota. Am J Gastroenterol 2010;105:289–97.

30. Boualit M, Salleron J, Turck D, et al. Long-term outcome after first intestinal resection in pediatric-onset Crohn's disease: a population-based study. Inflamm Bowel Dis 2012. http://dx.doi.org/10.1002/ibd.23004.

31. Efron JE, Young-Fadok TM. Preoperative optimization of Crohn's disease. Clin Colon Rectal Surg 2007;20(4):303–8.

32. Zerbib P, Koriche D, Truant S, et al. Pre-operative management is associated with low rate of post-operative morbidity in penetrating Crohn's disease. Aliment Pharmacol Ther 2010;32(3):459–65.

33. Huprich JE, Rosen MP, Fidler JL, et al. ACR appropriateness criteria on Crohn's disease. J Am Coll Radiol 2010;7(2):94–102.

34. Jensen MD, Kjeldsen J, Rafaelsen SR, et al. Diagnostic accuracies of MR enterography and CT enterography in symptomatic Crohn's disease. Scand J Gastroenterol 2011;46(12):1449–57.

35. Bruining DH, Siddiki HA, Fletcher JG, et al. Benefit of computed tomography enterography in Crohn's disease: effects on patient management and physician level of confidence. Inflamm Bowel Dis 2012;18(2):219–25.

36. Dasari BV, McKay D, Gardiner K. Laparoscopic versus open surgery for small bowel Crohn's disease. Cochrane Database Syst Rev 2011;(1):CD006956.

37. Tilney HS, Constantinides VA, Heriot AG, et al. Comparison of laparoscopic and open ileocecal resection for Crohn's disease: a metaanalysis. Surg Endosc 2006; 20(7):1036–44.

38. Young-Fadok TM, Wolff BG, Meagher A, et al. Surgical management of ileosigmoid fistulas in Crohn's disease. Dis Colon Rectum 1997;40(5):558–61.

39. Melton GB, Stocchi L, Wick EC, et al. Contemporary surgical management for ileosigmoid fistulas in Crohn's disease. J Gastrointest Surg 2009;13(5): 839–45.

40. Michelassi F, Stella M, Balestracci T, et al. Incidence, diagnosis, and treatment of enteric and colorectal fistulae in patients with Crohn's disease. Ann Surg 1993; 218(5):660–6.

41. Fazio VW, Marchetti F, Church M, et al. Effect of resection margins on the recurrence of Crohn's disease in the small bowel. A randomized controlled trial. Ann Surg 1996;224(4):563–71 [discussion: 571–3].

42. Simillis C, Purkayastha S, Yamamoto T, et al. A meta-analysis comparing conventional end-to-end anastomosis vs. other anastomotic configurations after resection in Crohn's disease. Dis Colon Rectum 2007;50(10):1674–87.

43. Choy PY, Bissett IP, Docherty JG, et al. Stapled versus handsewn methods for ileocolic anastomoses. Cochrane Database Syst Rev 2011;(9):CD004320.

44. McLeod RS, Wolff BG, Ross S, et al. Recurrence of Crohn's disease after ileocolic resection is not affected by anastomotic type: results of a multicenter, randomized, controlled trial. Dis Colon Rectum 2009;52(5):919–27.

45. Tzivanakis A, Singh JC, Guy RJ, et al. Influence of risk factors on the safety of ileocolic anastomosis in Crohn's disease surgery. Dis Colon Rectum 2012; 55(5):558–62.

46. Canedo J, Lee SH, Pinto R, et al. Surgical resection in Crohn's disease: is immunosuppressive medication associated with higher postoperative infection rates? Colorectal Dis 2011;13(11):1294–8.

47. Kunitake H, Hodin R, Shellito PC, et al. Perioperative treatment with infliximab in patients with Crohn's disease and ulcerative colitis is not associated with an increased rate of postoperative complications. J Gastrointest Surg 2008;12(10): 1730–6 [discussion: 1736–7].

48. El-Hussuna A, Andersen J, Bisgaard T, et al. Biologic treatment or immunomodulation is not associated with postoperative anastomotic complications in abdominal surgery for Crohn's disease. Scand J Gastroenterol 2012;47(6): 662–8.

49. Ali T, Yun L, Rubin DT. Risk of post-operative complications associated with anti-TNF therapy in inflammatory bowel disease. World J Gastroenterol 2012;18(3): 197–204.

50. Poritz LS, Gagliano GA, McLeod RS, et al. Surgical management of entero and colocutaneous fistulae in Crohn's disease: 17 years' experience. Int J Colorectal Dis 2004;19(5):481–5 [discussion: 486].

51. Uchino M, Ikeuchi H, Matsuoka H, et al. Clinical features and management of duodenal fistula in patients with Crohn's disease. Hepatogastroenterology 2012;59(113):171–4.

52. Manganiotis AN, Banner MP, Malkowicz SB. Urologic complications of Crohn's disease. Surg Clin North Am 2001;81(1):197–215, x.

53. Brenner HI, Fishman EK, Harris ML, et al. Musculoskeletal complications of Crohn's disease: the role of computed tomography in diagnosis and patient management. Orthopedics 2000;23(11):1181–5.

54. Jaffe TA, Gaca AM, Delaney S, et al. Radiation doses from small-bowel follow-through and abdominopelvic MDCT in Crohn's disease. AJR Am J Roentgenol 2007;189(5):1015–22.

55. Jacobson S. Early postoperative complications in patients with Crohn's disease given and not given preoperative total parenteral nutrition. Scand J Gastroenterol 2012;47(2):170–7.

56. Rombeau JL, Barot LR, Williamson CE, et al. Preoperative total parenteral nutrition and surgical outcome in patients with inflammatory bowel disease. Am J Surg 1982;143(1):139–43.

57. Yamamoto T, Fazio VW, Tekkis PP. Safety and efficacy of strictureplasty for Crohn's disease: a systematic review and meta-analysis. Dis Colon Rectum 2007;50(11):1968–86.

58. Reese GE, Nanidis T, Borysiewicz C, et al. The effect of smoking after surgery for Crohn's disease: a meta-analysis of observational studies. Int J Colorectal Dis 2008;23(12):1213–21.

59. Koutroubakis IE. Venous thromboembolism in hospitalized inflammatory bowel disease patients: the magnitude of the problem is staggering. Am J Gastroenterol 2008;103(9):2281–3.

60. Sachdeva A, Dalton M, Amaragiri SV, et al. Elastic compression stockings for prevention of deep vein thrombosis. Cochrane Database Syst Rev 2010;(7): CD001484.

61. McNally MP, Burns CJ. Venous thromboembolic disease in colorectal patients. Clin Colon Rectal Surg 2009;22(1):34–40.

62. Tan JJ, Tjandra JJ. Laparoscopic surgery for Crohn's disease: a meta-analysis. Dis Colon Rectum 2007;50(5):576–85.

63. Milsom JW, Hammerhofer KA, Bohm B, et al. Prospective, randomized trial comparing laparoscopic vs. conventional surgery for refractory ileocolic Crohn's disease. Dis Colon Rectum 2001;44(1):1–8 [discussion: 8–9].

64. Maartense S, Dunker MS, Slors JF, et al. Laparoscopic-assisted versus open ileocolic resection for Crohn's disease: a randomized trial. Ann Surg 2006;243(2): 143–9 [discussion: 150–3].

65. Alves A, Panis Y, Bouhnik Y, et al. Factors that predict conversion in 69 consecutive patients undergoing laparoscopic ileocecal resection for Crohn's disease: a prospective study. Dis Colon Rectum 2005;48(12):2302–8.

66. Resegotti A, Astegiano M, Farina EC, et al. Side-to-side stapled anastomosis strongly reduces anastomotic leak rates in Crohn's disease surgery. Dis Colon Rectum 2005;48(3):464–8.

67. Ikeuchi H, Kusunoki M, Yamamura T. Long-term results of stapled and hand-sewn anastomoses in patients with Crohn's disease. Dig Surg 2000;17(5):493–6.

68. Alexander-Williams J, Fielding JF, Cooke WT. A comparison of results of excision and bypass for ileal Crohn's disease. Gut 1972;13(12):973–5.

69. Murray JJ, Schoetz DJ Jr, Nugent FW, et al. Surgical management of Crohn's disease involving the duodenum. Am J Surg 1984;147(1):58–65.

70. Yamamoto T, Bain IM, Connolly AB, et al. Outcome of strictureplasty for duodenal Crohn's disease. Br J Surg 1999;86(2):259–62.

71. Shapiro M, Greenstein AJ, Byrn J, et al. Surgical management and outcomes of patients with duodenal Crohn's disease. J Am Coll Surg 2008;207(1):36–42.

72. Worsey MJ, Hull T, Ryland L, et al. Strictureplasty is an effective option in the operative management of duodenal Crohn's disease. Dis Colon Rectum 1999; 42(5):596–600.

73. Katariya RN, Sood S, Rao PG, et al. Stricture-plasty for tubercular strictures of the gastro-intestinal tract. Br J Surg 1977;64(7):496–8.

74. Lee EC, Papaioannou N. Minimal surgery for chronic obstruction in patients with extensive or universal Crohn's disease. Ann R Coll Surg Engl 1982;64(4):229–33.

75. Dietz DW, Laureti S, Strong SA, et al. Safety and long-term efficacy of strictureplasty in 314 patients with obstructing small bowel Crohn's disease. J Am Coll Surg 2001;192(3):330–7 [discussion: 337–8].

76. Roy P, Kumar D. Strictureplasty. Br J Surg 2004;91(11):1428–37.
77. Michelassi F. Side-to-side isoperistaltic strictureplasty for multiple Crohn's strictures. Dis Colon Rectum 1996;39(3):345–9.
78. Michelassi F, Taschieri A, Tonelli F, et al. An international, multicenter, prospective, observational study of the side-to-side isoperistaltic strictureplasty in Crohn's disease. Dis Colon Rectum 2007;50(3):277–84.
79. Yamamoto T, Keighley MR. Long-term results of strictureplasty for ileocolonic anastomotic recurrence in Crohn's disease. J Gastrointest Surg 1999;3(5): 555–60.
80. Yamamoto T, Allan RN, Keighley MR. Strategy for surgical management of ileocolonic anastomotic recurrence in Crohn's disease. World J Surg 1999;23(10): 1055–60 [discussion: 1060–1].
81. Hassan C, Zullo A, De Francesco V, et al. Systematic review: endoscopic dilatation in Crohn's disease. Aliment Pharmacol Ther 2007;26(11–12):1457–64.
82. Laureti S, Fazio VW. Obstruction in Crohn's disease: strictureplasty versus resection. Curr Treat Options Gastroenterol 2000;3(3):191–202.
83. Marier JF, Mouksassi MS, Gosselin NH, et al. Population pharmacokinetics of teduglutide following repeated subcutaneous administrations in healthy participants and in patients with short bowel syndrome and Crohn's disease. J Clin Pharmacol 2010;50(1):36–49.
84. Uchino M, Ikeuchi H, Bando T, et al. Risk factors for short bowel syndrome in patients with Crohn's disease. Surg Today 2012;42(5):447–52.
85. Lal S, Teubner A, Shaffer JL. Review article: intestinal failure. Aliment Pharmacol Ther 2006;24(1):19–31.
86. Buchman AL. Etiology and initial management of short bowel syndrome. Gastroenterology 2006;130(2 Suppl 1):S5–15.
87. Nehra V, Camilleri M, Burton D, et al. An open trial of octreotide long-acting release in the management of short bowel syndrome. Am J Gastroenterol 2001; 96(5):1494–8.
88. Rankin GB, Watts HD, Melnyk CS, et al. National cooperative Crohn's disease study: extraintestinal manifestations and perianal complications. Gastroenterology 1979;77(4 Pt 2):914–20.
89. Lakatos L, Pandur T, David G, et al. Association of extraintestinal manifestations of inflammatory bowel disease in a province of western Hungary with disease phenotype: results of a 25-year follow-up study. World J Gastroenterol 2003; 9(10):2300–7.
90. Rothfuss KS, Stange EF, Herrlinger KR. Extraintestinal manifestations and complications in inflammatory bowel diseases. World J Gastroenterol 2006;12(30): 4819–31.
91. Larsen S, Bendtzen K, Nielsen OH. Extraintestinal manifestations of inflammatory bowel disease: epidemiology, diagnosis, and management. Ann Med 2010;42(2): 97–114.
92. Bernstein CN. Inflammatory bowel diseases as secondary causes of osteoporosis. Curr Osteoporos Rep 2006;4(3):116–23.
93. Ephgrave K. Extra-intestinal manifestations of Crohn's disease. Surg Clin North Am 2007;87(3):673–80.

Rectal Prolapse

Genevieve B. Melton, MD, MA*, Mary R. Kwaan, MD, MPH

KEYWORDS

- Rectal prolapse • Rectopexy
- Perineal proctosigmoidectomyl perineal rectosigmoidectomy

KEY POINTS

- Rectal prolapse remains a common problem, most often in elderly women with concomitant pelvic floor difficulties.
- Clinical evidence in the literature is fair with respect to surgical repair options, but it seems that patients with acceptable health status benefit from an abdominal approach for treatment of rectal prolapse and have a lesser risk of recurrence.
- Both laparoscopic and robotic approaches also seem promising for abdominal rectopexy with or without resection, although long-term follow-up data is in progress.
- Further prospective studies are needed to improve understanding of the natural history of this disease and the functional outcomes after repair of rectal prolapse.

INTRODUCTION

Rectal prolapse (procidentia) is a socially debilitating condition where the full thickness of the rectal wall protrudes from the anus. Patients with rectal prolapse may concomitantly also experience fecal incontinence and other defecatory difficulties. Moschowitz[1] in the nineteenth century postulated that rectal prolapse was caused by a defect in the pelvic floor fascia, resulting in a sliding hernia with increasing intra-abdominal pressure. The more current prevailing theory, suggested by Broden and Snellman,[2] is that rectal prolapse is a true intussusception of the rectum onto itself through the anal sphincters.

As opposed to mucosal prolapse (**Fig. 1**) or internal intussusception of the rectum, this article focuses solely on considerations with full-thickness rectal prolapse where concentric rings of rectum prolapse externally either spontaneously or with bearing down. Rather than exhaustively covering the topic of rectal prolapse, this article specifically examines areas where special consideration should be paid by surgeons in treatment planning, outcome optimization, and proper counseling of patients. Specifically, this article examines abdominal versus perineal approaches, sigmoid resection with rectopexy versus rectopexy versus mobilization alone, ventral versus

Division of Colon and Rectal Surgery, University of Minnesota, 420 Delaware Street South East, MMC 450, Minneapolis, MN 55455, USA
* Corresponding author.
E-mail address: gmelton@umn.edu

Surg Clin N Am 93 (2013) 187–198
http://dx.doi.org/10.1016/j.suc.2012.09.010
0039-6109/13/$ – see front matter © 2013 Elsevier Inc. All rights reserved.

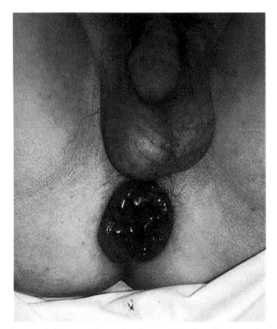

Fig. 1. Mucosal prolapse with acute thrombosis—notice the absence of concentric rings seen in the full-thickness rectal prolapse. (*Courtesy of* W. Brian Sweeney, MD).

posterior rectopexy, minimally invasive approaches, division versus preservation of the lateral ligaments with posterior rectopexy, and recurrence. In framing these topics, it is highly important to note that along with patient-specific factors that must be considered in planning treatment options, each surgeon must also take into account familiarity with different operative approaches and techniques. This article does not specifically cover functional outcomes after rectal prolapse repair because, in general, they are highly variable.

Although the study has finished accruing patients, the multicenter Prolapse Surgery: Perineal or Rectopexy (PROSPER) trial has yet to report any interim or long-term results. This large prospective study compares the abdominal with perineal approaches, suture rectopexy with and without resection, and perineal proctosigmoidectomy with the Delorme procedure.[3] This much-anticipated large prospective trial promises to advance future understanding of the treatment of rectal prolapse.

ABDOMINAL VERSUS PERINEAL APPROACHES

Surgical procedures to address rectal prolapse can be broadly split into 2 larger categories—those performed using a perineal approach (**Fig. 2**) and those performed using an abdominal approach. Classically, perineal approaches have the advantage of being technically possible without general anesthetic, thus making them appealing for elderly patients or those with significant comorbidities (eg, severe cardiopulmonary disease). In these cases, a spinal (regional) anesthetic can be considered (although this technique usually precludes prone positioning[4]) or even sedation with a local anesthetic. The most common perineal procedures are perineal proctosigmoidectomy (Altemeier procedure) or mucosal sleeve resection (Delorme procedure). Abdominal

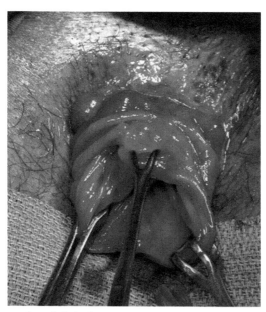

Fig. 2. Perineal approach to full-thickness rectal prolapse. (*Courtesy of* Scott R. Steele, MD.)

procedures for rectal prolapse include most commonly rectopexy with or without resection.

Because of the significant bias in patient selection associated with choosing a perineal versus an abdominal approach, only 1 prospective study, a randomized controlled trial by Deen and colleagues,[5] directly compared perineal proctosigmoidectomy and pelvic floor repair (levatorplasty) with abdominal rectopexy and pelvic floor repair (10 patients in each group) in elderly female patients with rectal prolapse and fecal incontinence. Recurrence rates were similar, with 1 rectal prolapse recurrence in the perineal group and 2 patients in both groups developing mucosal prolapse. Incontinence continued to be an issue in 6 of 10 patients in the perineal surgery group compared with 1 of 10 patients in the abdominal surgery group. Functional outcomes with anorectal physiology demonstrated an increase in mean maximum resting pressure in the abdominal surgery group and a decrease in the perineal surgery group (19.3 [15.28] cm H_2O abdominal vs -3.4 [13.75] cm H_2O perineal; $P = .003$) along with greater rectal compliance in the abdominal surgery compared with the perineal surgery group (3.9 [0.75] vs 2.2 [0.78] mL/cm H_2O; $P<.001$). More clinically significant, frequency of defecation with abdominal surgery was 1 (range, 1–3) daily compared with perineal surgery 3 (range, 1–6) daily. Unfortunately, because of the small size of this study, it is difficult to make significant broad-based conclusions, although several retrospective studies consistently have observed lower recurrence rates with abdominal repair versus perineal repair.[6–8]

Considerations with respect to variation in abdominal approach and repair in the setting of recurrent rectal prolapse are delineated later. For those patients in whom a perineal approach is most suitable, assessment of preoperative continence, other defecatory dysfunction, and the size of the prolapse should be considered with the choice of procedure (**Fig. 3**). In particular, in planning a perineal approach in a patient with preoperative incontinence, a levatorplasty in conjunction with perineal

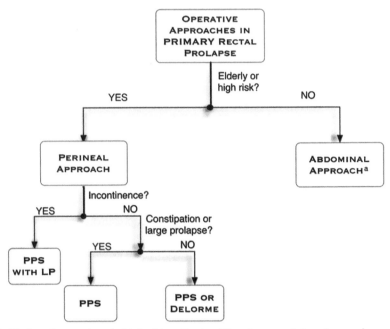

Fig. 3. Choice of procedure in high-risk patients with primary rectal prolapse where a perineal approach is most suitable. LP, levatorplasty; PPS, perineal proctosigmoidectomy. [a]Abdominal approach is discussed elsewhere in the text.

proctosigmoidectomy has been shown to result in better postoperative continence.[9–11] Similarly, although the Delorme procedure is suitable in the setting of small-sized rectal prolapse, a perineal proctosigmoidectomy may be more appropriate in the setting of large prolapse or significant constipation.

Although this seems a well-tolerated procedure, it is not without complications. Overall, morbidity varies among series, although reported in as high as 25%, including a few anastomotic problems. In a series of 103 patients from Washington University, 4 patients had an anastomotic leak or fistula, and 3 patients developed abscesses requiring drainage, with an overall morbidity of 8%.[10] A recent series from Cleveland Clinic Florida reported a leak rate of 3.2% and 1 (0.7%) anastomotic hemorrhage.[12] Pescatori and Zbar[13] also reported major postoperative bleeding in 2 of 38 (5%) patients undergoing perineal rectosigmoidectomy. Finally, in a recent National Surgical Quality Improvement Program (NSQIP) study of 706 patients undergoing a perineal procedure, the rate of postoperative sepsis was 2.7%, and the rate of return to the operating room was 2.4%. Mortality occurred in 1.4%.[14]

Recurrence rates with perineal proctosigmoidectomy are up to 10% in wide-ranging follow-up intervals,[6,12,14–21] with greater recurrence rates in studies reporting longer follow-up. With prolonged follow-up, unusual in recent published series, the recurrence rate is up to 26%.[22] Morbidity after the Delorme procedure is up to 32% in studies and is similar to perineal proctosigmoidectomy. Recurrence rates with a Delorme procedure are unfortunately higher and are between 7% and more than 20% when patients are followed up to a decade after surgery.[23–28] Perhaps because of differences in patient selection and mostly retrospective study design, postoperative constipation is not well reported as a significant functional problem.

RESECTION WITH RECTOPEXY VERSUS RECTOPEXY

Proponents of rectopexy with resection primarily use this procedure instead of recto-pexy alone, especially in the setting of a patient who has rectal prolapse with signifi-cant constipation and is an acceptable operative risk. Although the sigmoid resection provides some improvement of constipation symptoms, sigmoidectomy adds signifi-cant risk from the associated anastomosis. There are 2 prospective trials from the 1990s examining outcomes after rectopexy alone versus rectopexy with sigmoid resection.

Luukkonen and colleagues[29] compared patients with suture rectopexy and sigmoid resection versus suture rectopexy with mesh alone (15 patients per group). At 6-month follow-up, they observed no recurrent rectal prolapse and similar improvements in continence in those patients with preoperative incontinence along with observed improvement in resting anal pressures. Although the rectopexy-alone group and resection-rectopexy group observed the resolution of constipation in 7 and 3 patients, respectively, an additional 5 patients after rectopexy alone became postoperatively severely constipated. In contrast, McKee and colleagues[30] compared suture recto-pexy with resection versus suture rectopexy alone (9 patients per group) and reported no recurrence in either cohort at 3-month follow-up. There were 7 patients with the suture rectopexy alone and 2 patients in the resection groups with severe postopera-tive constipation, and incontinence outcomes were similar. Although they observed greater rectal compliance in the rectopexy alone group, no other anometric physiology or defecography changes were observed.

The recurrence rate for rectopexy in a series of 122 patients from the Cleveland clinic was 5.2% at 3.9 years.[22] With median follow-up of 48 months, a 9% recurrence rate was reported by Wilson and colleagues[31] after laparoscopic sutured nonresec-tional rectopexy. A multicenter review of 623 patients from 15 centers calculated a pooled 1-year, 5-year, and 10-year recurrence rate after abdominal rectopexy of 0.69%, 4.24%, and 28.9%, respectively. The majority of patients underwent recto-pexy alone, with 21% undergoing resection rectopexy. Despite the large number of patients, the investigators believed that the patients and procedures were likely too heterogenous to make strong conclusions.[32] Not surprisingly, however, recurrence rates most strongly correlated with longer follow-up intervals—highlighting the impor-tance of proper counseling regarding this potential occurrence.

Mortality rates for rectopexy alone are low, despite the older demographic that develops rectal prolapse. This low rate may reflect proper patient selection more than anything else, because more frail patients may undergo a perineal procedure. In a series of 154 patients from Germany, the mortality rate after laparoscopic resec-tion rectopexy was 1.3% (n = 2), due to ischemic small bowel in a trocar hernia and myocardial infarction in a second patient.[33] Major complications (mostly bleeding) occurred in 6% and minor complications in 19.5% of patients. There was one anasto-motic leak. In the NSQIP study, which included 569 patients whose prolapse surgery was performed via an abdominal approach (laparoscopic or open), organ space infec-tions (a proxy for bowel leak) occurred in 2.3% of patients, with 8.1% of these patients returning to the operating room.[14]

FIXATION WITH RECTOPEXY VERSUS MOBILIZATION WITHOUT FIXATION

There has been controversy as to whether mobilization alone is sufficient as a repair approach, although there have been 2 reports of good outcomes with minimal recur-rence using this technique.[34,35] A recent multicenter randomized controlled trial that compared mobilization of the rectum without rectopexy to suture rectopexy[36] has improved understanding of the relative long-term outcomes associated with this approach. The study compared 116 no-rectopexy patients who had rectal mobilizations with 136 rectopexy patients. The no-rectopexy patients had a greater rate of sigmoid resection, but otherwise the groups were alike. Although immediate operative outcomes were similar, 5-year actuarial recurrence rates were significantly greater in the no rectopexy group compared with the rectopexy group (8.6% vs 1.5%, $P = .003$). Although these results seem promising, in general the data lead to skepticism about the long-term function and durability of the mobilization only procedure.

VENTRAL VERSUS POSTERIOR REPAIR

Ventral rectopexy is described particularly for treatment of rectal intussception and less in the setting of isolated full-thickness rectal prolapse. In ventral rectopexy, the anterior wall of rectum is mobilized and mesh is placed anteriorly on the rectum with fixation to the sacrum. Although initial descriptions (Loygue and colleagues[37]) included both anterior and posterior mobilization, an alternate approach is to perform ventral rectopexy with posterior mobilization along the sacrum only to fix the mesh posteriorly. To date, there has been no published prospective study comparing posterior versus ventral rectopexy directly.

Also, although the literature for ventral rectopexy is somewhat complicated because it mixes rectal internal intussception and rectal prolapse patients, a recent systematic review demonstrated recurrence rates after ventral rectopexy to be good in the setting of full-thickness rectal prolapse (0–15%), although follow-up was short at approximately 1 year for many studies.[38] The series by D'Hoore and colleagues,[39] reporting on 42 patients with median follow-up of 5 years, found a recurrence in 5% of patients. Other reports demonstrate a wide range of complication rates (1.4%–47%) that include wound infections, hematomas, and urinary tract infections. Somewhat unique to this procedure, however, are additional complications related to the mesh, such as septicemia from the mesh, disc infection, and mesh erosion and detachment. Functional problems remain an issue, although half of the studies demonstrated improvement in constipation symptoms. It also seems that ventral rectopexy with posterior mobilization is associated more often with postoperative constipation compared with ventral rectopexy without posterior mobilization, where constipation outcomes are superior.[38] The speculation for this finding is that posterior mobilization, as with other mesorectal dissection procedures, can be associated with injury to autonomic nerves to the pelvis. Additionally, the degree of lateral dissection (which varies among cohorts) may also play a role in both function and recurrence (discussed later).

At its core, ventral rectopexy is a procedure that requires mesh placement to secure the repair. There are few recent reports of mesh erosion into the rectum or the vagina with this repair. There were no reports from the series by D'Hoore and colleagues,[39] from the series of 75 patients by Collinson and colleagues,[40] among 80 patients reported by Wijffels and colleagues,[4] or among 80 patients reported by Slawik and colleagues.[41] Only 1 mesh erosion among 73 patients who had repair with an Orr-Loygue technique was reported by Slawik and colleagues. Although this remains a concern, it seems less of an issue than originally believed.

PRESERVATION VERSUS DIVISION OF THE LATERAL LIGAMENTS WITH POSTERIOR RECTOPEXY

Preservation of the lateral ligaments with posterior rectopexy theoretically may benefit patients because this area carries autonomic nerves, which may preserve innervation to the rectum. Several prospective studies directly compare outcomes with division versus preservation of the lateral ligaments in the setting of posterior rectopexy for rectal prolapse. Overall, there was an increase in the 3 trials of recurrence with preservation versus division of the lateral ligaments (4/21 vs 0/23, OR 15). Speakman and colleagues[42] observed only 2 mucosal prolapse recurrences in the group with lateral ligament preservation compared with none in the lateral ligament division group. Mollen and colleagues[43] compared defecatory outcomes after preservation versus division of the lateral ligaments and reported delayed transit (with likely constipation) and found lower rates of constipation with preservation of the lateral ligaments (4/21 vs 10/23, OR 0.32).

Although these studies are small, difficult to combine, and difficult to accurately extrapolate outcomes from, it is highly important to counsel patients that postoperative constipation may occur after surgery. Furthermore, surgeons should consider preservation of the lateral ligaments on at least one side if sufficient mobilization and exposure is present while keeping the lateral ligaments intact.

LAPAROSCOPY AND OTHER MINIMALLY INVASIVE APPROACHES

Two prospective studies have compared laparoscopic versus open posterior rectopexy, both with the use of mesh. Solomon and colleagues[44] prospectively enrolled 39 patients and found that laparoscopy had longer operative times but was associated with less pain, shorter hospital stay, and similar recurrence rates. Both this study and one from Boccasanta and colleagues[45] demonstrated excellent outcomes with respect to recurrence, with only a single recurrence in the open group between both studies.

Additionally, several other observational retrospective studies have looked at laparoscopic rectopexy.[46–48] Laparoscopic rectopexy with or without resection seems safe and has low recurrence rates (0–6%). Similar to minimally invasive approaches in other colorectal disease, these results are essentially equivalent to open rectopexy and are associated with longer operative time and cost but less pain, shorter hospital stays, and less wound infection rates. In addition, a few studies have focused on robotic rectopexy and demonstrated longer operative time and greater cost but allow excellent visualization and suturing as well as equivalent operative outcomes to laparoscopy.[49–51] Due mostly to cost, the ultimate role of the robotic approach remains to be determined.

INCARCERATION AFTER RECTAL PROLAPSE

Reports of incarcerated or gangrenous rectal prolapse are rare (**Fig. 4**). Two recent case reports describe this acute event in patients who were not previously known to have rectal prolapse.[52,53] For an incarcerated prolapse without gangrene, patients should be treated with pain medication and placed in the Trendelenburg position and a generous application of sucrose should be applied to the prolapse with concurrent manual pressure. The hyperosmolarity of the sugar decreases the edema and often allows manual reduction of the prolapse. In many cases, an anal block with local anesthetic along with short-acting intravenous benzodiazepines may aid in successful reduction. Undoubtedly, this treatment approach is commonly applied and successful but infrequently reported. If successful reduction is not achieved expeditiously, then the patient usually requires a perineal rectosigmoidectomy (Altemeier procedure). A series of 8 patients with incarcerated rectal prolapse, 4 with gangrene, was reported by Ramanujam and Venkatesh in 1992.[54] This was the initial presentation of rectal prolapse for all patients. All were repaired with a perineal rectosigmoidectomy, and 2 patients suffered an anastomotic leak requiring a diverting colostomy. Patients

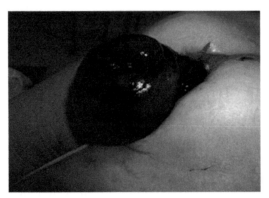

Fig. 4. Incarcerated rectal prolapse. (*Courtesy of* Isaac Felemovicius, MD).

presenting with gangrene should be strongly considered for a diverting colostomy after perineal rectosigmoidectomy, particularly if they have risk factors of poor healing or exhibit signs of early sepsis on presentation.

RECURRENT RECTAL PROLAPSE

Recurrent rectal prolapse can occur at both long-term and short-term follow-up. There are few studies examining patients with recurrent rectal prolapse, but these studies do lead to some interesting observations. Hool and colleagues[55] examined 24 patients with recurrent prolapse over a 30-year period at a single institution and found that many failures in the 29 surgical procedures were technical in nature (24 of 234 total patients, <10%). A large number of these followed Ripstein repair with mesh, but in more than 50% of cases, no cause for recurrence was identified. Median observed recurrence time was 2 years (one-third by 7 months).

Pikarsky and colleagues[56] analyzed recurrent rectal prolapse in 27 patients and matched these patients with a set of patients with primary rectal prolapse. They found that in follow-up, surgical outcomes with recurrent rectal prolapse were virtually identical to those with primary rectal prolapse at median 2-year follow-up. Fengler and colleagues[57] examined 14 patients with recurrent rectal prolapse at an average time of 14 months. After repair of the recurrence, patients were followed for 50 months. At that time, there was 1 death unrelated to surgery and none of the remaining patients recurred, whether an abdominal or a perineal repair was performed. Finally, Steele and colleagues[58] looked at 685 rectal prolapse patients, with 78 (11%) recurrent rectal prolapse patients, occurring at a median of 33 months. There were more

Table 1	
Management options for recurrent rectal prolapse	
Initial Operation	**Management Options**
Rectopexy	All options are technically acceptable
Rectopexy with resection	Redo rectopexy with or without resection Avoid perineal proctosigmoidectomy
Perineal proctosigmoidectomy	Redo perineal proctosigmoidectomy Rectopexy Avoid rectopexy with resection

re-recurrences in those with perineal repair compared with abdominal repair (19/51 vs 4/27, P = .03) at median 9 months. The investigators concluded that an abdominal approach should be attempted when the patient's risk profile allowed it, regardless of the number of prior repairs.

One important consideration in the setting of recurrent prolapse is to understand the nature of previous repairs. There is a technical risk of devascularizing the remaining rectal segment in either (1) a previous prolapse repair with sigmoid resection and rectopexy where a perineal approach could result in a segment of devascularized rectum between 2 anastomotic connections or (2) a previous perineal proctosigmoidectomy where an abdominal sigmoid resection with rectopexy could devascularize the distal rectum. Devascularization could result in stricture or necrosis with perforation. **Table 1** outlines potential options for patients with recurrent rectal prolapse.

SUMMARY

Rectal prolapse remains a common problem, most often in elderly women with concomitant pelvic floor difficulties. Clinical evidence in the literature is fair with respect to surgical repair options, but it seems that patients with acceptable health status benefit from an abdominal approach for treatment of rectal prolapse and seem to have a lesser risk of recurrence. Both laparoscopic and robotic approaches also seem promising for abdominal rectopexy with or without resection, although long-term follow-up data is in progress. Further prospective studies are needed to improve understanding of the natural history of this disease and the outcomes after repair of rectal prolapse.

REFERENCES

1. Moschowitz AV. The pathogenesis, anatomy and cure of prolapse of the rectum. Surg Gynecol Obstet 1912;15:7–21.
2. Broden B, Snellman B. Procidentia of the rectum studied with cineradiography. A contribution to the discussion of causative mechanism. Dis Colon Rectum 1968; 11(5):330–47.
3. The Prosper Trial Webpage. Available at: http://www.prosper.bham.ac.uk/index.shtml. Accessed May 12, 2012.
4. Wijffels N, Cunningham C, Dixon A, et al. Laparoscopic ventral rectopexy for external rectal prolapse is safe and effective in the elderly. Does this make perineal procedures obsolete? Colorectal Dis 2012;13(5):561–6.
5. Deen KI, Grant E, Billingham C, et al. Abdominal resection rectopexy with pelvic floor repair versus perineal rectosigmoidectomy and pelvic floor repair for full-thickness rectal prolapse. Br J Surg 1994;81(2):302–4.
6. Johansen OB, Wexner SD, Daniel N, et al. Perineal rectosigmoidectomy in the elderly. Dis Colon Rectum 1993;36(8):767–72.
7. Watts JD, Rothenberger DA, Buls JG, et al. The management of procidentia. 30 Years' experience. Dis Colon Rectum 1985;28(2):96–102.
8. Swinton NW, Palmer TE. The management of rectal prolapse and procidentia. Am J Surg 1960;99:144–51.
9. Zbar AP, Takashima S, Hasegawa T, et al. Perineal rectosigmoidectomy (Altemeier's procedure): a review of physiology, technique and outcome. Tech Coloproctol 2002;6(2):109–16.
10. Glasgow SC, Birnbaum EH, Kodner IJ, et al. Preoperative anal manometry predicts continence after perineal proctectomy for rectal prolapse. Dis Colon Rectum 2006;49(7):1052–8.

11. Ramanujam PS, Venkatesh KS. Perineal excision of rectal prolapse with posterior levator ani repair in elderly high-risk patients. Dis Colon Rectum 1988;31(9): 704–6.

12. Lee SH, Lakhtaria P, Canedo J, et al. Outcome of laparoscopic rectopexy versus perineal rectosigmoidectomy for full-thickness rectal prolapse in elderly patients. Surg Endosc 2011;25(8):2699–702.

13. Pescatori M, Zbar AP. Tailored surgery for internal and external rectal prolapse: functional results of 268 patients operated upon by a single surgeon over a 21-year period*. Colorectal Dis 2009;11(4):410–9.

14. Fleming FJ, Kim MJ, Gunzler D, et al. It's the procedure not the patient: the operative approach is independently associated with an increased risk of complications after rectal prolapse repair. Colorectal Dis 2011;14(3):362–8.

15. Altemeier WA, Culbertson WR, Schowengerdt C, et al. Nineteen years' experience with the one-stage perineal repair of rectal prolapse. Ann Surg 1971;173(6): 993–1006.

16. Friedman R, Muggia-Sulam M, Freund HR. Experience with the one-stage perineal repair of rectal prolapse. Dis Colon Rectum 1983;26(12):789–91.

17. Gopal KA, Amshel AL, Shonberg IL, et al. Rectal procidentia in elderly and debilitated patients. Experience with the Altemeier procedure. Dis Colon Rectum 1984;27(6):376–81.

18. Williams JG, Rothenberger DA, Madoff RD, et al. Treatment of rectal prolapse in the elderly by perineal rectosigmoidectomy. Dis Colon Rectum 1992;35(9):830–4.

19. Kim DS, Tsang CB, Wong WD, et al. Complete rectal prolapse: evolution of management and results. Dis Colon Rectum 1999;42(4):460–6 [discussion: 6–9].

20. Azimuddin K, Khubchandani IT, Rosen L, et al. Rectal prolapse: a search for the "best" operation. Am Surg 2001;67(7):622–7.

21. Glasgow SC, Birnbaum EH, Kodner IJ, et al. Recurrence and quality of life following perineal proctectomy for rectal prolapse. J Gastrointest Surg 2008; 12(8):1446–51.

22. Riansuwan W, Hull TL, Bast J, et al. Comparison of perineal operations with abdominal operations for full-thickness rectal prolapse. World J Surg 2010; 34(5):1116–22.

23. Uhlig BE, Sullivan ES. The modified delorme operation: its place in surgical treatment for massive rectal prolapse. Dis Colon Rectum 1979;22(8):513–21.

24. Monson JR, Jones NA, Vowden P, et al. Delorme's operation: the first choice in complete rectal prolapse? Ann R Coll Surg Engl 1986;68(3):143–6.

25. Senapati A, Nicholls RJ, Thomson JP, et al. Results of Delorme's procedure for rectal prolapse. Dis Colon Rectum 1994;37(5):456–60.

26. Oliver GC, Vachon D, Eisenstat TE, et al. Delorme's procedure for complete rectal prolapse in severely debilitated patients. An analysis of 41 cases. Dis Colon Rectum 1994;37(5):461–7.

27. Tobin SA, Scott IH. Delorme operation for rectal prolapse. Br J Surg 1994;81(11): 1681–4.

28. Graf W, Ejerblad S, Krog M, et al. Delorme's operation for rectal prolapse in elderly or unfit patients. Eur J Surg 1992;158(10):555–7.

29. Luukkonen P, Mikkonen U, Jarvinen H. Abdominal rectopexy with sigmoidectomy vs. rectopexy alone for rectal prolapse: a prospective, randomized study. Int J Colorectal Dis 1992;7(4):219–22.

30. McKee RF, Lauder JC, Poon FW, et al. A prospective randomized study of abdominal rectopexy with and without sigmoidectomy in rectal prolapse. Surg Gynecol Obstet 1992;174(2):145–8.

31. Wilson J, Engledow A, Crosbie J, et al. Laparoscopic nonresectional suture rectopexy in the management of full-thickness rectal prolapse: substantive retrospective series. Surg Endosc 2011;25(4):1062–4.
32. Raftopoulos Y, Senagore AJ, Di Giuro G, et al. Recurrence rates after abdominal surgery for complete rectal prolapse: a multicenter pooled analysis of 643 individual patient data. Dis Colon Rectum 2005;48(6):1200–6.
33. Laubert T, Bader FG, Kleemann M, et al. Outcome analysis of elderly patients undergoing laparoscopic resection rectopexy for rectal prolapse. Int J Colorectal Dis 2012;27(6):789–95.
34. Nelson R, Spitz J, Pearl RK, et al. What role does full rectal mobilization alone play in the treatment of rectal prolapse? Tech Coloproctol 2001;5(1):33–5.
35. Ananthakrishnan N, Parkash S, Sridhar K. Retroperitoneal colopexy for adult rectal procidentia. A new procedure. Dis Colon Rectum 1988;31(2):104–6.
36. Karas JR, Uranues S, Altomare DF, et al. No rectopexy versus rectopexy following rectal mobilization for full-thickness rectal prolapse: a randomized controlled trial. Dis Colon Rectum 2011;54(1):29–34.
37. Loygue J, Nordlinger B, Cunci O, et al. Rectopexy to the promontory for the treatment of rectal prolapse. Report of 257 cases. Dis Colon Rectum 1984;27(6):356–9.
38. Samaranayake CB, Luo C, Plank AW, et al. Systematic review on ventral rectopexy for rectal prolapse and intussusception. Colorectal Dis 2010;12(6):504–12.
39. D'Hoore A, Cadoni R, Penninckx F. Long-term outcome of laparoscopic ventral rectopexy for total rectal prolapse. Br J Surg 2004;91(11):1500–5.
40. Collinson R, Wijffels N, Cunningham C, et al. Laparoscopic ventral rectopexy for internal rectal prolapse: short-term functional results. Colorectal Dis 2010;12(2):97–104.
41. Slawik S, Soulsby R, Carter H, et al. Laparoscopic ventral rectopexy, posterior colporrhaphy and vaginal sacrocolpopexy for the treatment of recto-genital prolapse and mechanical outlet obstruction. Colorectal Dis 2008;10(2):138–43.
42. Speakman CT, Madden MV, Nicholls RJ, et al. Lateral ligament division during rectopexy causes constipation but prevents recurrence: results of a prospective randomized study. Br J Surg 1991;78(12):1431–3.
43. Mollen RM, Kuijpers JH, van Hoek F. Effects of rectal mobilization and lateral ligaments division on colonic and anorectal function. Dis Colon Rectum 2000;43(9):1283–7.
44. Solomon MJ, Young CJ, Eyers AA, et al. Randomized clinical trial of laparoscopic versus open abdominal rectopexy for rectal prolapse. Br J Surg 2002;89(1):35–9.
45. Boccasanta P, Rosati R, Venturi M, et al. Comparison of laparoscopic rectopexy with open technique in the treatment of complete rectal prolapse: clinical and functional results. Surg Laparosc Endosc 1998;8(6):460–5.
46. Heah SM, Hartley JE, Hurley J, et al. Laparoscopic suture rectopexy without resection is effective treatment for full-thickness rectal prolapse. Dis Colon Rectum 2000;43(5):638–43.
47. Ashari LH, Lumley JW, Stevenson AR, et al. Laparoscopically-assisted resection rectopexy for rectal prolapse: ten years' experience. Dis Colon Rectum 2005;48(5):982–7.
48. Kairaluoma MV, Viljakka MT, Kellokumpu IH. Open vs. laparoscopic surgery for rectal prolapse: a case-controlled study assessing short-term outcome. Dis Colon Rectum 2003;46(3):353–60.

49. Heemskerk J, de Hoog DE, van Gemert WG, et al. Robot-assisted vs. conventional laparoscopic rectopexy for rectal prolapse: a comparative study on costs and time. Dis Colon Rectum 2007;50(11):1825–30.
50. Munz Y, Moorthy K, Kudchadkar R, et al. Robotic assisted rectopexy. Am J Surg 2004;187(1):88–92.
51. Delaney CP, Lynch AC, Senagore AJ, et al. Comparison of robotically performed and traditional laparoscopic colorectal surgery. Dis Colon Rectum 2003;46(12): 1633–9.
52. Voulimeneas I, Antonopoulos C, Alifierakis E, et al. Perineal rectosigmoidectomy for gangrenous rectal prolapse. World J Gastroenterol 2010;16(21):2689–91.
53. Yildirim S, Koksal HM, Baykan A. Incarcerated and strangulated rectal prolapse. Int J Colorectal Dis 2001;16(1):60–1.
54. Ramanujam PS, Venkatesh KS. Management of acute incarcerated rectal prolapse. Dis Colon Rectum 1992;35(12):1154–6.
55. Hool GR, Hull TL, Fazio VW. Surgical treatment of recurrent complete rectal prolapse: a thirty-year experience. Dis Colon Rectum 1997;40(3):270–2.
56. Pikarsky AJ, Joo JS, Wexner SD, et al. Recurrent rectal prolapse: what is the next good option? Dis Colon Rectum 2000;43(9):1273–6.
57. Fengler SA, Pearl RK, Prasad ML, et al. Management of recurrent rectal prolapse. Dis Colon Rectum 1997;40(7):832–4.
58. Steele SR, Goetz LH, Minami S, et al. Management of recurrent rectal prolapse: surgical approach influences outcome. Dis Colon Rectum 2006;49(4):440–5.

Recurrent Pelvic Surgery

Sarah Y. Boostrom, MD, Eric J. Dozois, MD, FACS, FASCRS*

KEYWORDS

- Recurrent pelvic surgery • Reoperative pelvic surgery • Surgical approach

KEY POINTS

- Recurrent pelvic surgery is technically challenging and has the potential for major complications.
- The 5-year survival following recurrent pelvic surgery for recurrent rectal carcinoma is reported to be as high as 58%; however, morbidity is reported to be between 20% and 80%, with wound complications compromising most of the postoperative complications.
- Indications for recurrent pelvic surgery include recurrent rectal cancer, complications following ileal pouch–anal anastomosis for inflammatory bowel disease, and anastomotic leak following low pelvic anastomosis.
- The important role of an experienced multidisciplinary team in the evaluation process, the decisions regarding surgical approach, and in the performance of reoperative surgery cannot be overemphasized.

INTRODUCTION

Recurrent pelvic surgery is technically challenging and has the potential for major complications. This article addresses this complex topic in patients with both benign and malignant disease. In general, indications for recurrent pelvic surgery include recurrent rectal cancer, complications following ileal pouch–anal anastomosis (IPAA) for inflammatory bowel disease, and anastomotic leak following low pelvic anastomosis related to surgery for rectal cancer.

This article provides a perspective regarding a safe approach to patients who may require reoperative pelvic surgery for the indications listed earlier, with a particular focus on the work-up, technical approach, and the importance of an experienced multidisciplinary team. Within this overview, the advantages and disadvantages of surgical options and alternatives are presented in detail to facilitate management of these complex clinical situations and, most importantly, to benefit the patient's care.

The authors have no financial disclosures.
Division of Colon and Rectal Surgery, Mayo Clinic, 200 First Street Southwest, Rochester, MN 55905, USA
* Correspondence author.
E-mail address: dozois.eric@mayo.edu

Surg Clin N Am 93 (2013) 199–215
http://dx.doi.org/10.1016/j.suc.2012.09.016

surgical.theclinics.com

RECURRENT RECTAL CANCER

Many controversies exist regarding surgery for locally recurrent rectal cancer. These controversies include effectiveness and response to adjuvant chemoradiotherapy, the timing of resection, and the operative indications. These factors not only affect the prognosis of the patients, but they also affect patient selection and ultimately their outcomes. The selection of patients for recurrent pelvic operation includes a wide range of variables including the patient's fitness for surgery, the extent of recurrent disease, the presence of metastatic disease, and the intent of the resection (cure vs palliation). The extent and magnitude of the operation must be discussed with the patient. The possibility of a permanent colostomy and urostomy, and the complications of reoperative pelvic surgery such as hemorrhage, urinary and sexual dysfunction, and poor wound healing, should be reviewed in detail.

Indication and Patient Selection

Locally recurrent rectal cancer remains a significant problem, with the incidence of recurrence reportedly as high as 33%, despite modern management.[1–3] However, only approximately 20% of patients with recurrent disease may be amenable to repeat curative resection.[4] Despite the incidence of metastatic disease approaching 70%, up to 50% of patients with recurrent pelvic disease die with local disease only.[2,5–9] In addition, although most local recurrences occur within the first 2 to 3 years following initial curative resection, a small number do recur after longer periods of time.[10,11] The 5-year survival following recurrent pelvic surgery for recurrent rectal carcinoma is reported to be as high as 58%. However, morbidity is reported to be between 20% and 80%, with wound complications compromising most postoperative complications.[3,12,13]

Diagnostic Considerations

Patients being considered for resection should undergo evaluation and staging by a multidisciplinary team. Physical examination including rectal examination, vaginal examination in women, and inguinal nodal basin also contribute to the evaluation and aid in determining extent of recurrence and resectability. Evaluation of the remaining colon via endoscopy is imperative to rule out synchronous tumors and adequacy of bowel for reconstructing. Staging and evaluation of extent of local regional disease is best accomplished with computed tomography (CT) or magnetic resonance imaging (MRI). Positron emission tomography (PET) scan is useful to assist in distinguishing tumor recurrence from postradiation scar and to rule out distant metastatic disease. In the setting of recurrent pelvic tumor and prior treatment, MRI may better delineate the tumor in relation to the musculoskeletal anatomy.

Careful evaluation of all outside records, including operative notes, chemotherapy regimens, and radiation administered, provides valuable information for both perioperative and intraoperative management. In reoperative pelvic surgery, it is imperative that the technical details of any prior operations be thoroughly reviewed, as this decreases ambiguity at the time of reoperation.

Radiation history is important in the evaluation of patients with recurrent rectal carcinoma because treatment with chemoradiation is a significant part of the multidisciplinary management of recurrent disease. As maximum allowable dosages come into play, not only the history of prior radiation therapy, but the type and extent are crucial in decision making and treatment planning. In a multicenter study, Valentini and colleagues[14] reported an 8.5% complete pathologic response and a 29% downstaging following reirradiation. Das and colleagues[15] similarly reported an improved 3-year survival of up to 66% in patients retreated with chemoradiation before recurrent surgery compared with patients who did not receive retreatment. If additional external beam radiation is administered, plans for surgical intervention are expedited, thus allowing for the benefit of the synergistic effects of both external and intraoperative radiation.

Rationale for Surgery

Without any treatment, mean survival is approximately 8 months in patients with locally recurrent rectal cancer. Radiation and chemotherapy may alleviate symptoms, but 5-year survival remains poor at less than 5%.[16–19] Thus surgery remains the best chance for cure in patients with recurrent rectal cancer. In addition, management algorithms have changed, with a paradigm shift from palliation to cure in patients with locally advanced and even metastatic disease.

Standard resection of the recurrent tumor with gross tumor-free margins of resection and appropriate regional lymphadenectomy is the goal of reoperative surgery for pelvic recurrence.

Inherent to oncologic principles, the goal of surgery for recurrence is to remove the tumor with negative microscopic margins (R0 resection). However, recurrent rectal carcinomas are reported to have R1 and R2 resection rates of up to 58%. In the Mayo Clinic series, the reported curative negative resection margin was 45% of 394 patients who underwent surgical exploration for recurrent rectal carcinoma. These patients had a statistically significant improved 5-year survival of 37% compared with the 16% in patients in whom negative margins were not achieved.[20] MD Anderson similarly achieved negative margins in 76% of 85 patients undergoing resection for recurrent rectal cancer. The 5-year disease-free survival was 46% and multivariate regression analysis revealed that an R1 resection was associated with a negative prediction of survival.[21] Thus the evidence concludes that surgical margins remain the most significant factor for long-term survival when operating for recurrent rectal carcinoma.[2,20,21]

Anterior and Posterior Pelvic Exenteration

In some instances, recurrent rectal tumors are fixed to local regional pelvic structures (sacrum, bladder and prostate, or vagina) and en-bloc resection is necessary to achieve a negative margin resection. In patients with recurrent rectal carcinoma in which surrounding organs are involved, an anterior exenteration is required. This involves the en-bloc removal of all pelvic organs, leading to permanent end colostomy and a urostomy. When a negative margin resection is achieved in these patients, long-term survival can be achieved along with minimal morbidity and mortality after surgery. Stocchi and colleagues[22] reported 3-year and 5-year survival rates of 45% and 19%, respectively, in 82 patients who underwent en-bloc resection of organs involving the urinary tract. Postoperative mortality was 2% and morbidity was 39%, with urinary leak only comprising 6%.

When recurrence involves the sacrum, the technical aspects of the operation (posterior exenteration) are more challenging and morbidity and mortality are higher, although a survival benefit is seen when performed by an experienced team. As such, proper patient selection is important. Wanebo and colleagues[23] reported a 5-year overall survival of 31% and a 5-year disease-free survival of 23% in 53 patients who underwent abdominosacral resection for cure. Mortality was 8%, and the most common complication was wound or flap separation seen in 38%. Akasu and colleagues[24] reported on 40 patients who underwent abdominosacral resection for cure. R0 resections were achieved in 60% of patients. Morbidity and mortality were 61% and 2%, respectively, with a 5-year overall survival of 34% and 5-year disease-free survival of 24%. Sagar and colleagues[25] described 40 patients undergoing abdominosacral resection for recurrent rectal cancer and reported an R0 resection in 50%. Morbidity and mortality were 60% and 2.5%, respectively, with a mean disease-free survival of 55.6 months for the patients with an R0 resection. Although often considered a contraindication for surgery, Dozois and colleagues[26] reported an overall median survival of 31 months in 9 patients who underwent high sacrectomy (above the third sacral body) for recurrent rectal cancer.

Multimodality Approach Including Intraoperative Radiation Therapy

To improve surgical outcomes in patients with recurrent rectal tumors, a multimodality approach is used. A multimodality approach that includes chemotherapy and radiation (both before and after surgery) allows for optimal local control rates up to 73% and long-term survival of up to 40%.[2,12,20,27–30] This recent trend of collaboration among different specialties has been shown to be successful.

Intraoperative radiation (IORT) is used in to improve local control and has proved beneficial in both primary advanced rectal tumors and recurrent rectal cancer. A dose of IORT is biologically equivalent to 2 to 3 times the fractionated external radiation dose, and can be delivered either as intraoperative electron beam radiation or by high-dose brachytherapy. IORT is used when minimal gross disease remains or microscopic positive margins are suspected in the resection field. Advantages of IORT include the ability to visually control the target volume definition, the ability to homogeneously treat a controlled thickness of tissue, and the ability to protect uninvolved surrounding structures.[31] In most instances, surrounding structures may be mobilized out of the radiation field. However, nerves may not be easily mobilized and thus are the dose-limiting factor for intraoperative radiation. High-dose intraoperative brachytherapy, used at Memorial Sloan-Kettering and throughout areas of Europe, delivers radiation through the use of catheters. This method is more convenient for the surgical team and patient; however, it is more difficult to protect the surrounding vital structures and tissue. Both modalities of electron beam and brachytherapy have proved to provide similar survival.[20,32,33] Rutten and colleagues[32] reported on 62 patients treated with IORT for locally recurrent rectal cancer and described a 3-year survival rate of 49% with local control rates of 63%. In the largest series to date reported by Hahnloser and colleagues[20] at Mayo Clinic, of 304 patients who underwent resection of recurrent rectal cancer, IORT was performed in 33% of the 138 patients with an R0 resection and was performed in 52% of the 166 patients with R1 and R2 resections. The 5-year survival of the R0 group versus the R1/R2 group was 37% and 21%, respectively. Morbidity and mortality were 32% and 0.3%, respectively. Thus, it seems that patients receiving IORT for microscopically positive margins experience similar local control and survival compared with patients with R0 resections.

High-dose intraoperative brachytherapy, used in 74 patients at Memorial Sloan-Kettering, yielded 5-year local control, distant disease-free, local disease-free, and overall survival rates of 39%, 39%, 23%, and 23%, respectively. Similar to the intraoperative electron beam series, patients with negative margins of resection were reported to have 5-year local control rates of 43%, compared with 26% in those patients with microscopically positive margins. With regard to overall survival, a negative microscopic margin and the use of intraoperative brachytherapy again proved to be significant predictors of improved survival.[33]

Reconstructive Options

The empty pelvic space following extended resections for recurrent rectal cancer is associated with many complications, including abscess, bowel obstruction, fistulas, and wound breakdown. In addition, radiation remains an exacerbating factor for negatively affecting the healing of perineal wounds. Thus, vascularized tissue such as omentum or myocutaneous flaps is commonly used for filling the empty pelvis following resection. A series from MD Anderson reported significantly fewer complications in the 108 patients closed by tissue transfer compared with the 67 patients closed by primary closure following pelvic surgery.[34] A series from Memorial Sloan-Kettering on patients undergoing neoadjuvant chemoradiation and abdominoperineal resection similarly reported perineal wound complications of 15.8% in patients who underwent myocutaneous flap reconstruction compared with 44.1% complications in those without a vascularized flap.[35] Therefore, vascularized myocutaneous flaps are preferable in the reoperative pelvis in those undergoing extensive pelvic dissections, in those with large perineal wounds, and in those patients who have been treated with neoadjuvant or intraoperative radiation. Given the preference for myocutaneous flaps using the rectus muscle, it should be mentioned that, in surgical planning, a midline incision is preferred to a transverse to preserve rectus muscle as well as to facilitate a permanent ostomy.

Palliative Reoperative Pelvic Surgery

Palliative pelvic reoperative surgery may be necessary in select patients to relieve pain, treat necrotic abscesses following chemoradiation, relieve bowel obstruction, and to treat fistulas that negatively affect quality of life. Brophy and colleagues[36] reported 35 patients undergoing palliative exenteration procedures for recurrent pelvic carcinoma with refractory symptoms including pain, bleeding, obstruction, and fistulas. Operative morbidity and mortality were 47% and 3%, respectively. Median overall survival was 20 months and improvement in quality of life was reported in 88% of patients. Esnaola and colleagues[37] prospectively assessed pain in 45 patients with unresectable recurrent rectal cancer for which 30 patients underwent a palliative resection. Patients who did not undergo palliative resection reported significantly more pain beyond the third month of treatment.

COMPLICATIONS FOLLOWING IPAA

Reoperative pelvic surgery in patients with inflammatory bowel disease typically occurs in patients who have complications following IPAA for ulcerative colitis (UC). Postoperative complications, whether immediate or delayed, may require pelvic reoperation to control sepsis or revise/reconstruct a failing pouch. Pelvic sepsis may occur in approximately 25% of patients following IPAA and leads to pelvic fibrosis, pouch fibrosis, and eventual pouch dysfunction.[38,39] Although some patients ultimately require pouch excision with a permanent ileostomy, a small proportion of patients successfully undergoes reoperative pouch surgery with subsequent salvage.

Diagnostic Evaluation

When patient symptoms suggest complications in the pouch following surgery for UC, a thorough evaluation should be undertaken to clarify the source of the problem. Imaging, such as CT, is excellent to evaluate for pelvic infection and guide drainage if indicated. Pelvic MRI can be useful to elucidate fistula tracts as well as extent of sepsis. A pouchogram can be useful to assess the architecture of the pouch and for anastomotic leak. Pouchoscopy provides information about the health of the lining of the pouch and can determine whether Crohn disease is present. An examination under anesthesia may be necessary to complete the assessment of the pouch, ensure control of sepsis, and determine the strategy for pouch salvage. Confirming a diagnosis of Crohn disease is important because biologic therapy, such as infliximab, may convert a patient with Crohn disease to a surgical candidate or suppress the disease enough to allow a pouch revision to be more successful.[40,41]

Indications and Technical Approach

Although some minor reconstructive options may be performed transperineally, most major pouch reconstruction options require an abdominal approach with recurrent pelvic exploration. Reports of reoperative pouch reconstruction success vary from 48% to 93%, with success in large part depending on the patient's underlying disease (Crohn disease vs UC) and whether the complication is of mechanical versus infectious cause.[42] For example, patients with a history of pelvic sepsis or those with a delayed diagnosis of Crohn disease often experience minimal success from recurrent pelvic pouch surgery. Although perineal approaches such as ileal pouch advancement are well described, an abdominal approach is typically required as well to safely free the pouch from the sacrum and pelvic floor, especially in the setting of prior pelvic sepsis.[43,44] When reoperating in the setting of prior pelvic sepsis, excision of all infected tissue as well as control of all existing sinuses and fistulas is imperative to prevent recurrence.

Outcomes Following Pouch Salvage Surgery

Many technical approaches to pouch reoperation have been described with varying success.[45] Shawki and colleagues[46] reported on 76 patients who underwent reoperation for pouch complications (52 UC, 17 Crohn, 6 familial adenomatous polyposis, and 1 indeterminate colitis). The most common indication for reoperation was sepsis and sepsis-related complications. In 23 of their patients, a repeat pelvic operation was required for pouch revision, 7 patients underwent complete pouch reconstruction, and 16 patients underwent pouch revision. The pouch salvage rate in these patients was 69%. The most common reason for pouch failure was a diagnosis of Crohn disease and pelvic sepsis. MacLean and colleagues[47] described 63 combined abdominoperineal pouch reconstructions in 57 patients, of whom 30% underwent pouch reconstruction and 70% underwent revision. The primary indication for reoperation was pouch-vaginal fistula and pelvic sepsis. Pouch revision success was achieved in 67% of the patients. Mathis and colleagues[42] reported 51 patients with an initial diagnosis of UC, of whom 22 patients were subsequently proved to have Crohn disease. Sixty-five percent underwent pouch reoperation for infectious complications and 35% underwent reoperation for mechanical complications. Complete reconstruction was performed in 43% and partial revision in 57%. Pouch survival following reconstruction was 93% at 1 year and 89% at 5 years. Again, most (75%) failed pouches occurred in patients with a later diagnosis of Crohn disease. Pouch survival in patients with a mechanical indication was 91% compared with pouch survival of 79% in those with an infectious indication. Taken together, these results indicate that, although this is often technically demanding surgery, a significant proportion of pouches may be salvaged with an experienced team.

ANASTOMOTIC LEAK FOLLOWING LOW PELVIC ANASTOMOSIS

The overall incidence of anastomotic leak following low anterior resection ranges from 1% to 19%, and, when it occurs, it presents a significant challenge in management.[48–51] Apart from significant patient morbidity and sometimes mortality, resultant function is significantly worse, and the cost of treatment of the anastomotic leak has been shown to be substantial.[52–54] Of even more concern has been the finding that local recurrence is increased and survival is decreased following anastomotic leak in the setting of surgery for colorectal cancer.[55–58] Anastomotic leaks may also lead to chronic fibrosis and scarring, and thus ultimately lead to chronic complications including decreased neorectal capacitance, incontinence, or stricture.[49,59]

Clinical Presentation and CT-guided Drainage

The location of the anastomotic leak, specifically above or below the peritoneal reflection, typically dictates how a patient presents clinically. Patients with anastomotic leaks within the peritoneal cavity present with classic signs of hemodynamic compromise and peritonitis; however, patients with leaks very low in the pelvis may present subclinically and thus be difficult to detect. In general, patients with clinical deterioration, sepsis, or diffuse peritonitis, require immediate surgical intervention. Patients who are not systemically ill, and have subclinical anastomotic leaks, may not require immediate reoperation and can often be managed with CT-guided percutaneous drainage. A CT-guided or ultrasound-guided percutaneous drain may be used for simple diagnostic aspiration if the cavity is less than 3 cm, or left in place for continued drainage if the cavity is greater than 3 cm.

Management Algorithm

Management algorithms have been developed to address anastomotic leaks in an organized and systematic fashion.[60] In the management of an anastomotic leak in the pelvis, extensive peritoneal contamination, significant breakdown of the anastomosis, or evidence of ischemia require takedown of the anastomosis with complete diversion in the form of a colostomy or ileostomy. If the anastomosis ring is mostly intact and there are no signs of bowel ischemia, leaving the anastomosis alone, draining the area, and placing a proximal diverting loop ileostomy may salvage the anastomosis. Local repairs are typically not successful; however, an omental flap in addition to proximal diversion may assist in healing of the pelvic anastomosis. Other novel techniques including covered stents, vacuum-assisted closure device, or over-the-scope clips are in their early stages of use, and data remain sparse.[61,62]

The critical initial goal in patients requiring reoperation is to control sepsis. Salvage or reconstruction of the anastomosis will be most successful 6 to 12 months later. In very low anastomotic leaks, when the abscess cavity is thought to be in continuity, transanal drainage may be performed in the operating room under direct vision. In this instance, the anastomosis is opened and the abscess is drained, followed by placement of a catheter in the defect for irrigation. In the management of pelvic abscesses using drains, serial sinograms must reveal no fistula as well as resolution of the abscess cavity before confidence about its integrity is warranted. If, after many months, a persistent fistula remains in continuity with the bowel, an eventual operation may be required for anastomotic revision or diversion. A diverting proximal stoma is often required in conjunction with local measures to control sepsis.

When reoperative pelvic surgery is performed for a failed anastomosis, it is important to consider the tissue quality of the pelvic floor, remaining rectum or anus, and sphincter function. In highly motivated patients with good sphincter function, reoperation with attempt at coloanal anastomosis may lead to a successful outcome. In the setting of chronic pelvis sepsis, the remaining rectal stump is often fibrotic and a high risk for reanastomosis, but the anal canal typically remains soft and pliable, providing a good point for a coloanal anastomosis. Preoperative manometry is useful to assess sphincter function. Patients must also be aware that bowel length may limit the surgeon's ability to create a low anastomosis and that a permanent ostomy may be required. In addition, a diverting loop ileostomy is required for 3 months if a low pelvic anastomosis can be created.

Strategy for Maximizing Bowel Length for Coloanal Anastomotic Reconstruction

The surgeon operating on patients following a failed anastomosis in hopes of reestablishing continuity must be familiar with strategies to maximize bowel length. It is often necessary to bring the mid–descending colon down to the anus. Our algorithm includes first mobilizing fully the splenic flexure, separating the omentum from the transverse colon, then ligating the inferior mesenteric vein at a point just cephalad to where the left colic vein empties into it (at the inferior border of the pancreas); this is the most important step in maximizing bowel length. The areolar tissue between the Toldt and Gerota fascia must be completely separated for maximal length. If reach is still not possible, the middle colic artery can be ligated if the ileocolic and marginal arteries are intact. Should this still be a problem, the hepatic flexure may be mobilized and the colon either brought through an infraileocolic window or carefully brought down the right side without kinking the vasculature (**Fig. 1**).

TECHNICAL ASPECTS OF REOPERATIVE PELVIC SURGERY

The technical strategy of reoperative pelvic surgery is similar whether the indication is for recurrent malignancy, inflammatory bowel disease, or anastomotic leak. Reoperation in an irradiated pelvis; one with a large, locally advanced malignancy; or in patients with chronic pelvic sepsis can be a daunting undertaking. The surgical team, including the anesthesiologist, must be prepared for a long case and the potential for major blood loss. Warm intravenous fluids, adequate vascular access, and rapid fluid infusers are standard. A detailed briefing with the operating room staff before the operation better prepares all individuals involved in the case.

The patient is typically placed in the Lloyd-Davies position with all extremities safely padded to avoid nerve injuries. Bilateral ureteral stents are placed for ease of ureter identification during surgery. A lower midline incision is made and the abdomen is explored for evidence of unexpected metastatic disease. The low midline incision should be limited if possible to the level of the umbilicus, because this allows the abdominal wall to keep the small intestine safely packed cephalad as well as keeping it warm throughout the procedure.

The small bowel is often found to be adherent to pelvic structures or recurrent tumor. Any small bowel suspicious for adherence to tumor must be resected en-bloc. Once the small bowel is cleared from the pelvis, the ureters and gonadal vessels are identified and looped with a Silastic vessel loops. The course of the ureters is typically normal until the level of the pelvic brim and then is often more medial

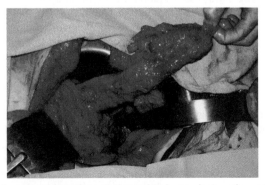

Fig. 1. The available colonic length past the pubic bone during the creation of a colonic pouch after using techniques for maximizing bowel length.

(toward the midline) than usual as they enter the pelvis. Identification of the ureters in the lower abdomen in an area of normal anatomy is a good strategy to get started.

It is helpful to identify stable landmarks, including the proximal ureters, the distal aorta, and common iliac vessels, before committing to the deeper pelvic dissection (**Fig. 2**). If dense fibrosis is encountered near the promontory, the iliac veins will be at especially high risk for injury. The most common vein injured in difficult pelvic dissections is the left common iliac vein because it is typically immobile, fragile, and courses from right to left across the midline with little protective tissue overlying. Apart from the left common iliac vein, other major risk zones for severe bleeding are the presacral veins and pelvic sidewalls. If possible, the surgeon should remain anterior to Waldeyer fascia when in the retrorectal space to avoid the presacral veins. In the event of presacral vein hemorrhage, strategies used to stop the bleeding include thumbtacks, argon beam coagulation, bone wax, packing, or a muscle patch.[63–65]

Ligation of the internal iliac veins and arteries may significantly decrease bleeding when sacral resection above the third sacral body is being performed. When dissection lateral and posterior to the iliac vessels is necessary, an in-depth knowledge of the vascular and neuromuscular anatomy is necessary to avoid injuries to the lateral sacral vessels and the lumbosacral and autonomic plexuses. Multiple anomalous variations occur in these largely unnamed vessels. Sequential ligation of the lateral sacral vessels using loop magnification decreases significant bleeding.

Early identification of correct tissue planes may be accomplished if dissection is begun posterior between the mesorectum and Waldeyer fascia. Next, lateral dissection is performed, followed by anterior dissection. The anterior dissection can be challenging if the bladder or uterus is densely adherent to the rectum. The anterior dissection plane lies between Denovillier fascia and the seminal vesicles in a man or vagina in a woman. In the case of recurrent rectal cancer, if anterior fixation is present, bladder, prostatic, or vaginal resection may be required. As dissection proceeds further distally, involvement of the vagina in women or the prostate in men may become evident. In women, minimal involvement of the posterior vaginal wall may be excised and repaired primarily; however, large defects typically require a reconstructive flap. Bladder involvement may require partial resection or may require complete resection. Minimal involvement of the bladder may allow for resection with primary repair; however, involvement of the bladder trigone or prostate requires complete removal of the organ. When resecting the bladder, the space of Retzius is dissected allowing for full mobilization of the organ. The blood supply to the bladder is taken by ligating the arteries and veins along the pelvic sidewall. The bilateral vasa are then identified and clipped.

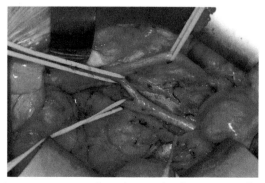

Fig. 2. Vascular and ureter exposure, dissection, and isolation in a difficult pelvic operation following radiation.

Bilateral ureters are then isolated, traced down to the bladder, and clipped and divided. The vesicular veins that drain the bladder into the internal iliac veins are easily torn and difficult to control as the vessels retract or tear back to the internal iliac system. Meticulous dissection with serial ligation typically avoids this problem. The endopelvic fascia is then incised and the dorsal venous complex is identified and ligated. Distal dissection continues until the urethra is encountered and subsequently transected. The technique described earlier, which is used for anterior pelvic exenteration, is used in the abdominal portion of posterior exenteration as well. However, it is important to obtain frozen section biopsies at the anticipated sacral transection margin to ensure adequate resection in the setting of malignancy.

Because dissection of the sacrum is more extensive, mobilization of vessels including the aorta, vena cava, and the iliac arteries and veins is often necessary. For sacral resections above the fourth sacral body, we ligate the internal iliac artery branches distal to the takeoff of the superior gluteal arteries. This method ensures preservation of blood flow to the gluteal region, which typically is used as reconstructive flaps (**Fig. 3**). In order to avoid venous congestion and inadvertent hemorrhage, internal iliac vein branches are ligated before dividing and ligating the main vessels. Lateral and middle sacral vein branches draining into the left common iliac vein and vena cava are then ligated and divided. Given the short retractable status of these venous branches, suture ligature is preferable. If an anterior-posterior approach is anticipated, a thick piece of Silastic mesh can be placed between the sacrum and the vessels and soft tissue structures (bladder, uterus, rectum flap), thus protecting against injury during the prone stage when blind osteotomies are performed (**Fig. 4**).

ROLE OF THE MULTIDISCIPLINARY SURGICAL TEAM

Whether for benign or malignant disease, recurrent pelvic surgery generally requires the expertise of an experienced multidisciplinary surgical team. Combining expertise improves operative efficiency and safety. Depending on the disease and extent, this operative team may consist of the colorectal surgeon in addition to specialists from the fields of gynecology, urology, vascular surgery, plastic and reconstructive surgery, neurosurgery, and orthopedics. Because of the potential for significant morbidity, and

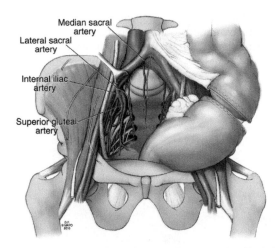

Fig. 3. Ligation of internal iliac artery branches distal to the takeoff of the superior gluteal arteries. (*Courtesy of* the Mayo Foundation, Rochester, MN; with permission.)

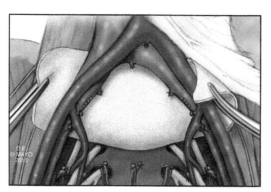

Fig. 4. Use of Silastic mesh between sacrum and vessels. (*Courtesy of* the Mayo Foundation, Rochester, MN; with permission.)

possible mortality, when performing reoperative pelvic surgery, patients should be referred to experienced centers for assessment and eventual surgery to decrease this risk. Reoperation for malignant disease is likely the most challenging of reoperative pelvic surgeries, and, when anterior, posterior, or total pelvic exenteration is required, the presence of multiple surgical specialists gives the patient the best chance at an optimal (negative margin) oncologic resection.

OPTIONS FOR SOFT TISSUE RECONSTRUCTION FOLLOWING REOPERATIVE PELVIC SURGERY

Reconstruction following recurrent pelvic surgery may involve vaginal reconstruction in women, closure of a large perineum defect, and filling dead space within the pelvic cavity. The following discussion provides an overview of soft tissue reconstructive options depending on what tissue is available and the size of the defect.

Omental Flap

The main advantages of an omental pedicle flap following pelvic exenteration are to fill the pelvic dead space and prevent small bowel from adhering to the raw surfaces left behind. The omentum is mobilized leaving either a right or left omental pedicle. Lengthening of the pedicle is maximized by detaching the gastroepiploic arcade from the stomach, thereby preserving the gastroepiploic pedicle on the omentum. The gastroepiploic artery and vein on the opposite side are subsequently divided and ligated. The right gastroepiploic vessels are preferred because they are larger and have more epiploic branches then the left. A window can be fashioned through the transverse mesocolon to allow a more direct route to the pelvis if additional length is required.

Vertical Rectus Abdominis Myocutaneous Flap

The vertical rectus abdominis myocutaneous flap (VRAM) provides a well-vascularized piece of tissue that can be transposed to the pelvis to fill the dead space and reconstruct the perineum. The VRAM flap is mobilized by raising a supraumbilical skin flap with underlying fat and rectus muscle. The anterior rectus sheath is taken with the flap; however, the posterior rectus sheath is left for abdominal wall closure. The blood supply to the VRAM is the deep inferior epigastric artery and vein, which are mobilized as a pedicle (**Fig. 5**). The flap is then sized according to the wound and transabdominal passage is performed by rotating the pedicle into the pelvis,

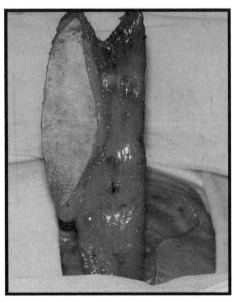

Fig. 5. Harvest of VRAM on pedicle after elevating from abdominal wall preparing for use in pelvic reconstruction.

taking care not to twist it. The flap is then secured to the perineum with the skin of the pedicle facing exterior.

Gluteus Maximus Myocutaneous Flap

The gluteus maximus flap, which is based on the inferior gluteal artery pedicle, can be constructed by local advancement or as a V-Y advancement myocutaneous flap. The technique, which involves dissection and advancement of the superior half of the muscle and overlying skin, consists of preparing 2 myocutaneous gluteus maximus flaps leaving 50% of the underlying muscle intact. Both flaps are then deepithelialized and 1 of the 2 flaps is advanced into the pelvic defect. The second flap is advanced toward the midline and sutured in layers to the first flap. This procedure results in filling of the pelvic dead space as well as a solid midline reconstruction. Both donor defects are then closed using a V-Y technique (**Fig. 6**).

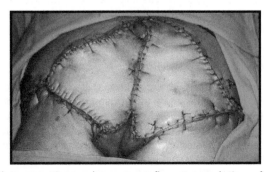

Fig. 6. Bilateral gluteus maximus advancement flap at completion of operation used to cover large perineal defect.

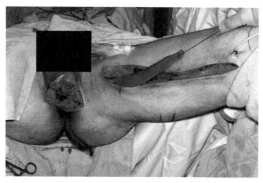

Fig. 7. Harvest of gracilis flap used for pelvic reconstruction following abdominoperineal resection.

Gracilis Flap

The gracilis muscle may be used to partially fill a pelvic defect to preserve the rectus muscle. However, the gracilis flap is smaller, has an inconsistent blood supply, and is difficult to rotate freely, thus it may not be the most suitable option for obliteration of a large pelvic dead space. A longitudinal incision is made over the muscle of the medial thigh and the muscle and skin are mobilized and rotated into the perineal wound. The blood supply depends on the proximal portion of the profunda femoris artery (**Fig. 7**).

SUMMARY

This article provides a comprehensive perspective on the approach to patients who may require reoperative pelvic surgery for a variety of benign and malignant indications. Reoperative pelvic surgery is technically demanding and has the potential for significant morbidity and mortality. The importance of an experienced multidisciplinary team in the evaluation process, the decisions regarding surgical approach, and in the performance of reoperative surgery cannot be overemphasized. With diligent preparation, good judgment, and an expert team, excellent outcomes can be expected in most patients.

REFERENCES

1. Wanebo HJ, Koness RJ, Vezeridis MP, et al. Pelvic resection of recurrent rectal cancer. Ann Surg 1994;220(4):586–95 [discussion: 595–7].
2. Pacelli F, Tortorelli AP, Rosa F, et al. Locally recurrent rectal cancer: prognostic factors and long-term outcomes of multimodal therapy. Ann Surg Oncol 2010; 17(1):152–62.
3. Bouchard P, Efron J. Management of recurrent rectal cancer. Ann Surg Oncol 2010;17(5):1343–56.
4. Sagar PM, Pemberton JH. Surgical management of locally recurrent rectal cancer. Br J Surg 1996;83(3):293–304.
5. McDermott FT, Hughes ES, Pihl E, et al. Local recurrence after potentially curative resection for rectal cancer in a series of 1008 patients. Br J Surg 1985;72(1):34–7.
6. Pilipshen SJ, Heilweil M, Quan SH, et al. Patterns of pelvic recurrence following definitive resections of rectal cancer. Cancer 1984;53(6):1354–62.
7. Rich T, Gunderson LL, Lew R, et al. Patterns of recurrence of rectal cancer after potentially curative surgery. Cancer 1983;52(7):1317–29.

8. Gunderson LL, Sosin H. Areas of failure found at reoperation (second or symptomatic look) following "curative surgery" for adenocarcinoma of the rectum. Clinicopathologic correlation and implications for adjuvant therapy. Cancer 1974;34(4):1278–92.
9. Mannaerts GH, Rutten HJ, Martijn H, et al. Abdominosacral resection for primary irresectable and locally recurrent rectal cancer. Dis Colon Rectum 2001;44(6): 806–14.
10. Palmer G, Martling A, Cedermark B, et al. A population-based study on the management and outcome in patients with locally recurrent rectal cancer. Ann Surg Oncol 2007;14(2):447–54.
11. Bakx R, Visser O, Josso J, et al. Management of recurrent rectal cancer: a population based study in greater Amsterdam. World J Gastroenterol 2008;14(39): 6018–23.
12. Heriot AG, Byrne CM, Lee P, et al. Extended radical resection: the choice for locally recurrent rectal cancer. Dis Colon Rectum 2008;51(3):284–91.
13. Jimenez RE, Shoup M, Cohen AM, et al. Contemporary outcomes of total pelvic exenteration in the treatment of colorectal cancer. Dis Colon Rectum 2003;46(12): 1619–25.
14. Valentini V, Morganti AG, Gambacorta MA, et al. Preoperative hyperfractionated chemoradiation for locally recurrent rectal cancer in patients previously irradiated to the pelvis: a multicentric phase II study. Int J Radiat Oncol Biol Phys 2006; 64(4):1129–39.
15. Das P, Delclos ME, Skibber JM, et al. Hyperfractionated accelerated radiotherapy for rectal cancer in patients with prior pelvic irradiation. Int J Radiat Oncol Biol Phys 2010;77(1):60–5.
16. Kramer T, Share R, Kiel K, et al. Intraoperative radiation therapy of colorectal cancer. In: Abe M, editor. Intraoperative radiation therapy. New York: Pergamon Press; 1991. p. 308–10.
17. Cummings BJ, Rider WD, Harwood AR, et al. Radical external beam radiation therapy for adenocarcinoma of the rectum. Dis Colon Rectum 1983;26(1):30–6.
18. Danjoux CE, Gelber RD, Catton GE, et al. Combination chemo-radiotherapy for residual, recurrent or inoperable carcinoma of the rectum: E.C.O.G. study (EST 3276). Int J Radiat Oncol Biol Phys 1985;11(4):765–71.
19. Rhomberg W, Eiter H, Hergan K, et al. Inoperable recurrent rectal cancer: results of a prospective trial with radiation therapy and razoxane. Int J Radiat Oncol Biol Phys 1994;30(2):419–25.
20. Hahnloser D, Nelson H, Gunderson LL, et al. Curative potential of multimodality therapy for locally recurrent rectal cancer. Ann Surg 2003;237(4):502–8.
21. Bedrosian I, Giacco G, Pederson L, et al. Outcome after curative resection for locally recurrent rectal cancer. Dis Colon Rectum 2006;49(2):175–82.
22. Stocchi L, Nelson H, Sargent DJ, et al. Is en-bloc resection of locally recurrent rectal carcinoma involving the urinary tract indicated? Ann Surg Oncol 2006; 13(5):740–4.
23. Wanebo HJ, Antoniuk P, Koness RJ, et al. Pelvic resection of recurrent rectal cancer: technical considerations and outcomes. Dis Colon Rectum 1999; 42(11):1438–48.
24. Akasu T, Yamaguchi T, Fujimoto Y, et al. Abdominal sacral resection for posterior pelvic recurrence of rectal carcinoma: analyses of prognostic factors and recurrence patterns. Ann Surg Oncol 2007;14(1):74–83.
25. Sagar PM, Gonsalves S, Heath RM, et al. Composite abdominosacral resection for recurrent rectal cancer. Br J Surg 2009;96(2):191–6.

26. Dozois EJ, Privitera A, Holubar SD, et al. High sacrectomy for locally recurrent rectal cancer: can long-term survival be achieved? J Surg Oncol 2011;103(2):105–9.
27. Mannaerts GH, Rutten HJ, Martijn H, et al. Comparison of intraoperative radiation therapy-containing multimodality treatment with historical treatment modalities for locally recurrent rectal cancer. Dis Colon Rectum 2001;44(12):1749–58.
28. Haddock MG, Gunderson LL, Nelson H, et al. Intraoperative irradiation for locally recurrent colorectal cancer in previously irradiated patients. Int J Radiat Oncol Biol Phys 2001;49(5):1267–74.
29. Bussieres E, Gilly FN, Rouanet P, et al. Recurrences of rectal cancers: results of a multimodal approach with intraoperative radiation therapy. French Group of IORT. Intraoperative Radiation Therapy. Int J Radiat Oncol Biol Phys 1996; 34(1):49–56.
30. Shoup M, Guillem JG, Alektiar KM, et al. Predictors of survival in recurrent rectal cancer after resection and intraoperative radiotherapy. Dis Colon Rectum 2002;45(5):585–92.
31. Fraass BA, Miller RW, Kinsella TJ, et al. Intraoperative radiation therapy at the National Cancer Institute: technical innovations and dosimetry. Int J Radiat Oncol Biol Phys 1985;11(7):1299–311.
32. Rutten HJ, Mannaerts GH, Martijn H, et al. Intraoperative radiotherapy for locally recurrent rectal cancer in The Netherlands. Eur J Surg Oncol 2000;26(Suppl A): S16–20.
33. Alektiar KM, Zelefsky MJ, Pat PB, et al. High-dose-rate intraoperative brachytherapy for recurrent colorectal cancer. Int J Radiat Oncol Biol Phys 2000;48(1): 219–26.
34. Khoo AK, Skibber JM, Nabawi AS, et al. Indications for immediate tissue transfer for soft tissue reconstruction in visceral pelvic surgery. Surgery 2001;130(3): 463–9.
35. Chessin DB, Hartley J, Cohen AM, et al. Rectus flap reconstruction decreases perineal wound complications after pelvic chemoradiation and surgery: a cohort study. Ann Surg Oncol 2005;12(2):104–10.
36. Brophy PF, Hoffman JP, Eisenberg BL. The role of palliative pelvic exenteration. Am J Surg 1994;167(4):386–90.
37. Esnaola NF, Cantor SB, Johnson ML, et al. Pain and quality of life after treatment in patients with locally recurrent rectal cancer. J Clin Oncol 2002;20(21):4361–7.
38. Scott NA, Dozois RR, Beart RW Jr, et al. Postoperative intra-abdominal and pelvic sepsis complicating ileal pouch-anal anastomosis. Int J Colorectal Dis 1988;3(3): 149–52.
39. Williams NS, Johnston D. The current status of mucosal proctectomy and ileoanal anastomosis in the surgical treatment of ulcerative colitis and adenomatous polyposis. Br J Surg 1985;72(3):159–68.
40. Matzke GM, Kang AS, Dozois EJ, et al. Mid pouch stricturoplasty for Crohn's disease after ileal pouch-anal anastomosis: an alternative to pouch excision. Dis Colon Rectum 2004;47(5):782–6.
41. Colombel JF, Ricart E, Loftus EV, et al. Management of Crohn's disease of the ileoanal pouch with infliximab. Am J Gastroenterol 2003;98(10):2239–44.
42. Mathis KL, Dozois EJ, Larson DW, et al. Outcomes in patients with ulcerative colitis undergoing partial or complete reconstructive surgery for failing ileal pouch-anal anastomosis. Ann Surg 2009;249(3):409–13.
43. Fazio VW, Tjandra JJ. Pouch advancement and neoileoanal anastomosis for anastomotic stricture and anovaginal fistula complicating restorative proctocolectomy. Br J Surg 1992;79(7):694–6.

44. Fazio VW, Tjandra JJ. Transanal mucosectomy. Ileal pouch advancement for anorectal dysplasia or inflammation after restorative proctocolectomy. Dis Colon Rectum 1994;37(10):1008–11.

45. Fazio VW, Wu JS, Lavery IC, et al. Repeat ileal pouch-anal anastomosis to salvage septic complications of pelvic pouches: clinical outcome and quality of life assessment. Ann Surg 1998;228(4):588–97.

46. Shawki S, Belizon A, Person B, et al. What are the outcomes of reoperative restorative proctocolectomy and ileal pouch-anal anastomosis surgery? Dis Colon Rectum 2009;52(5):884–90.

47. MacLean AR, O'Connor B, Parkes R, et al. Reconstructive surgery for failed ileal pouch-anal anastomosis: a viable surgical option with acceptable results. Dis Colon Rectum 2002;45(7):880–6.

48. Golub R, Golub RW, Cantu R Jr, et al. A multivariate analysis of factors contributing to leakage of intestinal anastomoses. J Am Coll Surg 1997;184(4):364–72.

49. Heald RJ, Leicester RJ. The low stapled anastomosis. Br J Surg 1981;68(5):333–7.

50. Vignali A, Fazio VW, Lavery IC, et al. Factors associated with the occurrence of leaks in stapled rectal anastomoses: a review of 1,014 patients. J Am Coll Surg 1997;185(2):105–13.

51. Petersen S, Freitag M, Hellmich G, et al. Anastomotic leakage: impact on local recurrence and survival in surgery of colorectal cancer. Int J Colorectal Dis 1998;13(4):160–3.

52. Fielding LP, Stewart-Brown S, Blesovsky L, et al. Anastomotic integrity after operations for large-bowel cancer: a multicentre study. Br Med J 1980;281(6237):411–4.

53. Ansari MZ, Collopy BT, Hart WG, et al. In-hospital mortality and associated complications after bowel surgery in Victorian public hospitals. Aust N Z J Surg 2000;70(1):6–10.

54. Braga M, Vignali A, Zuliani W, et al. Laparoscopic versus open colorectal surgery: cost-benefit analysis in a single-center randomized trial. Ann Surg 2005;242(6):890–5 [discussion: 895–6].

55. Branagan G, Finnis D. Prognosis after anastomotic leakage in colorectal surgery. Dis Colon Rectum 2005;48(5):1021–6.

56. Merkel S, Wang WY, Schmidt O, et al. Locoregional recurrence in patients with anastomotic leakage after anterior resection for rectal carcinoma. Colorectal Dis 2001;3(3):154–60.

57. Chang SC, Lin JK, Yang SH, et al. Long-term outcome of anastomosis leakage after curative resection for mid and low rectal cancer. Hepatogastroenterology 2003;50(54):1898–902.

58. Walker KG, Bell SW, Rickard MJ, et al. Anastomotic leakage is predictive of diminished survival after potentially curative resection for colorectal cancer. Ann Surg 2004;240(2):255–9.

59. Nesbakken A, Nygaard K, Lunde OC. Outcome and late functional results after anastomotic leakage following mesorectal excision for rectal cancer. Br J Surg 2001;88(3):400–4.

60. Phitayakorn R, Delaney CP, Reynolds HL, et al. Standardized algorithms for management of anastomotic leaks and related abdominal and pelvic abscesses after colorectal surgery. World J Surg 2008;32(6):1147–56.

61. Geiger TM, Miedema BW, Tsereteli Z, et al. Stent placement for benign colonic stenosis: case report, review of the literature, and animal pilot data. Int J Colorectal Dis 2008;23(10):1007–12.

62. Glitsch A, von Bernstorff W, Seltrecht U, et al. Endoscopic transanal vacuum-assisted rectal drainage (ETVARD): an optimized therapy for major leaks from extraperitoneal rectal anastomoses. Endoscopy 2008;40(3):192–9.
63. Kandeel A, Meguid A, Hawasli A. Controlling difficult pelvic bleeding with argon beam coagulator during laparoscopic ultra low anterior resection. Surg Laparosc Endosc Percutan Tech 2011;21(1):e21–3.
64. Civelek A, Yegen C, Aktan AO. The use of bonewax to control massive presacral bleeding. Surg Today 2002;32(10):944–5.
65. Harrison JL, Hooks VH, Pearl RK, et al. Muscle fragment welding for control of massive presacral bleeding during rectal mobilization: a review of eight cases. Dis Colon Rectum 2003;46(8):1115–7.

Laparoscopy in Colorectal Surgery

Anjali S. Kumar, MD, MPH[a],*, Sang W. Lee, MD[b]

KEYWORDS

- Laparoscopy • Colorectal surgery • Complications

KEY POINTS

- Laparoscopic colorectal surgery may be comparable to open techniques when considering oncological and long-term follow-up outcomes.
- Although fewer perioperative complications and faster postoperative recovery are regularly mentioned when studies of laparoscopy are presented, a minimally invasive approach does possess a unique set of complications and should be well understood as the technique gains widespread acceptance.
- Complications resulting from conversion of procedures from laparoscopic-to-open, especially in reactive conversion in response to an unexpected intra-abdominal finding or injury may lead to worse outcomes than complications from open surgery alone, but conversion rates themselves, are significantly lower in experienced hands, and in high-volume centers.

INTRODUCTION

As the worldwide adoption of minimally invasive techniques such as laparoscopy for the treatment of colon and rectal surgical conditions gains momentum, it is not only important to embrace the advantages, but also to understand its limitations and complications. Minimally invasive approaches encompass an ever-expanding litany of options, including advanced endoscopic procedures, single-port access laparoscopy, or robotic surgery, each with its own distinctive features. Although it may be too early to categorize and characterize the complications unique to each of them as it applies to colorectal disease, complications and consequences of laparoscopic colorectal surgery have a robust body of published data to draw from.

Although the results from the first 3 large, multicenter, prospective, randomized trials of laparoscopy in colorectal surgery for malignancy (Clinical Outcomes of

Financial disclosures: Nothing to disclose.

[a] Section of Colon and Rectal Surgery, MedStar Washington Hospital Center, Georgetown University School of Medicine, 106 Irving Street, Northwest, Suite 2100 N, Washington, DC 20010-2975, USA; [b] Division of Colon and Rectal Surgery, NY Presbyterian Hospital, Weill-Cornell Med College, 525 East 68th Street Box 172, New York, NY 10021, USA

* Corresponding author.

E-mail address: askumarmd@gmail.com

Surg Clin N Am 93 (2013) 217–230

http://dx.doi.org/10.1016/j.suc.2012.09.006

surgical.theclinics.com

Surgical Therapy [COST],[1] Colon Cancer Laparoscopic or Open Resection [COLOR],[2] Medical Research Council Conventional versus Laparoscopic-Assisted Surgery in Colorectal Cancer [MRC-CLASICC][3]) demonstrate a noninferiority of a laparoscopic approach compared with open colectomy regarding metrics such as oncological outcomes, long-term follow-up studies and meta-analyses of data from these 3 pivotal trials raise some concern that laparoscopy may be more prone to intraoperative and postoperative complications. Indeed, there are several considerations unique to laparoscopy as it applies to all disease processes, including colorectal. In this article, we discuss several of them. Beginning with initial entry into the abdomen, we detail troubles related to injury from trocar insertion, as well as the potential late complications from trocars, such as hernias and port-site recurrences. Moving on to complications that are a result of intra-abdominal surgery and reconstruction, we review overall differences in rates of intraoperative complications from laparoscopy, differences in leak rates, and the long-term outcomes of intracorporeal and extracorporeal anastomoses, as well as laparoscopic injury to the genitourinary tract. Finally, we focus on the impact of conversion from laparoscopy-to-open on patient outcomes.

COMPLICATIONS RELATED TO TROCARS
Insertion

A critical difference between laparoscopic and open techniques is the need in laparoscopy to gain entry into the abdominal cavity with minimal violation of the anterior peritoneum. Typically, trocars of 3 to 15 mm are inserted, and once peritoneal entry is confirmed, the abdomen can be insufflated to create domain for visualization and adequate inspection for injury. There are a variety of insertion techniques, including Hasson open cut down, Veress needle (**Fig. 1**) followed by stepwise expansion, and optical trocars. Each of these has its own proponents along with individual learning curves. Although some surgeons use the same technique routinely, others cite various

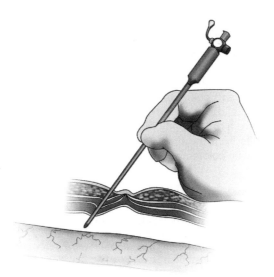

Fig. 1. Veress needle used to obtain access to the abdomen in order to insufflate the peritoneal cavity. It is passed blindly into the abdomen. Although it has a retracting, rounded tip which shields the needle, there is still significant risk of injury to underlying bowel, especially if it is fixed in a position just under the needle's insertion point.

patient-specific factors for deciding which method to use. For example, multiple prior midline incisions may prompt a left upper quadrant Veress-aided entry, whereas in a morbidly obese patient an optical trocar may provide advantages. As such, the reported complication rates are widely variable in the literature. Lal and colleagues,[4] in a series of more than 6000 consecutive laparoscopic cases, reported a 0% visceral or vascular complication rate when an open cut down technique was used for first trocar placement. Of note, only 8% of their patient population had prior abdominal surgery, highlighting the safety in virgin abdomens.

When looking specifically at laparoscopic colectomy cases, an absence of standardization among trocar insertion techniques in multicenter randomized trials has led to some difficulty in reliably assessing complication rates related to trocar insertion. In a comprehensive meta-analysis by Van der Voort and colleagues,[5] the incidence of bowel injury during a laparoscopic procedure was reported to be 0.13% (430 of 329,935 cases reviewed). The incidence of bowel injury in their review was 0.22% (66 of 29,532 cases reviewed). The small bowel was the most common site of injury (55%) followed by the colon at 38%. Not surprisingly, Veress needle insertion was the most common mechanism of injury (42%), occurring even more often than thermal injuries during laparoscopic dissection and manipulation (26%). A history of prior abdominal surgery or adhesions was a significant risk factor for injury, accounting for 69% of the cases of bowel injury.

A dreaded complication of trocar insertion is missed intestinal injury. In their review, only 67% of the injuries were identified within 24 hours of the operative procedure, resulting in a mortality rate of 3.6%. Therefore, extreme diligence is needed during trocar insertion and during the dissection to avoid inadvertent damage that may result in increased morbidity and mortality. Additionally, to help minimize the risk of a missed injury, a brief laparoscopic abdominal exploration before port removal may be performed to look for signs of injury (ie, succus, bilious staining, serosal tears). Concern of injury needs to be investigated adequately and addressed immediately, even if it requires conversion to open.[6]

In general, gaining access under direct vision, especially in cases in which patients are at higher risk of trocar-related injury, is recommended. Additionally, in patients in whom dense adhesions are suspected, choosing an entry site away from the prior incision may help to avoid injury. More than anything, having experience and an understanding of the potential difficulties of whatever method is chosen will likely minimize untoward outcomes.

Bleeding Port Sites

Abdominal wall bleeding may complicate any laparoscopic procedure. Piercing or laceration of vessels traversing the abdominal wall during trocar placement is generally the cause, and can be evident immediately or go unrecognized, complicating the operation and the postoperative course. Planned and careful trocar placement can prevent most injuries, thereby avoiding severe morbidity. The literature in colorectal surgery rarely mentions bleeding from trocar sites as a complication of laparoscopy, but we can learn from experiences of other laparoscopic procedures. By far, the most common minor vascular injury during laparoscopic cholecystectomy is to the inferior epigastric vessels, reported to occur in up to 2.5% of cases.[7] Interestingly, a German group studied the course of the inferior epigastric arteries and the ascending branch of the deep circumflex iliac artery in human cadavers, and measured the vessels relative to abdominal wall and bony structures. When compared with the morphometric locations of trocar incision sites most commonly recommended in laparoscopic literature, about half of the sites recommended for trocar placement were in high-risk areas for arterial injury.[8] Transillumination techniques to visualize the path of vessels can be helpful to avoid direct injury, but may be possible only in patients with a lean body habitus. Rates of clinically significant bleeding or abdominal wall hematoma from trocar injury are not specifically reported in the randomized clinical trials of laparoscopic colorectal surgery. Insertion lateral to the rectus sheath is felt to decrease potential injury to the epigastric vessels, (**Fig. 2**) although it has not been directly investigated. Additionally, this may compromise ideal port placement. Yet, when injury at the port site causes significant bleeding, suture placement around the trocar site, using a suture passer device with the trocar still in place, can result in tamponade and ligation of the injured vessel. Other methods to control bleeding include standard electrocautery or port removal with direct suture ligation. Occasionally, the skin incision must also be extended to view the bleeding site and achieve hemostasis.

Adhesions and Port-site Hernias

One of the obvious advantages of laparoscopic abdominal surgery is the decrease in complications related to a large midline incision. It stands to reason that intra-abdominal adhesions in laparoscopic intestinal surgery would be greatly reduced in the absence of a midline incision; however, it has been difficult to document this advantage, because investigators must rely on rates of readmissions and reoperations. Taylor and colleagues[9] analyzed long-term outcome data from patients enrolled in the MRC-CLASICC trial. They looked at readmission from both adhesive intestinal obstruction and incisional hernia in patients undergoing laparoscopic-assisted and open surgery for colorectal cancer. There was a relatively low rate of readmissions

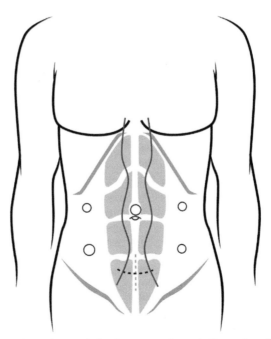

Fig. 2. Because the epigastric vessels (*red*) traverse through the rectus abdominus muscles, insertion of trocars lateral to the rectus sheath is felt to decrease potential injury to the epigastric vessels.

as a result of intestinal adhesive disease (11/411), with no significant difference between laparoscopic and open groups. Incisional and port-site hernia rates were higher than adhesive intestinal obstruction rates (36/411), with 9% of hernias seen in the open group versus 8.6% of hernias in the laparoscopic group (no significant difference). They did, however, show an increase in rates of both adhesions and hernia complications among patients whose procedure was converted from a laparoscopic approach to open. Other investigators have cited wound infections, nontangential abdominal wall insertion, failure to close port fascial incisions larger than 5 to 7 mm, and tension at the umbilical port site as risk factors for the development of port-site hernias.[10–12]

Port-site Tumor Recurrence

Port-site tumor recurrence is an isolated metastasis of cancer at the trocar insertion site following laparoscopic resection of cancer. Reported rates of port-site tumor recurrences early in the experience of laparoscopic surgery for colon cancer were as high as 21%.[13] This raised serious concern regarding its safety, and slowed the use of laparoscopic techniques in treating colon cancer. The etiology of port wound cancer formation is unclear. Experimental animal studies suggest that it is likely to be related to poor surgical technique causing exfoliation of tumor cells, resulting in direct seeding rather than "aerosolization" of tumor cells.[14,15] It should be pointed out that wound tumor recurrence can also occur after open surgery for colon cancer. A large retrospective study of patients with colon cancer found the incidence of incisional tumor to be 0.68%,[16] highlighting the concerns regarding the increased rates in the initial reports of laparoscopic colectomy.

All of the large prospective randomized controlled trials comparing patients who underwent laparoscopic versus open resection for colon cancer reported their long-anticipated oncologic outcomes results. In 2007, Fleshman and colleagues[17] reported tumor recurrence rates based on the National Cancer Institute's COST trial's 5-year follow-up data. Wound tumor recurrences were similar for the 2 groups: 0.5% in the open and 0.9% in the laparoscopic groups. In 2008, Lacy and colleagues[18] reported similar results based on the Barcelona MRC-CLASICC trial. In this study, with median follow-up of 95 months, only 1 of 106 laparoscopic patients developed port-site tumor metastasis. In comparison, none of the open patients developed wound metastases. In 2009, the European randomized controlled study, the COLOR trial reported their rates of tumor recurrences. The median follow-up of this study was 53 months. Port tumor recurrences were found in 7 (1.3%) of 534 laparoscopic patients and in 2 (0.4%) of 542 open colectomy patients ($P = .09$). In the laparoscopic group, 5 of the 7 tumors were at trocar sites, whereas 2 were at the extraction sites.[19] Even in the latest Cochrane Database Systematic Review comparing the long-term results of laparoscopic versus open resections for colorectal cancer that included 12 randomized controlled trials and 3346 patients, there were no differences in the occurrence of port-site or wound-site differences between the 2 approaches ($P = .16$).[20]

Some investigators claim that use of wound protectors to prevent port-site recurrence can decrease tumor-seeding rates,[21] whereas others insist that because port-site metastasis is a sign of more widespread metastatic disease, that local factors have little to do with port-site recurrences when proper surgical technique in tumor handling follows rigorous oncological principles.[22]

It appears that the previously unexpected high rates of port tumor recurrences are not observed in the latest updates of all large randomized controlled trials. Now that we have studies that clearly justify the use of laparoscopic surgery for colon cancer, increasingly more colon cancer surgeries are being performed laparoscopically. As more surgeons attempt laparoscopic colon cancer surgeries for the first time, proper training and observance of safe, oncologically sound principles are essential in preventing the resurgence of high port-site tumor recurrence.

INTRA-ABDOMINAL COMPLICATIONS

There are differing assessments of the relative risks of intra-abdominal complications during laparoscopy versus open colorectal surgery. A meta-analysis of randomized controlled trials evaluating laparoscopic versus open surgery for any colorectal indication was performed by Sammour and colleagues[23] using the Cochrane Collaboration tool to compare intraoperative complication rates of laparoscopic and equivalent open colorectal resection. Intra-abdominal complications were categorized per event as follows: total complications, hemorrhage, bowel injury, and solid organ injury. Although complete data were obtained from only 10 of the 30 randomized clinical trials considered (including articles on hand-assisted resection), the analysis resulted in a large number of cases analyzed (total, n = 4055; laparoscopic, n = 2159, open, n = 1896). The total intraoperative complication rate was higher in the laparoscopic group (odds ratio [OR] 1.37, $P = .010$). When they broke down the types of injuries, there was no difference in the rate of intraoperative hemorrhage or solid organ injury, but a higher rate of bowel injury was observed in the laparoscopic group (OR 1.88, $P = .020$). In contrast, Ohtani and colleagues[24] published in the same year a meta-analysis of randomized clinical trials for surgery on colorectal cancer alone. They found no significant differences in overall perioperative complications or anastomotic leakage between laparoscopic and open groups. In addition, cancer outcomes were similar between the 2 groups.

Mechanisms for potential injuries and strategies to prevent them are addressed by the Society of Gastrointestinal and Endoscopic Surgeons (SAGES). SAGES has created 2 certified courses related to laparoscopic safety and training: Fundamentals of Laparoscopic Surgery (FLS) and Fundamentals for the Use of Surgical Energy (FUSE). Some of the intra-abdominal injury preventions strategies that they discuss include the following: (1) during exchange of instruments, direct visualization of the instruments during entry is important to avoid bowel injury; (2) crush or laceration injury to the intestines can result when retracting a loop of intestines using a bowel grasper and inadvertently pulling it into the trocar, so caution should be exercised during any retraction maneuvers; (3) tips of all sharp instruments should be within view and guarded at all times[25]; (4) although using monopolar energy devices, some disposable trocars can act as insulators and create capacitance, which can create unexpected discharge of current to the intestines.[26]

Leak Rates Relative to Technique of Anastomoses

Laparoscopic-assisted colon resection has been shown to result in earlier return of bowel function, decreased postoperative pain, decreased length of stay, and decreased morbidity when compared with open resection.[27,28] Unique to colectomy, as opposed to solid organ resection, is the requirement to create a patent anastomosis in tissue with an inherently high bacterial load. Therefore, it is important to understand the differences in complication rates relative to the technique used to form the anastomosis. These complications should be further subdivided according to anatomic location within the bowel, as the anatomy, mesenteric mobility, and bacterial load differ by location along the lower gastrointestinal tract. As we design randomized trials to study complication profiles, we must stratify these differences according to type and location of anastomosis, as we do in this section.

Data for intracorporeal versus extracorporeal anastomosis complication rates among patients who underwent right hemicolectomy were reported by Scatizzi and colleagues[29] in a case-control design. Forty consecutive patients who underwent laparoscopic right hemicolectomy for curative intent with intracorporeal anastomosis (totally laparoscopic colectomy [TLC]) for adenocarcinoma, were compared with 40 matched patients who underwent laparoscopic right hemicolectomy with extracorporeal anastomosis (laparoscopic-assisted colectomy [LAC]). There were no differences between groups in terms of operating time (median 150 minutes), histopathological results, surgical site complications (5% for LAC and 2.5% for TLC), nonsurgical site complications (2.5% for LAC and 5% for TLC), or hospitalization (median 5 days). Incision length was significantly shorter for TLC ($P<.05$), although interestingly this decrease did not correlate with differences in the use of postoperative analgesics. There were 6 postoperative cases of vomiting with reinsertion of the nasogastric tube in the LAC group, and only 1 case in the TLC group ($P<.05$), leading to a higher rate of early regular diet tolerance. Single-surgeon reviews from the United States involving a series of cases wherein most cases were right colectomies, have shown similar results.[30] Another Italian study on right hemicolectomy intracorporeal anastomosis was conducted by Hellan and colleagues.[31] This was a prospective study of 80 consecutive cases that also showed no significant differences in median length of stay, number of removed lymph nodes or blood loss, or operative time. They looked specifically at postoperative ileus, which occurred in 22% of patients who had intracorporeal anastomoses versus 16% who had extracorporeal anastomoses. This study reported in good detail the types of anastomotic complications experienced. Twisting of the mesentery (n = 2), anastomotic volvulus (n = 1), or leak (n = 1) occurred in 4 patients in the extracorporeal group compared with 1 minor anastomotic leak in the intracorporeal group. Among left colectomies with colorectal anastomoses, the impact of an intracorporeal double-stapled anastomosis by a single surgeon was studied by Bergamaschi and Arnaud[32] in a series of 54 consecutive patients. Specimens were delivered in a plastic bag via the suprapubic port, which also permitted placement of a 33-mm anvil of a circular stapler into the colon for the end-to-end or side-to-end anastomosis. Minor intraoperative complications occurred in 3.7%, whereas minor postoperative complications occurred in 9.2%. Looking at comparative studies, an excellent prospective observational multicenter study conducted in Europe involving 24 centers in Germany, Austria, and Switzerland accrued more than 1000 consecutive patients undergoing laparoscopic colorectal procedures. They specifically reported the anastomotic insufficiency rates in the various sections of the bowel compared with open colorectal surgery. Among 626 operations performed for benign indications and 517 for cancer, 91% involved the sigmoid colon or rectum and 406 used an intracorporeal double-stapled technique. Leakage rate was very low overall, reported at 4.25% (colon 2.9%; rectum 12.7%), approximating what is seen with conventional colorectal surgery. They further stratified leak rates by location in the rectum. They observed a leakage rate of 24.1% for rectal anastomoses less than 10 cm from the anal verge versus 6.8% in the upper rectum (greater than 10 cm from the anal verge). Even in the presence of a low pelvic anastomotic leak, however, surgical reintervention was required in only 1% of the cases.[33] In summary, when controlling for factors that lead to anastomotic insufficiency, such as tension, blood supply, and anatomic location, anastomotic leakage rates in laparoscopic restorative colectomy cases versus open are expected to be similar. This is supported by further meta-analyses[34] that demonstrated laparoscopy in rectal cancer was associated with significant benefits, including lower late morbidity rates in addition to shorter length of stay; reduced ileus; and lower estimated blood loss, transfusion rate, and wound infections.

Injury to the Genitourinary Tract

Iatrogenic injury to the urinary tract during colorectal surgery can be a source of significant morbidity. Fortunately, the incidence of ureteral injury during laparoscopy appears to be low, reported to be approximately 1% to 5%.[35] However, iatrogenic ureteric injuries have increased markedly during the past 2 decades, according to one of the most comprehensive studies to date by Parpala-Spårman and colleagues.[36] In their retrospective review, a total of 72 genitourinary injuries were recorded. There was an incremental increase in complications among the 3 successive 7-year periods from 1986 to 2006. Of note, only 11% of the injuries occurred in association with a defined urological procedure. Their study points an alarming finger to laparoscopic technique as the leading cause of injury and potentially the incremental increase in injury rates. Among those who experienced a ureteral injury, 56% had undergone a laparoscopic procedure, as opposed to 33% who had open surgery. Fortunately, the overwhelming majority of injuries were in the lower ureter (89%), and were managed by ureteroneocystotomy in half of all cases. Despite this, the complication rate from repair was also high, at 36%. One of the major contributing factors of morbidity was a delay in diagnosis, which occurred in 79% (median time to diagnosis was 6 days). Urologic injuries were mostly secondary to gynecologic procedures (64%), and this has remained uniform across the literature. General surgical procedures, including colorectal resections, accounted for 25%. In the United States, investigators from the Mt. Sinai Medical Center[37] conducted one of the largest reviews of ureteral injury with respect to laparoscopic colorectal procedures. Among a group of 5729 patients who underwent colectomy, 14 ureteral injuries occurred, resulting in a 0.244% incidence of iatrogenic ureteral injury. Consistent with the Scandinavian data, a significant increase in ureteral injuries occurred after laparoscopic versus open procedures (0.66% vs 0.15%, $P = .007$). Half of the patients who experienced injury had undergone prior abdominal operations. Operative indications for colon resection were not associated with incidence of injury (inflammatory bowel disease, malignant neoplasm, and diverticulitis; n = 7, 4, and 2, respectively), but the study may have been underpowered to detect this difference. As shown in open surgery, the use of a ureteral stent did not necessarily avoid injury but helped with identification.

Although most cases of ureteral injury occur in patients without significant risk factors, it stands to reason and has been shown that the incidence of urinary tract injuries increases in patients with prior pelvic operations, inflammatory bowel disease, infection, and in patients with extensive neoplasms that can cause distortion of normal surgical planes. Mechanisms of injury include ligation, transection, devascularization, and energy induced.[38] Early identification of urinary tract injuries is paramount in minimizing morbidity and preservation of renal function and these data demonstrate that there must be a high index of suspicion, especially during laparoscopic operations, and particularly among patients with the risk factors listed previously.

Ureteral intubation does carry a degree of added morbidity and cost,[39] so *routine* use of ureteral stents can lead to increased overall postoperative morbidity and added operative time, but stent placement in *select* patients who are at high risk may help in early identification of injury.

CONVERSION

Conversion from laparoscopic to open surgery is affected by variety of patient-related, as well as surgeon-related factors. Patient-related factors include dense interloop adhesions, high body mass index, advanced tumor with local invasion, and inflammatory conditions.[40] Regardless of surgeon's level of skill and experience, the possibility of conversion to open approach during laparoscopic surgery is unavoidable. Conversion should be considered as a solution to limitation of safety of laparoscopic surgery rather than complication, and more often than not reflects good surgical judgment.[41]

The rates of conversion vary considerably among reported series. Not surprisingly, rates of conversion from laparoscopic to open colectomy in all 3 first large multicenter prospective trials (COST, COLOR, MRC-CLASICC) were somewhat high, ranging from 17% to 29 %.[16–18] Although many of these trials included highly skilled laparoscopic surgeons, the increased rate of conversion may reflect a cautious attitude of surgeons performing a new surgical technique with a potentially harmful outcome; however, it also may reflect relative inexperience of the participating surgeons at the time in the setting of colectomy. In fact, the conversion rate in the MRC-CLASICC trial decreased from 38% in the first year to 16% in the sixth year of patient recruitment.[17]

There has been a significant controversy over whether conversion to the open approach during laparoscopic colectomy has negative impact on patient outcomes. Multiple studies have shown that patients who were converted during laparoscopic colectomies when compared with those who had successful laparoscopic colectomies had longer operative time, increased blood loss, higher wound infection rate, and longer length of stay.[39,42] With this in mind, it is not surprising that short-term benefits associated with laparoscopic surgery disappear when patients are converted to open surgery.

What is alarming is that some studies suggest converted patients may have potentially worse outcomes when compared with those who underwent standard open surgery. There are a limited number of studies that compared outcomes of patients who were converted with those who had open surgery. Gonzalez and colleagues[43] showed greater blood loss and longer length of stay when converted cases were compared with nonconverted laparoscopic colectomy but no difference when compared with open surgery. Similarly, Casillas and colleagues[44] did not find any significant difference in operating room time, length of stay, or morbidity rates between converted patients and open patients. Hewett and colleagues[45] recently reported results from an Australasian randomized study comparing laparoscopic with open surgery for cancer. In this study, converted cases had longer operative time, longer hospitalization, and higher infection rate than laparoscopic or open cases. Discrepancy in results between these studies may be related to difference in definition of conversion regarding incision length and clinical situations. Because there is no standardized definition, we may be comparing different groups of patients.[46]

Belizon and colleagues,[41] reported that clinical impact of conversion also depends on whether the case is converted early (<30 minutes) or late. After initial laparoscopic assessment of risk for conversion, early proactive conversion is likely to result in favorable outcome in high-risk patients. In contrast, reactive conversion, undertaken late in the operation (>30 minutes), in response to intraoperative complications, such as enterotomy or bleeding, are likely to result in poorer outcomes. Most studies do not differentiate between early versus late, or proactive versus reactive conversions. Selection bias certainly may play a large role in the outcomes of these studies. What is likely a more important learning principle is that early conversion based on initial laparoscopic intraoperative findings may be critical in avoiding complications in patients who are at high risk of conversion.

Studies have also shown that laparoscopic colectomies for left-sided pathologies and inflammatory process are much more likely to be converted.[40] In a series of patients with sigmoid diverticulitis,[47] however, hand-assisted laparoscopic colectomy was shown to be much less likely to result in conversion and higher postoperative complications, and rather result in similar other short-term outcomes when compared with straight laparoscopy. Advantages associated with hand-assisted laparoscopy were more dramatic when dealing with complicated diverticulitis (abscess or fistula). A cogent argument can be made for routine use of hand-assisted laparoscopic surgery for certain indications, such as sigmoid diverticulitis, although this is certainly open to debate.[48]

Conversion may also have a significant impact on the long-term oncologic outcomes of patients who are undergoing laparoscopic surgery for cancer. Fleshman and colleagues[18] reported significantly lower 5-year overall survival rate for converted patients in comparison with the open surgery patients; however, the patients who had a conversion had a significantly higher rate of advanced stage cancers. Chan and colleagues[49] also reported significantly lower disease-free survival and worse recurrence rate in converted patients when compared with the laparoscopic patients. This study was retrospective in nature and had a relatively small number of patients who had undergone conversion. Selection bias likely played a significant role in the outcomes in both of these studies. Recently Rottoli and colleagues[50] performed a case-controlled study in which they compared long-term oncologic outcomes of patients who underwent conversions with patients who had open surgery. They case-matched the patients for age, American Society of Anesthesiologists physical status classification system, year of surgery, tumor location, and tumor stage. The investigators found that long-term mortality among the patients who underwent conversions were significantly lower in the conversion group when compared with patients who underwent laparoscopic or open surgery. This was because of a significantly higher rate of comorbidities in the converted group; however, there was no significant difference in the 5-year cancer-specific survival rates among the 3 groups.

In summary, although the literature regarding the impact of laparoscopic conversion to open surgery on outcomes is variable, it clearly shows noninferiority compared with open in terms of oncologic outcomes. The surgeon's experience likely plays a significant role. Recently reported conversion rates by more experienced laparoscopic centers appear to be significantly lower (<10%).[51] As further experience in laparoscopic colectomy becomes commonplace in training environments, this rate may likely decrease even further.[52]

SUMMARY

Laparoscopic colorectal surgery, and the complications and consequences therein, is an evolving subject. In this summary we have demonstrated that laparoscopy offers safe surgery in experienced hands, noninferior to open with regard to oncological metrics, and likely beneficial in many others. Although fewer perioperative complications and faster postoperative recovery are regularly mentioned when studies of laparoscopy are presented,[53] a minimally invasive approach does possess a unique set of complications and should be well understood as the technique gains widespread acceptance. As our body of evidence grows, especially from large multicenter randomized trials, we will be interested to see the evolution of outcomes when comparing laparoscopic and open approaches for colorectal procedures. Even in the past few years, we have seen the use of laparoscopy increase in complex procedures and difficult disease processes, such as inflammatory bowel disease, whereas traditional metrics, such as operative times, are falling. Complications resulting from conversion of procedures from laparoscopic-to-open, especially in reactive conversion in response to a an unexpected intra-abdominal finding or injury may lead to worse outcomes than complications from open surgery alone, but conversion rates themselves are significantly lower in experienced hands, and in high-volume centers

(24% vs 24% vs 9% in low-volume, medium-volume, and high-volume centers, respectively; P <.001).[54] In addition, early proactive conversion in patients who are higher risk may further minimize the risk. Therefore, as centers and surgeons become more experienced, we can likely expect these complication rates to drop even further. Excellent exposure and magnification of anatomic structures in the narrow pelvic cavity by laparoscopy seem to facilitate pelvic dissection laparoscopically, although we do not know yet whether they confer a reduction in morbidity. We will look to the long-term follow-up data from randomized clinical trials of laparoscopic rectal surgery to further understand the advantages and disadvantages of this advanced technique.

ACKNOWLEDGMENTS

The authors gratefully acknowledge the contributions of Kirthi Kolli, MBBS, and Jasna Coralic, MD, who provided invaluable editorial assistance in the completion of this work. We also thank Christopher D. Jones (Dark Matter Media, Allentown, PA) for the illustrations used in this manuscript.

REFERENCES

1. Guillou PJ, Quirke P, Thorpe H, et al. Short-term endpoints of conventional versus laparoscopic-assisted surgery in patients with colorectal cancer (MRC CLASICC trial): multicentre, randomized controlled trial. Lancet 2005;365(9472):1718–26.
2. Clinical Outcomes of Surgical Therapy Study Group. A comparison of laparoscopically assisted and open colectomy for colon cancer. N Engl J Med 2004; 350(20):2050–9.
3. Veldkamp R, Kuhry E, Hop WC, et al. Colon cancer Laparoscopic or Open Resection Study Group (COLOR). Laparoscopic surgery versus open surgery for colon cancer: short-term outcomes of a randomised trial. Lancet Oncol 2005;6(7):477–84.
4. Lal P, Vindal A, Sharma R, et al. Safety of open technique for first-trocar placement in laparoscopic surgery: a series of 6,000 cases. Surg Endosc 2012; 26(1):182–8.
5. Van der Voort M, Heijnsdijk EA, Gouma DJ. Bowel injury as a complication of laparoscopy. Br J Surg 2004;91:1653–8.
6. Ostrzenski A. Laparoscopic intestinal injury: a review and case presentation. J Natl Med Assoc 2001;93:440–3.
7. Merlin TL, Hiller JE, Maddern GJ, et al. Systematic review of the safety and effectiveness of methods used to establish pneumoperitoneum in laparoscopic surgery. Br J Surg 2003;90:668–79.
8. Balzer KM, Witte H, Recknagel S, et al. Anatomic guidelines for the prevention of abdominal wall hematoma induced by trocar placement. Surg Radiol Anat 1999; 21(2):87–9.
9. Taylor GW, Jayne DG, Brown SR, et al. Adhesions and incisional hernias following laparoscopic versus open surgery for colorectal cancer in the CLASICC trial. Br J Surg 2010;97(1):70–8.
10. Pamela D, Roberto C, Francesco LM, et al. Trocar site hernia after laparoscopic colectomy: a case report and literature review. ISRN Surg 2011;2011:725601 [Epub 2011 May 29].
11. Skipworth JR, Khan Y, Motson RW, et al. Incisional hernia rates following laparoscopic colorectal resection. Int J Surg 2010;8(6):470–3 [Epub 2010].

12. Bevan KE, Venkatasubramaniam A, Mohamed F, et al. Respect for the laparoscopic port site: lessons in diagnosis, management, and prevention of port-site hernias following laparoscopic colorectal surgery. J Laparoendosc Adv Surg Tech A 2010;20(5):451–4.
13. Wexner SD, Cohen SM. Port site metastases after laparoscopic colorectal surgery for cure of malignancy. Br J Surg 1995;82:295–8.
14. Lee SW, Gleason NR, Bessler M, et al. Port site tumor recurrence rates in a murine model of laparoscopic splenectomy decreased with increased experience. Surg Endosc 2000;14(9):805–11.
15. Lee SW, Southall J, Allendorf J, et al. Traumatic handling of tumor independent of pneumoperitoneum increases port site tumor implantation rate of colon cancer in a murine model. Surg Endosc 1998;12(6):824–34.
16. Hughes ES, McDermott FT, Poglase AL, et al. Tumor recurrence in the abdominal wall scar tissue after large-bowel cancer surgery. Dis Colon Rectum 1983;26(9):571–2.
17. Fleshman J, Sargent DJ, Green E, et al, The Clinical Outcomes of Surgical Therapy Study Group. Laparoscopic colectomy for cancer is not inferior to open surgery based on 5-year data from the COST Study Group trial. Ann Surg 2007;246(4):655–62 [discussion: 662–4].
18. Lacy AM, Delgado S, Castells A, et al. The long-term results of the UK MRC CLASICC Trial Group. J Clin Oncol 2007;25(21):3061–8.
19. Buunen M, Veldkamp R, Hop WC, et al, Colon Cancer Laparoscopic or Open Resection Study Group. Survival after laparoscopic surgery versus open surgery for colon cancer: long-term outcome of a randomized clinical trial. Lancet Oncol 2009;10(1):44–52.
20. Kuhry E, Schwenk WF, Gaupset R, et al. Long-term results of laparoscopic colorectal cancer resection. Cochrane Database Syst Rev 2008;(2):CD003432.
21. Nakagoe T, Sawai T, Tsuji T, et al. Minilaparotomy wound edge protector (Lap-Protector): a new device. Surg Today 2001;31(9):850–2.
22. Seow-Choen F, Wan WH, Tan KY. The use of a wound protector to prevent port site recurrence may not be totally logical. Colorectal Dis 2009;11(2):123–5 [Epub 2008].
23. Sammour T, Kahokehr A, Srinivasa S, et al. Laparoscopic colorectal surgery is associated with a higher intraoperative complication rate than open surgery. Ann Surg 2011;253(1):35–43.
24. Ohtani H, Tamamori Y, Arimoto Y, et al. A meta-analysis of the short- and long-term results of randomized controlled trials that compared laparoscopy-assisted and conventional open surgery for colorectal cancer. J Cancer 2011;2:425–34 [Epub 2011 Aug 1].
25. Available at: http://www.flsprogram.org/. Accessed October 12, 2012.
26. Feldman L, Fuchshuber P, Jones DB. The SAGES manual on the fundamental use of surgical energy (FUSE). California: Springer; 2012.
27. Schwenk W, Haase O, Neudecker J, et al. Short-term benefits for laparoscopic colorectal resection. Cochrane Database Syst Rev 2005;(3):CD003145.
28. Ohtani H, Tamamori Y, Arimoto Y, et al. A meta-analysis of the short- and long-term results of randomized controlled trials that compared laparoscopy-assisted and open colectomy for colon cancer. J Cancer 2012;3:49–57 [Epub 2012].
29. Scatizzi M, Kröning KC, Borrelli A, et al. Extracorporeal versus intracorporeal anastomosis after laparoscopic right colectomy for cancer: a case-control study. World J Surg 2010;34(12):2902–8.

30. Grams J, Tong W, Greenstein AJ, et al. Comparison of intracorporeal versus extracorporeal anastomosis in laparoscopic-assisted hemicolectomy. Surg Endosc 2010;24(8):1886–91.
31. Hellan M, Anderson C, Pigazzi A. Extracorporeal versus intracorporeal anastomosis for laparoscopic right hemicolectomy. JSLS 2009;13(3):312–7.
32. Bergamaschi R, Arnaud JP. Intracorporeal colorectal anastomosis following laparoscopic left colon resection. Surg Endosc 1997;11(8):800–1.
33. Köckerling F, Rose J, Schneider C, et al. Laparoscopic colorectal anastomosis: risk of postoperative leakage. Results of a multicenter study. Laparoscopic Colorectal Surgery Study Group (LCSSG). Surg Endosc 1999;13(7):639–44.
34. Trastulli S, Cirocchi R, Listorti C, et al. Laparoscopic versus open resection for rectal cancer: a meta-analysis of randomized clinical trials. Colorectal Dis 2012. [Epub ahead of print]. http://dx.doi.org/10.1111/j.1463-1318.2012.02985.x.
35. Nam YS, Wexner SD. Clinical value of prophylactic ureteral stent indwelling during laparoscopic colorectal surgery. J Korean Med Sci 2002;17(5):633–5.
36. Parpala-Spårman T, Paananen I, Santala M, et al. Increasing numbers of ureteric injuries after the introduction of laparoscopic surgery. Scand J Urol Nephrol 2008; 42(5):422–7.
37. Palaniappa NC, Telem DA, Ranasinghe NE, et al. Incidence of iatrogenic ureteral injury after laparoscopic colectomy. Arch Surg 2012;147(3):267–71.
38. Delacroix SE Jr, Winters JC. Urinary tract injures: recognition and management. Clin Colon Rectal Surg 2010;23(2):104–12.
39. Fanning J, Fenton B, Jean GM, et al. Cost analysis of prophylactic intraoperative cystoscopic ureteral stents in gynecologic surgery. J Am Osteopath Assoc 2011; 111(12):667–9.
40. Gervaz P, Pikarsky A, Utech M, et al. Converted laparoscopic colorectal surgery. Surg Endosc 2001;15(8):827–32.
41. Belizon A, Sardinha CT, Sher E, et al. Converted laparoscopic colectomy: what are the consequences? Surg Endosc 2006;20:947–51.
42. Marusch F, Gastinger I, Schneider C, et al. Importance of conversion for results obtained with laparoscopic colorectal surgery. Dis Colon Rectum 2001;44(2):207–14.
43. Gonzalez R, Smith CD, Mason E, et al. Consequences of conversion in laparoscopic colorectal surgery. Dis Colon Rectum 2006;49:197–204.
44. Casillas S, Delaney CP, Senagore AJ, et al. Does conversion of a laparoscopic colectomy adversely affect patient outcome? Dis Colon Rectum 2004;47:1680–5.
45. Hewett PJ, Allardyce RA, Bagshaw PF, et al. Short-term outcomes of the Australasian randomized clinical study comparing laparoscopic and conventional open surgical treatments for colon cancer: the ALCCaS Trial. Ann Surg 2008;248(5): 728–38.
46. Shawki S, Bashankaev B, Denoya P, et al. What is the definition of "conversion" in laparoscopic colorectal surgery? Surg Endosc 2009;23:2321–6.
47. Lee SW, Yoo J, Dujovny N, et al. Laparoscopic vs. hand-assisted laparoscopic sigmoidectomy for diverticulitis. Dis Colon Rectum 2006;49(4):464–9.
48. Pendlimari R, Touzios JG, Azodo IA, et al. Short-term outcomes after elective minimally invasive colectomy for diverticulitis. Br J Surg 2011;98(3):431–5. http://dx.doi.org/10.1002/bjs. 7345 [Epub 2010 Nov 25].
49. Chan AC, Poon JT, Fan JK, et al. Impact of conversion on the long-term outcome in laparoscopic resection of colorectal cancer. Surg Endosc 2008;22:2625–30.
50. Rottoli M, Stocchi L, Geisler DP, et al. Laparoscopic colorectal resection for cancer: effects of conversion on long-term oncologic outcomes. Surg Endosc 2012;26(7):1971–6 PMID 22237758.

51. Milsom JW, Oliveira O, Trencheva K, et al. Long-term outcomes of patients undergoing curative laparoscopic surgery for mid and lower rectal cancer. Dis Colon Rectum 2009;52(7):1215–22.
52. Steele SR, Stein SL, Bordeianou LG, et al. The impact of practice environment on laparoscopic colectomy utilization following colorectal residency: a survey of the ASCRS Young Surgeons. Colorectal Dis 2012;14(3):374–81. http://dx.doi.org/10.1111/j.1463-1318.2011.02614.x.
53. Künzli BM, Friess H, Shrikhande SV. Is laparoscopic colorectal cancer surgery equal to open surgery? An evidence-based perspective. World J Gastrointest Surg 2010;2(4):101–8.
54. Kuhry E, Bonjer HJ, Haglind E, et al. Impact of hospital case volume on short-term outcome after laparoscopic operation for colonic cancer. Surg Endosc 2005;19(5):687–92.

Controversies in the Care of the Enterocutaneous Fistula

Kurt G. Davis, MD[a], Eric K. Johnson, MD[b],*

KEYWORDS

- Enterocutaneous fistula • Enteroatmospheric fistula • Abdominal wall reconstruction
- Complications

KEY POINTS

- The entities of enterocutaneous fistula (ECF) and enteroatmospheric fistula (EAF) remain a formidable challenge to surgeons facing affected patients.
- Awareness of its causes, contributing factors, potential preventive measures, and various management strategies are crucial to achieving optimal outcomes in the care of these patients.
- Due to a lack of high-quality evidence supporting any particular regimen of care, the surgeon is required to exercise skillful judgment in treating these individuals.

BACKGROUND AND OVERVIEW

The appearance of enteric contents from an abdominal incision is a devastating complication and can be emotionally distressing for both the patient and the operative surgeon. ECFs range from easily controlled low-output colocutaneous fistulas to high-output EAFs requiring prolonged nutritional support, specialized wound care, and complex reoperative surgery. These patients frequently face complications, and a well-organized multidisciplinary approach must be implemented in their

Disclosure: Dr Johnson has served as a speaker for Cook Biotech, Bloomington, IN.
The authors' team includes military service members and employees of the US Government. This work was prepared as part of their official duties. Title 17 U.S.C. 105 provides that "Copyright protection under this title is not available for any work of the United States Government." Title 17 U.S.C. 101 defines a US Government work as a work prepared by a military service member or employee of the US Government as part of that person's official duties. The views expressed in this presentation are those of the authors and do not reflect the official policy of the Department of the Army, the Department of Defense, or the US Government.
[a] Section of Colon and Rectal Surgery, Department of Surgery, 5005 North Piedras Street, William Beaumont Army Medical Center, Fort Bliss, TX 79920, USA; [b] Section of Colon and Rectal Surgery, Department of Surgery, 9040A Fitzsimmons Drive, Madigan Army Medical Center, Joint Base Lewis-McChord, Tacoma, WA 98431, USA
* Corresponding author. Section of General Surgery, Department of Surgery, JBLM, Tacoma, WA 98431.
E-mail address: doktrj@gmail.com

Surg Clin N Am 93 (2013) 231–250
http://dx.doi.org/10.1016/j.suc.2012.09.009
0039-6109/13/$ – see front matter Published by Elsevier Inc.

management to improve outcomes. Furthermore, in a hospital setting with limited resources, consideration should be given to having these patients evaluated in a center with specialized experience in dealing with ECFs. A great deal of controversy surrounds nearly every aspect of the care of these patients. A dearth of homogenous patient populations and the preponderance of case reports and case series make this situation unlikely to change soon.

It is important to highlight up front that the presence of an ECF is accompanied by a significant risk of mortality, reported between 5% and 20%,[1,2] with the variability owing to the heterogeneity of this cohort of patients. In addition to the significant mortality rates, the morbidity associated with ECFs is excessive. A prolonged hospital course, as well as extensive postoperative rehabilitation, often with nutritional supplementation, is common. The cost to the health care system and the psychological impact on the patient are difficult to quantify. However, ample data show increased intensive care unit length of stay, hospital length of stay, and hospital cost.[3]

A postoperative ECF (**Fig. 1**) seldom poses a diagnostic dilemma. It is defined as an abnormal communication between a bowel lumen and the skin and is frequently defined based on anatomic origin or cause.[4] It most commonly results from prior abdominal operations but can occur from trauma, Crohn disease, diverticulitis, malignancy, hernia mesh erosions, and, less commonly, intra-abdominal infections such as tuberculosis, typhoid, and actinomycoses.[3–5] Postoperative ECFs most commonly result from operations for malignancy, inflammatory bowel disease, or adhesiolysis, as well as emergency abdominal procedures.[6]

ECFs are arbitrarily classified as low or high output based on the amount of drainage in a 24-hour period. Less than 200 mL/d is considered low output, greater than 500 mL/d is classified as high output, and the intermediate group is defined as such. Adequate quantification of volume output is critical not only in defining the fistula but also in predicting the likelihood of closure and in planning for any subsequent surgical intervention.[7,8]

A significant subset of ECFs close with nonoperative treatment, including control of any infectious source, nutritional support, and appropriate wound care. It has been demonstrated that patients with high-output fistulas have a higher mortality, and there is some evidence, albeit less clear, that these fistulas demonstrate a lower likelihood of spontaneous closure.[9,10] Medical students are taught the familiar but still useful acronym "FRIENDS" to delineate those fistulas less likely to close spontaneously.

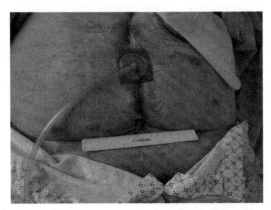

Fig. 1. Patient with a postoperative enterocutaneous fistula being managed with negative pressure wound therapy.

The presence of a Foreign body, prior Radiation exposure, the diagnosis of Inflammatory bowel disease or ongoing Infection, the presence of an Epithelialized fistula tract, a Neoplasm, the presence of a Distal obstruction or Sepsis/Steroids all make it unlikely for these fistulas to close spontaneously.[11] Based on multiple studies, only around a third of ECFs heal without additional reoperative therapy.[1] However, every attempt should be made to use nonoperative techniques to maximize the chances that spontaneous closure can occur.

Once the diagnosis of an ECF is made, the priority is control of sepsis and fluid resuscitation.[12] These patients are generally several days into their postoperative course and have often been receiving inadequate or no nutritional supplementation secondary to a prolonged ileus. In addition, they may have already experienced protein loss and catabolism and frequently have sepsis from a localized wound infection or deep abscess.[13] If the patient has a high-output fistula, consideration should be made for placing a urinary catheter and aggressively resuscitating the patient with crystalloids. Electrolyte levels should also be monitored and replaced as necessary.

Abdominal computed tomography should be performed soon after the diagnosis is made. This procedure is critical not only for assisting in the anatomic delineation of the fistula but also for excluding intra-abdominal sources of sepsis. Any intra-abdominal abscess should be drained with radiological assistance if possible.[14] This procedure is necessary in more than 10% of patients,[15] and allows egress of the intestinal contents lateral to the abdominal incision, which can ameliorate or delay return to the operating room.

NUTRITION

Nutritional disturbances are present in 50% to 90% of patients with an ECF and contribute significantly to the overall morbidity and mortality.[16,17] Adequate nutrition is essential for these patients but much more difficult to achieve in practice. Before the development of parenteral nutrition, there was a significantly reduced mortality in patients who could tolerate a 3000-kcal/d diet.[18]

One of the most significant advances in the treatment of ECF was the development of parenteral nutrition in the 1960s. Although initial reports demonstrated up to a 70% spontaneous fistula closure rate and a mortality of 6% solely with the use of intravenous alimentation, these results have not been replicated.[19,20] What has been shown as the fistula closure rate is twice as likely to occur spontaneously in patients receiving nutritional supplementation.[21,22] For patients with long-standing small-bowel fistulas, supplemental copper, folic acid, and vitamin B12 may be necessary, as trace minerals and vitamins also become depleted.[6]

Traditional surgical dogma based on early reports using hyperalimentation states that bowel rest along with total parenteral nutrition (TPN) leads to a higher incidence of spontaneous closure of an ECF. This teaching is based on the principle that this therapy results in a reduction in secretions within the gastrointestinal tract, thereby reducing fistula output and leading to a more rapid time to resolution.[1] The average time standard for spontaneous closure of ECFs on parenteral nutrition is 25 days,[1] although they may take up to 12 weeks. However, most studies in the literature involve heterogeneous patient populations and are predominantly retrospective in nature, making it difficult to compare and contrast the various studies and predict accurately the timing and rate of spontaneous closure.[15]

There is insufficient evidence to demonstrate that parenteral nutrition is superior to enteral nutrition with regards to spontaneous closure rates. The concern that enteral nutrition contributes to or worsens fistula output is likely unfounded,[23] and enteral nutrition has actually demonstrated a lower fistula formation rate in patients with trauma managed with an open abdomen.[24] More appropriately, parenteral nutrition should be reserved for patients who do not tolerate enteral feedings secondary to postoperative ileus or have an inability to maintain adequate nutrition via the enteral route.[5] Enteral nutrition is the preferred route of administration for nutrition unless there is a clear contraindication to enteral feedings.

It continues to be a difficult task to accurately assess the nutritional status of patients with ECFs. These patients frequently receive significant volume resuscitation, making accurate determinations based on weight impossible. The prolonged half-life of albumin makes it an impractical tool for use in these patients. Transferrin has a serum half-life of 8 days, making it better suited for use in these rapidly improving patients.[19] It has been demonstrated that a decrease in transferrin levels is associated with increased mortality and significantly lower rates of spontaneous fistula closure.[25] Serum transferrin has also been shown to predict which patients will have more favorable outcomes following surgical management.[26] In addition, techniques involving bioelectric impedence analysis (measurement of body composition) have been demonstrated to have some validity but have not found widespread use.[27]

Some investigators have also advocated routine nasogastric tube decompression.[13] The dogma contends that by decreasing the secretions from the oropharynx, the esophagus, and the stomach, there is a resultant decrease in the fistula output, aiding in spontaneous closure. In reality, the placement of a nasogastric tube to decompress the stomach likely contributes little to the management of the patient with an ECF, unless an ileus is present, but undoubtedly contributes to the discomfort of the patient.

MEDICAL MANAGEMENT

Somatostatin is a naturally occurring hormone principally produced by the delta cells of the pancreas. Somatostatin and its analogues have an inhibitory effect on digestion through reduction in enteric secretions, suppression of gastrointestinal hormones, decreased rate of gastric emptying, and splanchnic vasoconstriction.[28,29] Based on these inhibitory properties, it is no surprise that somatostatin has been advocated for use in the management of ECFs. By reducing the volume of output, it is thought that somatostatin may expedite spontaneous fistula closure. Owing to the short half-life of somatostatin (1–2 minutes), which requires continuous infusion, several longer-acting analogues have been developed.[30] Octreotide has been widely used in the treatment of ECFs, and with a half-life of 113 minutes, it allows intermittent subcutaneous dosing.[31]

Somatostatin and associated analogues have been used in adjunct in the conservative management of ECFs.[28] When combined with TPN, there seems to be a synergistic effect on the reduction in the levels of gastrointestinal effluents and an improvement in fistula closure rates.[29] However, a definitive evaluation of the efficacies of somatostatin and its analogues for the treatment of ECFs is difficult. The literature is limited by the large number of case reports and small patient series, whereas the few controlled trials comparing these drugs with placebo are weakened by the small size and heterogeneity of the patient populations.

The clinical efficacy of this therapy is measured by examining 3 parameters: fistula output volume, time to closure, and fistula closure rates. A medication that reduces fistula output would be beneficial to a patient with a high-output fistula with regards not only to prognosis but also to improved quality of life. Investigations have demonstrated that both somatostatin and octreotide are effective in reducing the fistula volume output, with some reports of a 70% reduction in output after the first day of treatment.[29,32–34] The time to closure is important, as it directly relates to the length of stay, medical cost, and complications. Although the literature is not unanimous on the benefits of somatostatin or octreotide on closure time, several controlled trials have demonstrated a significant improvement.[32,35–38] Therefore, there seems to be a positive effect on closure time of ECFs from these medications. On the other hand, most studies have shown that somatostatin and its analogues have no effect on the actual rate of closure in patients administered these medications along with conservative therapy.[28,34,37,38] Although this may seem like a failure of conservative therapy, it is more likely related to the nature of the individual fistula, such as its location or the presence of a distal obstruction, foreign body, or malignancy.

In addition to somatostatin, there are other pharmacologic adjuncts that have been used primarily or in conjunction with other therapies. Proton pump inhibitors and H2 receptor antagonists have been shown to decrease gastric secretions and have therefore been advocated by some investigators in an attempt to reduce the output from ECFs.[3,6,13] However, there is no evidence that these medications either decrease fistula output or increase the rate of spontaneous fistula closure.

In patients with Crohn disease, there has been a documented rate of ECF closure following the administration of 6-mercaptopurine and cyclosporine.[39,40] In addition, there has been some interest in the use of infliximab, a primary monoclonal antibody to tumor necrosis factor alpha, in patients with a Crohn disease–related fistula.[41,42] Although most patients evaluated had perianal fistulas, there are some encouraging preliminary results using infliximab in patients with ECFs as well. These treatments are obviously for use in an isolated patient population with inflammatory bowel disease and not for postoperative fistulas, as sepsis would preclude their use.

In addition, there have been case reports of ECFs being successfully treated with fibrin glue or fistula plugs.[3,13,43] These options are certainly attractive to surgeons searching for less-invasive means of treating these patients; however, there is little evidence that these treatments are justified. Although they add no additional morbidity, cost remains a factor.

WOUND CARE

Enteric contents coming in direct contact with the skin, in particular small bowel effluent, can result in significant skin breakdown, excoriation (**Fig. 2**), maceration, and severe pain and discomfort for the patient.[44] It is of primary importance to adequately control the effluent. For low-output fistulas, nothing more than a simple gauze dressing may be required. However, with high-output fistulas, the benefit of a skilled enterostomal therapist is invaluable.[44]

Vacuum-assisted devices for wound closure have been counted as both the solution and potentially the cause of ECFs. When these devices were first used in the treatment of patients with open abdomens, multiple reports were made of fistula formation as the result of applying negative pressure directly on the intestine.[45] A prospective randomized study of patients undergoing vacuum-assisted fascial closure versus mesh closure showed a significantly higher incidence of ECF associated with the vacuum-assisted device.[46] In addition, patients who were treated with a vacuum-assisted device for an existing ECF showed an increase in the development of new fistulas,[47] raising significant concerns regarding its use in these patient populations. The role of negative pressure wound therapy (NPWT) in both the management and etiology of ECF remains controversial; however, there are patients who can benefit from this therapy, yet selection remains difficult.[3,48,49] Negative pressure dressings have been without a doubt a significant advance in the care of complex wounds.

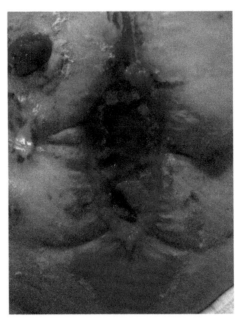

Fig. 2. This patient developed a postoperative deep enteroatmospheric fistula. There is obvious skin irritation and excoriation from poor control of the fistula effluent.

Manufacturers have devised alternate sponges and recommended decreasing the amount of suction applied to the wound bed in an attempt to decrease the incidence of ECF. A small series has demonstrated improved wound contracture and healing and there have been isolated reports of faster healing when using these devices, yet there remains no definitive answer regarding vacuum assistance.

ENTEROATMOSPHERIC FISTULA

Although EAF (**Fig. 3**) can be viewed as part of the spectrum of ECF, it has several unique characteristics that deserve discussion under a separate heading. In this discussion, coloatmospheric fistula and EAF have been grouped under the same heading of EAF. Unlike many postsurgical complications, EAF is often obvious when it occurs. One is typically in a situation in which a patient is being managed with an open abdomen for at least several days. Despite the best efforts to ensure that the exposed bowel is kept moist and that trauma to the viscera is avoided, a small erosion occurs in a segment of hollow viscera, leading to drainage of intestinal content into the wound. Any attempt to perform simple suture closure of the bowel is ill advised, as it almost always fails and results in a larger opening in the bowel wall.

EAF occurs most commonly in the setting of an open abdomen related to trauma and damage control laparotomy, decompressive laparotomy in the setting of high intra-abdominal pressure, or elective surgery "gone wrong," with resulting anastomotic leak or missed enterotomy. It also develops in patients who present with an acute abdominal septic process, in whom abdominal closure cannot be achieved at the completion of laparotomy secondary to bowel edema, and in those with large fascial dehiscences where remaining fascial quality prohibits effective abdominal wall closure, resulting in the open abdomen.

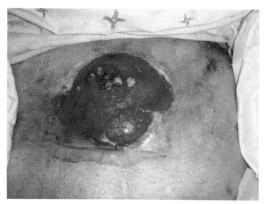

Fig. 3. This patient developed a superficial enteroatmospheric fistula after adhesiolysis and ventral hernia repair. Despite prolonged nonoperative care and repeated attempts at surgical reconstruction, the fistula recurred and persists.

Resolution of an EAF, either spontaneously or operatively, involves a lengthy and labor-intensive process. This process can be arbitrarily broken down into phases of treatment, as has been done by many investigators.[4,50] Regardless of the specifics of any particular management scheme, they all tend to be based on a few sound tenets: recognition and stabilization, anatomic definition/decision, and definitive surgery if needed.[4] This management scheme is similar to that used in the care of an ECF. Major differences are encountered in terms of effluent control, potential prevention, and the complexity of reconstructive surgery. The remainder of this article addresses the above-mentioned issues with specific attention dedicated to several areas of controversy surrounding the management of EAF.

PREVENTION

It is important to stress that the best way to approach an EAF is to prevent its occurrence altogether (**Fig. 4**). Although this disastrous event may be unavoidable, there are clearly factors that increase its risk such as having an open abdomen for a prolonged time. Some believe that the risk of EAF formation is also increased in patients who have an open abdomen for reasons other than trauma; however, a 2010 report showed that this is not true.[51] Every attempt should be made to close the open abdomen as soon as possible. Although there is an obvious lack of randomized data proving that an increased duration of bowel exposure to the outside environment results in an increased rate of EAF formation, this is clearly the consensus.[52,53] A report published in 2005 reviewing complications experienced in 344 damage-control laparotomies showed a higher rate of complications, including EAF, if the abdomen was left open longer than 8 days.[54]

The abdomen may not simply be closed at a time of the surgeon's choosing. Typically, one has to wait for resolution of visceral edema so that fascial closure can be achieved without leading to intra-abdominal hypertension. There are several reported techniques to potentially reduce the rate of EAF formation in the abdomen left open, and there are also several methods reported to decrease time to closure in these patients. Schecter and colleagues[55] advocate covering the viscera with a nonadherent drape and performing a skin-only closure as an intermediate when fascial reapproximation is not possible. Although this seems intuitive, it is based more on expert

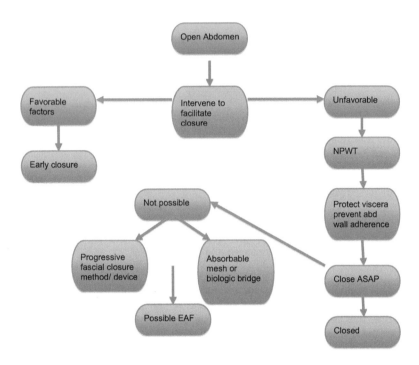

This algorithm is not meant to be exclusive of other methods. It is simply a suggested system of management

Fig. 4. Algorithm of one scheme that may be useful in preventing fistulization in the patient managed with an open abdomen.

opinion than on any data and may result in repetitive trauma to the skin if multiple reoperations are required before definitive closure.

The planned ventral hernia (PVH) approach uses absorbable polyglactin mesh to create a fascial bridge, effectively covering the bowel. If enough skin is available, it can be closed over drains placed between the absorbable mesh and the skin, resulting in a closed peritoneal cavity but a guaranteed ventral hernia in the future. This method was once popular but has fallen to a less-favored position because of the availability of NPWT, biologic meshes, and other early fascial closure techniques. The use of NPWT devices in close contact with the bowel is somewhat controversial. Initial success was tempered by concern over creating EAFs and the potential of promoting anastomotic leakage. Several later reports have either refuted these concerns or have even compared NPWT to absorbable mesh closure in patients with an open abdomen and have shown superior results in the NPWT group.[56–58] On the downside, a prospective randomized trial comparing NPWT closure to the use of absorbable mesh in this setting showed a higher rate of fistula formation in the NPWT group (21% vs 5%), but this was not statistically significant given the small number of patients in the trial.[46]

One issue that can plague any effort to achieve early fascial closure is progressive retraction of the rectus and oblique muscles laterally while the abdomen is left open (**Fig. 5**). Even with a reduction in visceral edema, this retraction continues to occur until the linea alba is reapproximated in the midline. Although there are many techniques available to prevent abdominal wall retraction, some have been shown in the literature to assist in achieving early (faster) abdominal wall closure.[59–63] All these methods have in common the use of some sort of mesh material fixed to fascial edges with

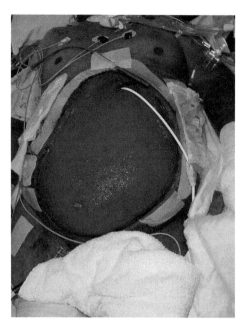

Fig. 5. One cost associated with leaving the abdomen open for a prolonged period. Unopposed lateral forces from the oblique muscles results in a large rectus diastasis.

progressive tightening at the midline as visceral edema resolves. NPWT is used as an outer wound dressing over the top of the mesh bridge to control fluids and exudate. A key aspect of these techniques is the use of a nonadherent layer or sheet over the viscera inside the peritoneal cavity to prevent adhesions to the anterior abdominal wall that would otherwise potentially result in a frozen abdomen.

In cases in which several days have passed and early closure seems impractical, one may choose to use biologic mesh bridges to achieve fascial "closure" with either skin reapproximation over drains or NPWT over top of the biologic graft. Although this has been shown to result in a high rate of incisional hernia formation,[64,65] it achieves the goal of closure over the viscera and has been shown to result in a low rate of bowel fistulization.[66] It is imperative that an experienced member of the surgical team be present during dressing changes for the patient with an open laparotomy wound. This practice can ensure the avoidance of trauma to the underlying viscera and the early recognition of areas of deserosalization that are likely precursors of an EAF. Girard and colleagues[67] reported securing of human acellular dermal matrix sheets to areas of intestinal deserosalization with fibrin glue. This procedure was done in 2 patients thought to be at risk for EAF, which ultimately did not occur in either. The use of this method has also been reported to be successful in closing small EAFs.[68,69]

As previously stated, nutritional optimization is central to the care of a patient with a gastrointestinal fistula. However, it is also a key component in the prevention of EAF. A patient with an open abdomen is in an extreme catabolic state with increased nutritional requirements. The benefits of enteral nutrition over parenteral nutrition are well established in surgical patients, and the use of early (less than or equal to 4 days after laparotomy) enteral nutrition has been shown to result in a statistically significant reduction in the rate of EAF as well as a faster time to abdominal closure.[70]

EFFLUENT CONTROL/SKIN PROTECTION

A poorly controlled EAF is a nightmare for patients and everyone involved in their care. It is a source of embarrassment and discomfort for the patient and frustration for the surgeon and results in the consumption of a tremendous amount of nursing and disposable medical resources. Early control of EAF output is critical, as contact between the skin and drainage results in significant skin damage that may limit options for subsequent control. A sound first step is to stop any and all oral intake. Bowel rest likely does not eliminate EAF output but significantly reduces the quantity. Use of a nasogastric tube for intermittent suction may also aid in reducing the quantity of the effluent, although again, this plays an indeterminate role. In most cases, NPWT has already been used, and simple continuation of this is all that is needed to obtain early control. EAFs that result in higher effluent output often overwhelm NPWT systems, resulting in the requirement for dressing changes on a daily basis or even more frequently. This situation can overwhelm both manpower and resources, requiring advanced methods of control (**Figs. 6** and **7**). The involvement of an enterostomal therapist or experienced wound care team cannot be overemphasized.[71] If the patient is being cared for in a facility without these resources, transfer to a higher level of care should certainly be considered.

There are several options available for skin protection using any of a variety of topical skin barriers. The enterostomal therapist/wound care team is familiar with the available options, and these materials should be used early. Fistuloclysis is a feeding strategy used with proximal EAFs, in which the effluent is reinstilled into the distal limb of the fistula. To refeed biliopancreatic secretions, they must be effectively controlled and collected. This process may be possible through the use of

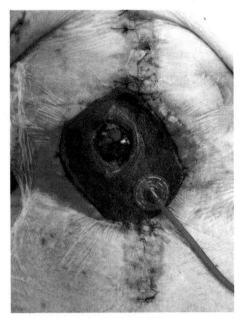

Fig. 6. A useful modification of an NPWT system. Sponge material is fashioned into a "donut" that is used to "dam" off the fistula, allowing effective effluent control with improved healing of the surrounding tissues. Stoma paste and powder can be used to improve isolation of the fistula.

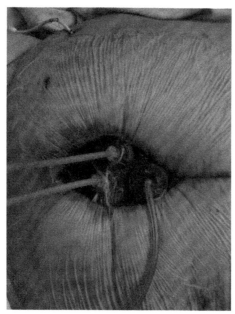

Fig. 7. In this case, the team has used baby bottle nipples and soft drainage tubes to isolate two2 enteroatmospheric fistulas in combination with a negative pressure dressing.

nasogastric tubes and NPWT systems but often is a difficult task. Poor control of gastrointestinal secretions leads to a frustrated patient and nursing staff and ultimately causes the fistula to remain open.

Aggressive effort toward the above-mentioned goals is warranted immediately and may require considerable thought. Several investigators have developed methods and systems, simply out of need, to address these concerns.[72–78] Creation of a "floating stoma" has been reported and may be useful in specific circumstances.[79] All these methods address a few simple ideas: "dam off" the EAF from the surrounding bowel or granulation tissue, provide NPWT to the surrounding tissues to assist with healing and exudate control, protect the surrounding skin to assist with dressing adherence and use in future surgery, and prevent trauma to the underlying viscera to eliminate the potential for additional EAF. Any system that can address all these concerns is effective, but none specifically designed for the purpose of EAF control has been marketed. It therefore requires considerable effort from the care team to design a custom device for a particular patient and to ensure its effective use on a daily basis.

In cases in which effluent control is simply impossible with NPWT-based wound care systems, the only remaining option may be the use of what amounts to a large stoma appliance, or wound manager (**Fig. 8**).[78] These devices can be custom cut to the size and shape of the open wound and function much like a standard ostomy appliance. They come in a variety of sizes and are marketed by at least 2 companies. If the surrounding skin is in good shape, a watertight seal is maintained, with effective collection of effluent in a large pouch. Despite continued contact with gastrointestinal secretions, granulation tissue continues to form over the underlying viscera, and the wound contracts over time. The wound appliance should be replaced with a fresh one as needed or every 4 to 5 days, much like and ostomy appliance is managed. Changes should be as infrequent as possible to avoid irritation or damage to the underlying skin.

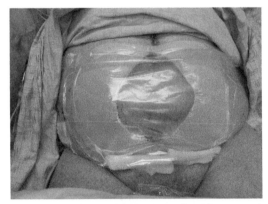

Fig. 8. When all other methods of control fail, a wound appliance can be custom fashioned to the shape of the wound to collect effluent. It functions much like a standard ostomy appliance.

TIMING OF SURGERY

Selection of the appropriate time to perform surgical reconstruction of an EAF that does not close spontaneously is critical. This area is controversial at best, and there are no level I data to support any specific period of delay before an attempt at closure of an EAF or abdominal wall reconstruction (AWR). Most experienced surgeons agree that a wait of at least 3 months after the initial laparotomy or fistula formation would be advised before any attempt at operative repair. This period allows for intra-abdominal adhesions to soften, inflammatory processes to resolve, and reduction in the risk of iatrogenic bowel injury during the reparative procedure. In patients who have had split-thickness skin grafting directly over the bowel, one would typically defer definitive surgery until the graft was no longer adherent to the underlying viscera; this is determined with a simple "pinch" test (**Fig. 9**) by pinching the skin graft between the index finger and thumb to see if it lifts freely from the intestine underneath. In general, this takes longer than 3 months and can take up to a year before conditions are ideal for proceeding with surgery.

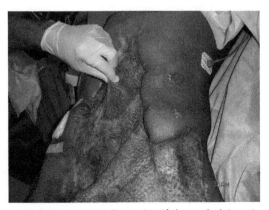

Fig. 9. The "pinch" test is being used to determine if the underlying viscera is free from the previously placed split-thickness skin graft.

Various investigators have reported delays that range between 2 and 929 days from initial temporary abdominal closure to attempted definitive reconstruction,[80–83] with mean times to attempted reconstruction of 311 days,[81] 184 days,[82] and 585 days.[83] Owing to the retrospective nature of these studies, it is difficult to relate the success of a reconstructive effort with the timing of surgery, but it is clear that a waiting period of 6 months or longer is common. Contrary to these reports, another investigator suggests that a delay of longer than 12 months may be associated with increased loss of domain, thereby making a tension-free repair more difficult, leading to an increased recurrence.[80] These studies included many patients who did not have EAFs but simply required AWR after management with a PVH strategy after an open abdomen. It is clear that any reconstructive attempt must be well planned and that the timing is intimately related to the resolution of inflammation, softening of the surrounding tissues, improvement in nutritional status, and overall fitness of the patient. Surgical judgment based on these multiple factors is likely the key to success.

ABDOMINAL WALL RECONSTRUCTION

What often really sets EAF apart from ECF is the extent of the associated abdominal wall defect and consideration of how to address this aspect. Reconstruction of the abdominal wall is a complex and high-risk procedure and is a necessary component of the surgical treatment of EAF in most cases. When performing definitive surgery for EAF or ECF, one immediate goal is to obtain closure of the abdomen over the visceral repair. Exposure of the bowel to the environment is one factor that likely leads to the formation of an EAF and must be avoided at all costs. The approach to closure of the abdominal wall is dictated in part by the decision to stage the repair or not. There is no ideal technique or simple approach to AWR. Component separation techniques (CST) and flap reconstructions tend to be technically demanding and are associated with an increased incidence of wound problems depending on the approach used. However, they can provide a functional AWR. Simple mesh underlay closure of fascial defects effects an acceptable hernia repair but often leaves the patient with a large area of laxity on the anterior abdominal wall. The lack of a functional anterior abdominal wall may limit their physical activity in the future, and the finished appearance may be cosmetically inferior. It is important to consider a patient's functional status and expectations when determining the approach to be used for AWR/hernia repair.

The CST originally popularized by Ramirez and colleagues[84] involves separating the rectus muscle from the posterior rectus sheath and the external oblique muscle from the internal oblique muscle, resulting in medial advancement of approximately 5 cm at the epigastrium, 10 cm at the waistline, and 3 cm in the suprapubic region unilaterally. This procedure is coupled with mesh reinforcement and restores a dynamic and functional abdominal wall. There are several reports in the literature on the success of CST in the management of large ventral hernias, revealing rates of hernia recurrence from 6% to 52%.[84–97] It may seem intuitive, but it is worth stating that larger hernia defects are more likely to recur and are more likely to require mesh-bridging techniques whether or not CST is used. Ideally, CST is used to facilitate reapproximation of the rectus complex in the midline with some sort of mesh buttress. Some defects are so large that bridging is still required even after performance of component separation. One can expect higher recurrence rates in these scenarios.

A randomized comparison of CST to prosthetic mesh closure with an expanded polytetrafluoroethylene (PTFE) patch in 39 patients[92] showed that wound complications were more frequent in the prosthetic group and 38% of the patients with wounds closed with mesh required its removal later because of infectious complications.

Recurrent hernia was noted in 52% of those undergoing CST and in 36% of those with prosthetic repair. Although it is difficult to draw definitive conclusions from this small study, the 2 methods were statistically equivalent in this group. Several minor modifications of the CST technique have been reported in the literature with varying success rates.[88,89,95,98] All these reports involved either single cases or small groups of patients. There has been a surge of interest in the use of the posterior CST[95] likely related to the ability to exploit the retrorectus space for placement of mesh reinforcement. Many of those who were major proponents of the classic anterior CST have shifted to the posterior approach.

Use of CST may assist in AWR by increasing abdominal domain. Comparisons of preoperative and postoperative CT scans of the abdomen and pelvis after CST repair of large abdominal wall hernias with associated loss of domain have shown significant increases in the intra-abdominal volume without any significant change in diaphragmatic height.[99] It may be possible to restore lost domain without the unfavorable result of pulmonary compromise secondary to a loss of thoracic volume.

One of the major criticisms of the anterior CST approach is the large bilateral skin flaps that result from the dissection necessary for exposure during the procedure. Flap complications comprise most of the wound occurrences noted in this procedure. Several approaches have been devised to avoid the seroma and potential infections that are common. The use of fibrin sealant has been shown to reduce seroma and wound infection rates in patients undergoing traditional anterior CST.[96] Placing numerous "quilting" mattress sutures has been described to eliminate dead space with the potential decrease in seroma formation but has not been studied prospectively. Rosen and colleagues[97] described the use of a laparoscopic CST in 7 patients that altogether eliminates the large flaps created using the open technique. The technique is similar to that used in totally extra-peritoneal pre-peritoneal (TEPP) laparoscopic inguinal hernia repair. Release of Scarpa fascia should also be performed with this approach, although care must be taken not to divide the linea semilunaris itself. After performance of the CST portion of the case laparoscopically, the midline may be reconstructed using either a laparoscopic or open approach; that would be necessary in all patients with EAF treated with a single-stage procedure. Short-term follow-up of patients treated with this technique has shown acceptable outcomes. Laparoscopic CST has been shown to be inferior for mobility in a porcine model, as it yielded only 86% of the medial mobilization of the rectus that was achieved with the open technique.[100] In cadavers, both have been shown to be equivalent.[101] Another minimally invasive method of achieving a lateral release has been described by creating small tunnels from the midline incision instead of large flaps.[102] Although this technique involves approach through a large midline incision, it avoids the creation of large flaps with their attendant wound morbidity, potentially making it ideal in the case of single-stage repair of EAF. Laparoscopic and other minimally invasive approaches to component separation are new and no randomized comparisons of these techniques to traditional techniques have been undertaken. These approaches are likely useful in achieving the goal of a functional abdominal wall while avoiding some of the morbidity associated with extensive open procedures.

SUMMARY

The entities of ECF and EAF remain a formidable challenge to surgeons facing affected patients. Awareness of its causes, contributing factors, potential preventive measures, and various management strategies are crucial to achieving optimal outcomes in the care of these complex patients. Owing to a lack of high-quality evidence supporting any particular regimen of care, the surgeon is required to exercise skillful judgment in treating these individuals.

REFERENCES

1. Sepehripour S, Papagrigoriadis S. A systematic review of the benefit of total parenteral nutrition in the management of enterocutaneous fistulas. Minerva Chir 2010;65(5):577–85.
2. Martinez JL, Luque-de-Leon E, Mier J, et al. Systematic management of postoperative enterocutaneous fistulas: factors related to outcomes. World J Surg 2008;32(3):436–43 [discussion: 44].
3. Draus JM Jr, Huss SA, Harty NJ, et al. Enterocutaneous fistula: are treatments improving? Surgery 2006;140(4):570–6 [discussion: 6–8].
4. Schecter WP. Management of enterocutaneous fistulas. Surg Clin North Am 2011;91(3):481–91.
5. Memon AS, Siddiqui FG. Causes and management of postoperative enterocutaneous fistulas. J Coll Physicians Surg Pak 2004;14(1):25–8.
6. Evenson AR, Fischer JE. Current management of enterocutaneous fistula. J Gastrointest Surg 2006;10(3):455–64.
7. Edmunds LH Jr, Williams GM, Welch CE. External fistulas arising from the gastro-intestinal tract. Ann Surg 1960;152:445–71.
8. Levy E, Frileux P, Cugnenc PH, et al. High-output external fistulae of the small bowel: management with continuous enteral nutrition. Br J Surg 1989;76(7): 676–9.
9. Campos AC, Andrade DF, Campos GM, et al. A multivariate model to determine prognostic factors in gastrointestinal fistulas. J Am Coll Surg 1999;188(5): 483–90.
10. Soeters PB, Ebeid AM, Fischer JE. Review of 404 patients with gastrointestinal fistulas. Impact of parenteral nutrition. Ann Surg 1979;190(2):189–202.
11. Reber HA, Roberts C, Way LW, et al. Management of external gastrointestinal fistulas. Ann Surg 1978;188(4):460–7.
12. Schecter WP, Hirshberg A, Chang DS, et al. Enteric fistulas: principles of management. J Am Coll Surg 2009;209(4):484–91.
13. Hwang RF, Schwartz RW. Enterocutaneous fistulas: current diagnosis and management. Curr Surg 2000;57(5):443–5.
14. Fazio VW. Intestinal fistula. Atlas of colorectal surgery. New York: Churchill Livingstone; 1996. p. 363–77.
15. Lynch AC, Delaney CP, Senagore AJ, et al. Clinical outcome and factors predictive of recurrence after enterocutaneous fistula surgery. Ann Surg 2004;240(5): 825–31.
16. Berry SM, Fischer JE. Enterocutaneous fistulas. Curr Probl Surg 1994;31(6): 469–566.
17. Makhdoom ZA, Komar MJ, Still CD. Nutrition and enterocutaneous fistulas. J Clin Gastroenterol 2000;31(3):195–204.
18. Chapman R, Foran R, Dunphy JE. Management of intestinal fistulas. Am J Surg 1964;108:157–64.
19. Dudrick SJ, Maharaj AR, McKelvey AA. Artificial nutritional support in patients with gastrointestinal fistulas. World J Surg 1999;23(6):570–6.
20. Aguirre A, Fischer JE, Welch CE. The role of surgery and hyperalimentation in therapy of gastrointestinal-cutaneous fistulae. Ann Surg 1974;180(4): 393–401.

21. Sitges-Serra A, Jaurrieta E, Sitges-Creus A. Management of postoperative enterocutaneous fistulas: the roles of parenteral nutrition and surgery. Br J Surg 1982;69(3):147–50.
22. Zera RT, Bubrick MP, Sternquist JC, et al. Enterocutaneous fistulas. Effects of total parenteral nutrition and surgery. Dis Colon Rectum 1983;26(2):109–12.
23. Chaudhry CR. The challenge of enterocutaneous fistulae. MJAFI 2004;60(3):235–68.
24. Dubose JJ, Lundy JB. Enterocutaneous fistulas in the setting of trauma and critical illness. Clin Colon Rectal Surg 2010;23(3):182–9.
25. Lubana PS, Aggarwal G, Aggarwal H, et al. Serum transferrin levels - a predictive marker of spontaneous closure and mortality in patients with enterocutaneous fistulae. Arab J Gastroenterol 2010;11:212–4.
26. Kuvshinoff BW, Brodish RJ, McFadden DW, et al. Serum transferrin as a prognostic indicator of spontaneous closure and mortality in gastrointestinal cutaneous fistulas. Ann Surg 1993;217(6):615–22 [discussion: 22–3].
27. Cox-Reijven PL, van Kreel B, Soeters PB. Bioelectrical impedance measurements in patients with gastrointestinal disease: validation of the spectrum approach and a comparison of different methods for screening for nutritional depletion. Am J Clin Nutr 2003;78(6):1111–9.
28. Hesse U, Ysebaert D, de Hemptinne B. Role of somatostatin-14 and its analogues in the management of gastrointestinal fistulae: clinical data. Gut 2001;49(Suppl 4):iv11–21.
29. di Costanzo J, Cano N, Martin J, et al. Treatment of external gastrointestinal fistulas by a combination of total parenteral nutrition and somatostatin. JPEN J Parenter Enteral Nutr 1987;11(5):465–70.
30. Sheppard M, Shapiro B, Pimstone B, et al. Metabolic clearance and plasma half-disappearance time of exogenous somatostatin in man. J Clin Endocrinol Metab 1979;48(1):50–3.
31. Jenkins SA, Nott DM, Baxter JN. Fluctuations in the secretion of pancreatic enzymes between consecutive doses of octreotide: implications for the management of fistulae. Eur J Gastroenterol Hepatol 1995;7(3):255–8.
32. Torres AJ, Landa JI, Moreno-Azcoita M, et al. Somatostatin in the management of gastrointestinal fistulas. A multicenter trial. Arch Surg 1992;127(1):97–9 [discussion: 100].
33. Barnes SM, Kontny BG, Prinz RA. Somatostatin analog treatment of pancreatic fistulas. Int J Pancreatol 1993;14(2):181–8.
34. Hild P, Dobroschke J, Henneking K, et al. Treatment of enterocutaneous fistulas with somatostatin. Lancet 1986;2(8507):626.
35. Emory RE Jr, Ilstrup D, Grant CS. Somatostatin in the management of gastrointestinal fistulas. Arch Surg 1992;127(11):1365.
36. Sancho JJ, di Costanzo J, Nubiola P, et al. Randomized double-blind placebo-controlled trial of early octreotide in patients with postoperative enterocutaneous fistula. Br J Surg 1995;82(5):638–41.
37. Hernandez-Aranda JC, Gallo-Chico B, Flores-Ramirez LA, et al. Treatment of enterocutaneous fistula with or without octreotide and parenteral nutrition. Nutr Hosp 1996;11(4):226–9 [in Spanish].
38. Pederzoli P, Bassi C, Falconi M, et al. Conservative treatment of external pancreatic fistulas with parenteral nutrition alone or in combination with continuous intravenous infusion of somatostatin, glucagon or calcitonin. Surg Gynecol Obstet 1986;163(5):428–32.

39. Korelitz BI, Present DH. Favorable effect of 6-mercaptopurine on fistulae of Crohn's disease. Dig Dis Sci 1985;30(1):58–64.
40. Hanauer SB, Smith MB. Rapid closure of Crohn's disease fistulas with continuous intravenous cyclosporin A. Am J Gastroenterol 1993;88(5):646–9.
41. Present DH, Rutgeerts P, Targan S, et al. Infliximab for the treatment of fistulas in patients with Crohn's disease. N Engl J Med 1999;340(18):1398–405.
42. Viscido A, Habib FI, Kohn A, et al. Infliximab in refractory pouchitis complicated by fistulae following ileo-anal pouch for ulcerative colitis. Aliment Pharmacol Ther 2003;17(10):1263–71.
43. Satya R, Satya RJ. Successful treatment of an enterocutaneous fistula with an anal fistula plug after an abdominal stab wound. J Vasc Interv Radiol 2010; 21(3):414–5.
44. Lundy JB, Fischer JE. Historical perspectives in the care of patients with enterocutaneous fistula. Clin Colon Rectal Surg 2010;23(3):133–41.
45. Fischer JE. A cautionary note: the use of vacuum-assisted closure systems in the treatment of gastrointestinal cutaneous fistula may be associated with higher mortality from subsequent fistula development. Am J Surg 2008; 196(1):1–2.
46. Bee TK, Croce MA, Magnotti LJ, et al. Temporary abdominal closure techniques: a prospective randomized trial comparing polyglactin 910 mesh and vacuum-assisted closure. J Trauma 2008;65(2):337–42 [discussion: 42–4].
47. Rao M, Burke D, Finan PJ, et al. The use of vacuum-assisted closure of abdominal wounds: a word of caution. Colorectal Dis 2007;9(3):266–8.
48. Erdmann D, Drye C, Heller L, et al. Abdominal wall defect and enterocutaneous fistula treatment with the vacuum-assisted closure (V.A.C.) system. Plast Reconstr Surg 2001;108(7):2066–8.
49. Cro C, George KJ, Donnelly J, et al. Vacuum assisted closure system in the management of enterocutaneous fistulae. Postgrad Med J 2002;78(920):364–5.
50. Polk TM, Schwab CW. Metabolic and nutritional support of the enterocutaneous fistula patient: a three-phase approach. World J Surg 2012;36(3):524–33.
51. Kritayakirana K, Maggio PM, Brundage S, et al. Outcomes and complications of open abdomen technique for managing non-trauma patients. J Emerg Trauma Shock 2010;3(2):118–22.
52. Bjorck M, D'Amours SK, Hamilton AE. Closure of the open abdomen. Am Surg 2011;77(Suppl 1):S58–61.
53. Fabian TC. Damage control in trauma: laparotomy wound management acute to chronic. Surg Clin North Am 2007;87(1):73–93.
54. Miller RS, Morris JA Jr, Diaz JJ Jr, et al. Complications after 344 damage-control open celiotomies. J Trauma 2005;59(6):1365–71.
55. Schecter WP, Ivatury RR, Rotondo MF, et al. Open abdomen after trauma and abdominal sepsis: a strategy for management. J Am Coll Surg 2006;203(3): 390–6.
56. Prichayudh S, Sriussadaporn S, Samorn P, et al. Management of open abdomen with an absorbable mesh closure. Surg Today 2011;41(1):72–8.
57. Stevens P. Vacuum-assisted closure of laparostomy wounds: a critical review of the literature. Int Wound J 2009;6(4):259–66.
58. Shaikh IA, Ballard-Wilson A, Yalamarthi S, et al. Use of topical negative pressure in assisted abdominal closure does not lead to high incidence of enteric fistulae. Colorectal Dis 2010;12(9):931–4.
59. Hedderich GS, Wexler MJ, McLean AP, et al. The septic abdomen: open management with Marlex mesh with a zipper. Surgery 1986;99(4):399–408.

60. Acosta S, Bjarnason T, Petersson U, et al. Multicentre prospective study of fascial closure rate after open abdomen with vacuum and mesh-mediated fascial traction. Br J Surg 2011;98(5):735–43.

61. Koss W, Ho HC, Yu M, et al. Preventing loss of domain: a management strategy for closure of the "open abdomen" during the initial hospitalization. J Surg Educ 2009;66(2):89–95.

62. Vertrees A, Greer L, Pickett C, et al. Modern management of complex open abdominal wounds of war: a 5-year experience. J Am Coll Surg 2008;207(6): 801–9.

63. Kafie FE, Tessier DJ, Williams RA, et al. Serial abdominal closure technique (the "SAC" procedure): a novel method for delayed closure of the abdominal wall. Am Surg 2003;69(2):102–5.

64. Blatnik J, Jin J, Rosen M. Abdominal hernia repair with bridging acellular dermal matrix - an expensive hernia sac. Am J Surg 2008;196:47–50.

65. De Moya M, Dunham M, Inaba K, et al. Long-term outcome of acelluar dermal matrix when used for large traumatic open abdomen. J Trauma 2008;65:349–53.

66. Scott BG, Welsh FJ, Pham HQ, et al. Early aggressive closure of the open abdomen. J Trauma 2006;60(1):17–22.

67. Girard S, Sideman M, Spain DA. A novel approach to the problem of intestinal fistulization arising in patients managed with open peritoneal cavities. Am J Surg 2002;184(2):166–7.

68. Becker HP, Willms A, Schwab R. Small bowel fistulas and the open abdomen. Scand J Surg 2007;96(4):263–71.

69. Jamshidi R, Schecter WP. Biological dressings for the management of enteric fistulas in the open abdomen: a preliminary report. Arch Surg 2007;142(8): 793–6.

70. Collier B, Guillamondegui O, Cotton B, et al. Feeding the open abdomen. JPEN J Parenter Enteral Nutr 2007;31(5):410–5.

71. Harris C, Shannon R. An innovative enterostomal therapy nurse model of community wound care delivery: a retrospective cost-effectiveness analysis. J Wound Ostomy Continence Nurs 2008;35(2):169–83.

72. Wright A, Wright M. Bedside management of an abdominal wound containing an enteroatmospheric fistula: a case report. Ostomy Wound Manage 2011; 57(1):28–32.

73. Ramsay PT, Mejia VA. Management of enteroatmospheric fistulae in the open abdomen. Am Surg 2010;76(6):637–9.

74. Layton B, Dubose J, Nichols S, et al. Pacifying the open abdomen with concomitant intestinal fistula: a novel approach. Am J Surg 2010;199(4):e48–50.

75. Al-Khoury G, Kaufman D, Hirshberg A. Improved control of exposed fistula in the open abdomen. J Am Coll Surg 2008;206(2):397–8.

76. Goverman J, Yelon JA, Platz JJ, et al. The "fistula-VAC," a technique for management of enterocutaneous fistulae arising within the open abdomen: a report of 5 cases. J Trauma 2006;60(2):428–31.

77. O'Brien B, Landis-Erdman J, Erwin-Toth P. Nursing management of multiple enterocutaneous fistulae located in the center of a large open abdominal wound: a case study. Ostomy Wound Manage 1998;44(1):20–4.

78. Geoghegan J, Robert K. The Convatec Wound Manager: a new stoma appliance. Br J Clin Pract 1990;44(12):750–1.

79. Subramanian MJ, Liscum KR, Hirshberg A. The floating stoma: a new technique for controlling exposed fistulae in abdominal trauma. J Trauma 2002; 53:386–8.

80. Jernigan TW, Fabian TC, Croce MA, et al. Staged management of giant abdominal wall defects. Ann Surg 2003;238:349–57.

81. Joels CS, Vanderveer AS, Newcomb WL, et al. Abdominal wall reconstruction after temporary abdominal closure: a ten-year review. Surg Innov 2006;13: 223–30.

82. Dionigi G, Dionigi R, Rovera F, et al. Treatment of high output entero-cutaneous fistulae associated with large abdominal wall defects: single center experience. Int J Surg 2008;6:51–6.

83. Rodriguez ED, Bluebond-Langner R, Silverman RP, et al. Abdominal wall reconstruction following severe loss of domain: the R Adams Cowley Shock Trauma Center Algorithm. Plast Reconstr Surg 2007;120:669–80.

84. Ramirez OM, Ruas E, Dellon L. "Components separation" method for closure of abdominal-wall defects: an anatomic and clinical study. Plast Reconstr Surg 1990;86:519–26.

85. De Vries Reilingh TS, van Goor H, Charbon JA, et al. Repair of giant midline abdominal wall hernias: "components separation technique" versus prosthetic repair. World J Surg 2007;31:756–63.

86. Dragu A, Klein P, Unglaub F, et al. Tensiometry as a decision tool for abdominal wall reconstruction with component separation. World J Surg 2009;33: 1174–80.

87. Vargo D. Component separation in the management of the difficult abdominal wall. Am J Surg 2004;188:633–7.

88. Shabatian H, Lee D, Abbas MA. Components separation: a solution to complex abdominal wall defects. Am Surg 2008;74:912–6.

89. De Vries Reilingh TS, van Goor H, Rosman C, et al. "Components separation technique" for the repair of large abdominal wall hernias. J Am Coll Surg 2003;196:32–7.

90. Howdieshell TR, Proctor CD, Sternberg E, et al. Temporary abdominal closure followed by definitive abdominal wall reconstruction of the open abdomen. Am J Surg 2004;188:301–6.

91. Lowe JB, Lowe JB, Baty JD, et al. Risks associated with "components separation" for closure of complex abdominal wall defects. Plast Reconstr Surg 2003; 111:1276–83.

92. Ewart CJ, Lankford AB, Gamboa MG. Successful closure of abdominal wall hernias using components separation technique. Ann Plast Surg 2003;50: 269–74.

93. Carbonell AM, Cobb WS, Chen SM. Posterior components separation during retromuscular hernia repair. Hernia 2008;12:359–62.

94. Ennis LS, Young JS, Gampper TJ, et al. The "open-book" variation of component separation for repair of massive midline abdominal wall hernia. Am Surg 2003; 69:733–43.

95. Tobias AM, Low DW. The use of subfascial vicryl mesh buttress to aid in the closure of massive ventral hernias following damage-control laparotomy. Plast Reconstr Surg 2003;112:766–76.

96. Kingsnorth AN, Shahid MK, Valliattu AJ, et al. Open onlay mesh repair for major abdominal wall hernias with selective use of components separation and fibrin sealant. World J Surg 2008;32:26–30.

97. Rosen MJ, Jin J, McGee MF, et al. Laparoscopic component separation in the single-stage treatment of infected abdominal wall prosthetic removal. Hernia 2007;11:435–40.

98. Stark B, Strigård K. Definitive reconstruction of full-thickness abdominal wall defects initially treated with skin grafting of exposed intestines. Hernia 2007; 11:533–6.

99. Hadad I, Small W, Dumanian GA. Repair of massive ventral hernias with the separation of parts technique: reversal of the 'lost domain'. Am Surg 2009;75: 301–6.

100. Rosen MJ, Williams C, Jin J, et al. Laparoscopic versus open-component separation: a comparative analysis in a porcine model. Am J Surg 2007;194: 385–9.

101. Milburn ML, Shah PK, Friedman EB, et al. Laparoscopically assisted components separation technique for ventral incisional hernia repair. Hernia 2007;11: 157–61.

102. Maas SM, van Engeland M, Leeksma NG, et al. A modification of the "components separation" technique for closure of abdominal wall defects in the presence of an enterostomy. J Am Coll Surg 1999;189:138–40.

Colorectal Considerations in Pediatric Patients

David M. Gourlay, MD

KEYWORDS

- Pediatric colorectal disease • Hirschsprung disease
- Congenital anorectal malformations • Rectal prolapse • Meconium syndromes
- Intussusception • Pseudo-obstruction

KEY POINTS

- Many congenital anomalies treated in infancy predispose patients to constipation and fecal incontinence that, if inadequately managed, can lead to the need for further operative interventions later in life.
- Most colorectal procedures performed in newborn and pediatric patients are amenable to a minimally invasive approach.
- Almost all infants and toddlers and many pediatric patients have an open umbilical ring, making this an easy and safe point of initial access.
- The surgeon must pay close attention to intra-abdominal pressure and flow rates to prevent intra-abdominal hypertension as well as hypothermia.
- Until teenage years, circular stapling devices are often too large to be accommodated for a low rectal anastomosis, and hand-sewn techniques are used.

INTRODUCTION

The intent of this article is not to discuss all pediatric diseases of the colon and rectum, but rather those diseases a colorectal surgeon or general surgeon caring for these patients will either see in practice de novo or as an adult in long-term follow-up. Many congenital anomalies treated in infancy predispose patients to constipation and fecal incontinence that, if inadequately managed, can lead to the need for further operative interventions later in life. Many of the diseases discussed herein are commonly diagnosed in pediatric patients, but less common in adults and are therefore less familiar to the adult surgeon. The article is divided up based on the typical age of presentation and is intended to provide an overview of these diseases, their management, and long-term outcomes.

Division of Pediatric Surgery, Department of Surgery, Medical College of Wisconsin, 999 North 92nd Avenue, Suite 320, Milwaukee, WI 53226, USA
E-mail address: dgourlay@chw.org

Surg Clin N Am 93 (2013) 251–272
http://dx.doi.org/10.1016/j.suc.2012.09.017   **surgical.theclinics.com**

Neonatal Diseases

Hirschsprung disease

Etiology and presentation Hirschsprung disease is characterized by an absence of ganglion cells in the myenteric and submucosal plexuses, and occurs in approximately 1 in 5000 live births.[1] The absence of ganglion cells occurs as result of incomplete development and migration of neural crests cells within the intestine, leading to an aganglionic section of intestine lacking normal peristalsis. This failure of migration or development always occurs in a caudal to cranial direction, beginning in the internal anal sphincter and extending proximally for a variable length. Although a majority of patients with Hirschsprung disease have the aganglionic section limited to the rectosigmoid region, it may involve the entire colon as well as the small intestine in a small minority of patients. Hirschsprung disease may also be associated with areas of small and/or large intestine containing normal-appearing dysfunctional ganglion cells; this condition is referred to as intestinal neuronal dysplasia.

Most cases of Hirschsprung disease are sporadic, although approximately 10% will have a family history. Patients with a family history or associated syndromes more often have long-segment disease. There are several syndromes and genetic abnormalities associated with Hirschsprung disease including Down syndrome, multiple neuroendocrine neoplasia 2, and congenital central hypoventilation syndrome (Ondine's curse), among others. The commonality between Hirschsprung disease and these syndromes include genetic abnormalities in either the RET proto-oncogene or genes encoding for the endothelin receptors, among other possible candidates.

Hirschsprung disease presents in the first year of life in the majority of patients and presents with obstructive symptoms. It is important to keep in mind that the classic history of failure to pass meconium within the first 24 hours of life occurs in 95% of normal newborns, but only 10% of newborns with Hirschsprung disease. Physical examination reveals a normally located anus that, upon digital rectal examination, produces a memorable explosion of stool. Because of the obstruction, some newborns or infants present with enterocolitis as their first clinical symptoms. Hirschsprung enterocolitis can be life threatening, and should be considered in the differential diagnosis of any child with abdominal tenderness, leukocytosis, and bloody stools associated with this history of stooling difficulties.

In patients presenting later in life, Hirschsprung disease most commonly presents with profound constipation. A detailed history of stooling at birth and during infancy often demonstrates failure to pass meconium in the first 1–2 days of life along with an extended history of enemas and suppository use throughout infancy and childhood. As a consequence, these children often have a distended abdomen, are in the lower percentiles for weight by age, and have a rectum and colon full of stool on plain radiography.

In addition to plain radiographs, the diagnostic evaluation should include a rectal biopsy as well as a retrograde contrast study of the rectum and colon. Absence of ganglion cells and hypertrophied nerve trunks on rectal biopsy is diagnostic of Hirschsprung disease. Staining for acetylcholine esterase can assist in the diagnosis. In newborns and infants, suction rectal biopsy can be obtained at the bedside with minimal morbidity. One should provide the pathologist with 3–5 pieces of rectum-containing mucosa and submucosa from 1–2 cm above the dentate line to ensure an accurate diagnosis. In children beyond infancy, diagnosis is made by open rectal biopsy that involves a full-thickness, 1- to 2-cm strip of rectum taken from the posterior wall 1 cm above the dentate line. Retrograde contrast enema is helpful to exclude other diagnosis as well as provide an estimation of the transition zone. The classic findings (**Fig. 1**) include a transition zone characterized by proximal dilatation with a spastic distal segment, a rectosigmoid diameter ratio of less than 1, and retention of contrast for more than 24 hours. This classic radiologic description is often not apparent in the first few weeks of life; however, a contrast enema may still be useful to rule out other congenital abnormalities. These classic findings are also absent in older children, who commonly present with severe impaction causing dilatation of both the colon and rectum. Therefore, this should not be used alone to exclude the diagnosis of Hirschsprung disease in the absence of biopsy confirmation.

Anorectal manometry can be useful if the diagnosis remains in doubt. Anorectal manometry in patients with Hirschsprung disease demonstrates loss of the rectoanal inhibitory reflex (RAIR). The RAIR is a relaxation of the internal sphincteric complex that occurs normally with distension of the rectum. In patients with Hirschsprung disease, even after operative correction, the RAIR is absent. As part of the differential for this symptom complex, anal achalasia is included in the spectrum of Hirschsprung disease, and is characterized by the presence of ganglion cells on rectal biopsy, but with the absence of the RAIR on anorectal manometry.

Management The immediate management, whether in a newborn or child, is to evacuate the retained stool. In newborns and infants, this often easily accomplished with rectal irrigations of 10 mL/kg of normal saline 3–4 times per day using a soft rubber catheter. Feeding can resume once the obstructive picture has resolved. This regimen can easily be taught to parents to be used in the outpatient setting to prevent recurrent obstruction and allow for an elective, single-stage operation. Timing of the operation is debated, and there are advocates for performing surgical correction both in the immediate neonatal period as well as delayed until the infant is a few months of age. Two caveats to this controversy include those patients with either enterocolitis at presentation or long segment disease. Enterocolitis can be life threatening and requires

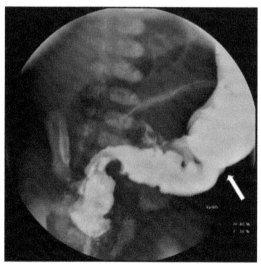

Fig. 1. An anteroposterior view of a retrograde contrast enema performed on a newborn with Hirschsprung disease. The arrow denotes the transition zone in the sigmoid colon. Note the proximal dilated sigmoid colon and the rectum in spasm giving a rectosigmoid ratio of less than 1.

prompt treatment with intravenous antibiotics, bowel rest, and rectal irrigations. In patients who do not immediately respond to this therapy, proximal diversion should be considered. Surgical pull-through should be delayed until several weeks after the enterocolitis has resolved. In addition, newborns who present with long segment disease often do not completely evacuate with rectal irrigations alone. Because they remain functionally obstructed, they require a leveling colostomy until definitive surgery at a later time.

Older children presenting with fecal impaction and diagnosed with Hirschsprung disease often require manual disimpaction. Water-soluble contrast enemas can be useful therapeutically to achieve complete disimpaction. These children may have such profound impaction they develop a nonfunctional mega-rectum requiring leveling colostomy at presentation. Whereas the aganglionic segment is often relatively short, it is typically difficult in these cases to determine function in the rectum and colon owing to the chronic dilatation. Therefore, definitive surgery is delayed for several weeks to months to allow for a better assessment of function of the defunctionalized colon and rectum by way of contrast studies to measure diameter and colonic motility studies to determine physiologic peristalsis.

Numerous operative procedures have been described for Hirschsprung, but the 3 most commonly performed are shown in **Fig. 2**. Each achieves the same goal: Removal of the aganglionic bowel with anastomosis of bowel containing ganglion cells to distal rectum while preserving the anal sphincter complex and anal canal. None of these procedures has consistently displayed better outcomes over the other, and in competent hands all have excellent outcomes. A full description of the operative procedure is not possible herein, but can be found elsewhere.[1] There are a few important principles that have a tremendous impact on long-term outcomes and must be obeyed. First, the anal canal and sphincteric complex must be left intact to avoid incontinence. Therefore, the anastomosis should be performed just above the dentate line. Second, the assistance of a competent pathologist to perform intraoperative frozen sections to assess the presence of ganglion cells is necessary to avoid leaving residual aganglionic bowel. The transition zone is often several centimeters long and irregular; therefore, the surgeon should provide the pathologist with multiple biopsies to ensure complete resection of the aganglionic bowel.[2] Each of the 3 procedures can

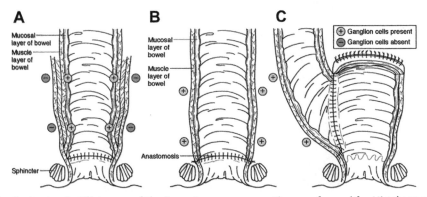

Fig. 2. Anatomic differences of the 3 most common operations performed for Hirschsprung disease. (*A*) The Soave procedure. (*B*) The Swenson procedure. (*C*) The Duhamel procedure. (*From* Dasgupta R, Langer JC. Hirschsprung disease. Curr Probl Surg 2004;41(12):949–88; with permission.)

be performed in a minimally invasive and single-stage fashion that employs a transanal anastomosis without diversion.

Early complications include those common to all operative procedures (bleeding, infection, injury to adjacent structures, anesthetic complications) as well as those specific to the bowel resection, including anastomotic leak and obstruction either owing to stricture or ischemia. These complications are the result of technical errors similar to those of any low anterior resection in an adult, and are managed in similar fashion.

Long-term outcomes and complications With appropriate care and informed patients/parents, most patients with Hirschsprung disease lead normal lives, with reasonably normal stool habits and a normal diet.[3] In 1 long-term follow-up study of adults treated surgically for Hirschsprung disease in childhood, 95% of adults reported to always have a sense of defecation and 92% reported the ability to distinguish the stool condition.[3] However, almost 10% reported severe periods of diarrhea, 5% reported severe constipation, and 5% severe soiling.

Most of these functional symptoms are in part related to the persistence of an aganglionic internal sphincter that predispose these patients to constipation and to overflow incontinence. This lack of normal anal sphincter function may increase the risk of enterocolitis in infants and toddlers, while increasing the risk of the development of a nonfunctional "mega-sigmoidrectum" in older children owing to untreated constipation. For all these reasons, long-term follow-up is necessary. Most symptoms of constipation can be treated without difficulty using stool softeners, enemas, and suppositories either occasionally or on a long-term basis. It must be emphasized to parents and older children that stooling at least once daily should be a benchmark and if not occurring should prompt a rectal irrigation or enema.

Postoperative enterocolitis Enterocolitis occurs in 17% to 50% of patients postoperatively and may not necessarily imply inadequate surgical treatment.[4] It is, however, uncommon after the age of 2 to 3 years. Treatment is as described. The surgeon should ensure the absence of a mechanical obstruction by performing a rectal examination and a contrast study. If recurrent enterocolitis occurs, the surgeon should consider further workup as described for obstructive complications.

Fecal incontinence True fecal incontinence should be uncommon provided the anal canal and sphincter complex are maintained during surgery. This is best determined by examination and anal–rectal manometry. Once diagnosed, these are not surgically correctable, and treatment may include use of a constipating bowel program and biofeedback training when the child is old enough. Most often, when fecal incontinence occurs, these structures are preserved and functional and incontinence is the result of fecal impaction and overflow incontinence. This is best identified by digital rectal examination and plain radiography to identify the presence of impacted stool. Treatment, once disimpaction has occurred, includes a bowel regimen as discussed to avoid further episodes of constipation. In those patients with long-standing constipation and a mega-sigmoidrectum, resection often alleviates refractory constipation. Permanent colostomy should be reserved for failures.

Obstructive symptoms Obstructive symptoms are common and most are self-limiting. Once mechanical obstruction is excluded with digital rectal examination and a retrograde contrast study, one should consider functional causes of obstruction. These include persistence of or acquired aganglionosis, a motility disorder, internal sphincter achalasia, and stool-holding behavior. An algorithm for the diagnostic workup and treatment is shown in **Fig. 3**. Intra-sphincteric injection of Botox in select patients with obstructive symptoms was reported to have a good response in 80% of patients to the initial treatment, although 69% required repeat treatment.[5] Children who fail to resolve their obstructive symptoms or who are lost to follow-up often present with mega-sigmoidrectum. In such cases, most require either permanent fecal diversion or preferably temporary diversion followed by resection of the mega-sigmoidrectum and a repeat pull-through procedure.

Meconium syndromes
Etiology and presentation Meconium syndromes include meconium ileus, meconium plug, and small left colon syndrome. Each is seen in the newborn period, although meconium ileus may result in a life-long intestinal disease. Each is associated with inspissated meconium in the intestine and present with signs and symptoms of obstruction in the neonatal period. The etiology of each disease is different and therefore is discussed separately.

    Meconium plug and small left colon syndrome Newborns with meconium plug are typically healthy, full-term newborns. Small left colon syndrome is occasionally used synonymously with meconium plug, but classically occurs in newborns of diabetic mothers. Both are believed to be the result of hypoperistalsis of the colon where the inspissated meconium is found. These 2 disease processes have similar presentations, treatment, and outcome. A water-soluble contrast enema in each case is diagnostic and therapeutic. Once the functional obstruction is resolved, no further long-term consequences should be expected and the newborn fed normally. Further episodes of constipation should prompt the surgeon to evaluate for Hirschsprung disease.

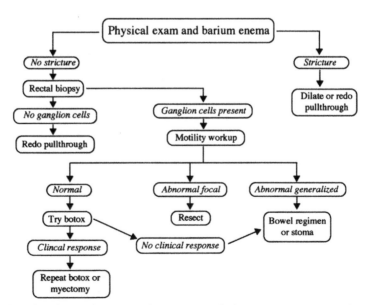

Fig. 3. Algorithm for evaluation and treatment of obstructive symptoms after surgical correction of Hirschsprung disease. (*From* Langer JC. Laparoscopic and transanal pull-through for Hirschsprung disease. Semin Pediatr Surg 2012;21(4):283–90; with permission.)

Meconium ileus Meconium Ileus is a consequence of a recessive genetic defect on the cystic fibrosis (CF) transmembrane receptor gene, of which there are now more than 800 different identified mutations. The incidence of CF in the United States is 1 in 2500 live births. Meconium ileus is the first presenting manifestation of CF in 10% to 20% affected newborns.[6] Each of the various genetic mutations in the CF transmembrane receptor gene results in abnormal chloride transport across epithelial cells affecting all organs with an epithelial lining. Although the respiratory manifestations of CF do not manifest until childhood, the pancreatic exocrine and intestine glandular function are often severely affected in utero. This results in secretion of hyperviscous mucus in combination with meconium containing high protein, low carbohydrate concentrations and low water content. This combination results in a thick and sticky meconium that is unable to pass through the ileocecal valve.

The presentation of meconium ileus can be classified as simple, complex, or meconium peritonitis. Often, these findings are noted in utero on ultrasonography and may prompt parental testing for the CF genetic mutation. Simple meconium ileus presents with signs and symptoms of intestinal obstruction without perforation. Digital rectal examination often yields pale white meconium. Plain radiographs classically have "soap bubbles" or a "ground glass" appearance. Complex meconium ileus and meconium peritonitis are the result of an in utero complication of simple meconium ileus: Volvulus or ischemia of the obstructed bowel leading to perforation. Often the perforation develops into a pseudocyst and/or atretic bowel. Depending on the timing of the in utero event, the newborn may present at birth clinically well (meconium ileus) or systemically ill (meconium peritonitis). In either case, newborns present with the signs, symptoms, and imaging findings of intestinal obstruction. Plain radiographs also demonstrate the presence of a pseudocyst—a very dilated, air-filled mass with microcalcifications. In a physiologically well newborn, a water-soluble contrast enema demonstrates a microcolon (owing to lack of use in utero) with inspissated pellets of meconium at the terminal ileum. Genetic testing for the CF transmembrane receptor genetic mutations recognizes more than 90% of the known mutations, but takes several days to return. The sweat chloride test is the diagnostic gold standard, yet again, is not diagnostically accurate until the newborn is 4 to 6 weeks of age, and does little in the acute period.[7]

Management Simple meconium ileus can almost always be managed nonoperatively. Proximal bowel decompression in combination with retrograde water-soluble contrast enema(s) to evacuate inspissated meconium can be successful in relieving the obstruction.[6,7] Provided the newborn remains physiologically well, this can be repeated over several days until complete evacuation of the inspissated meconium is accomplished. To aid in the clearance of inspissated meconium, one can use small volumes of 5 to 10% N-acetylcysteine via the orogastric tube 3 to 4 times daily.[7] Attempts at radiologic reduction are associated with a low risk of perforation; however, with prompt operative exploration, this has little impact on long-term outcome. Once the obstruction is relieved, enteral feeds and pancreatic enzyme replacement should be initiated.

Failed clearance of simple meconium ileus by radiologic means, complex meconium ileus, and meconium peritonitis require operative intervention. With simple meconium ileus, one should expect few if any adhesions. The goal of the operation is to completely evacuate the inspissated meconium. This can be often accomplished with a small distal enterotomy and lavage of the intestine with 1% N-acetylcysteine and expression of the meconium through the enterotomy.[7] Historically, a variety of different enterostomies have been proposed. Currently, simple closure of the enterotomy is most commonly practiced owing to the greater risk of complications associated with an enterostomy.[8] Enteral feeds and pancreatic enzyme replacement are started once the ileus has resolved. Recurrent inspissation occurs in upwards of 25% of patients and can be treated with water-soluble contrast enemas, as discussed.

Complex meconium ileus and meconium peritonitis tend to more often be associated with inflammatory adhesions. One should be prepared for blood transfusion and the need for temporary proximal diversion if the abdomen is too hostile. If possible, complete enterolysis, assessment of intestinal length and reestablishment of intestinal continuity after evacuation of all inspissated meconium should be the goal. This may require resection or tapering (in the case of in inadequate bowel length) of a bulbous nonfunctional proximal atretic segment. Enteral feeds and pancreatic enzyme replacement are started once the ileus has resolved. Temporary fecal diversion may be necessary, depending on the condition of the newborn during the operation. In the case of proximal diversion, successful reoperation is typically possible at 4 to 6 weeks postoperatively.

Long-term outcomes and complications Over the second part of the 20th century, mortality for surgically treated meconium ileus has decreased to nearly zero.[7] Long-term survival of patients with CF has also improved, with many surviving into the third and fourth decades of life.[9] Although most newborns with meconium ileus do well once the obstruction resolves and supplemental pancreatic enzymes are initiated, a life-long risk of gastrointestinal problems remains. These include pancreaticobiliary complications, intussusception, appendicitis, colon strictures, fibrosing colonopathy (FC), rectal prolapse, and meconium ileus equivalent.

Pancreaticobiliary complications Biliary cirrhosis, portal hypertension, and liver failure are not uncommon in older children with CF. Treatment is similar to that for other causes of liver failure. Pancreatic obstruction may lead to recurrent pancreatitis, and such complications should be treated in similar fashion to other diseases that cause obstruction of the pancreatic duct. Radiolucent gallstones are noted in 12% to 27% of patients with CF, and 4% will develop cholecystitis.[10] Treatment should be cholecystectomy.

Appendicitis The incidence of appendicitis is similar to that on non-CF patients.[11] Both acute and chronic appendicitis symptoms have been described in CF patients. Appendectomy is curative.

Meconium ileus equivalent Recurrence of obstruction from inspissated stool in children and adults is commonly referred meconium ileus equivalent or distal intestinal obstruction syndrome. Typically, this occurs after cessation of pancreatic enzymes, change in diet, or, at times, dehydration. Treatment is similar to simple meconium ileus, as discussed.[6,9] The inspissated stool can act as a lead point causing intussusception, and should be treated with radiologic or operative reduction in those cases that fail radiologic reduction.

Colonic obstruction Both colon strictures and FC present as distal intestinal obstructions, typically in children age 2 to 7 years of age who often have had a history of meconium ileus as newborns. Both are believed to be a consequence of high-dose, delayed-release pancreatic enzyme therapy.[7] These 2 entities were more common when higher doses of pancreatic enzymes were used and have become extremely rare in the current era. In the case of a colonic stricture, the process is focal. This is in contrast with FC, in which long segment fusiform luminal narrowing occurs primarily in the right colon that can extend to include the entire colon. These 2 complications are easily distinguished by contrast enema or colonoscopy. Crohn's disease has been reported to be 17-fold more common in CF patients with a similar presentation to FC, and therefore should be included the differential diagnosis. Segmental resection of an isolated stricture is often necessary and curative, although FC has traditionally been treated by partial or subtotal colectomy.[6,9] Surgical treatment should be accompanied by an appropriate reduction of pancreatic enzyme replacement.

Rectal prolapse Upwards of 30% of patients with CF develop rectal prolapse in early childhood. Of those children presenting with rectal prolapse, in 4% to 8% the prolapse is the first presenting sign of CF.[6] The surgeon being consulted for rectal prolapse in a young child should be prompted to rule out CF with a sweat chloride test. Prolapse most likely occurs as a consequence of frequent stools, colonic distension from malabsorption, and frequent coughing. Initiation of pancreatic enzyme therapy can be curative. Rectal sclerotherapy is highly successful[9,12] and rectopexy, as discussed, should be used for patients who fail nonoperative therapy.[13]

Anorectal malformations
Etiology and presentations Anorectal malformations (ARM) represent a spectrum of anomalies of the anus and rectum that range from anal stenosis to cloacal anomalies. The embryology and genetics that lead to ARM are complex and incompletely understood. It is believed the abnormalities leading to ARM occur as early as gestational weeks 3 through 8. This is when the bilaminary disk develops into ectodermal, mesodermal, and endodermal components forming the rudiments of the pelvic structures.[14] Likely, given the spectrum of ARM and associated anomalies, the ultimate phenotype depends on the timing of these abnormal events. Historically, ARM were described as "high," "intermediate," or "low," but are in fact better defined based on the exact anatomic anatomy: Rectoperineal fistula, rectrourethral fistula (boys), rectovestibular fistula (girls), rectovaginal fistula, rectobladder neck, imperforate anus without fistula, rectal stenosis/atresia, and persistent cloaca. Use of these definitions allows a better understanding of the anatomic deformity as well as an understanding of the appropriate treatment.

Most ARM are readily identifiable in the routine neonatal physical examination. However, it is not uncommon for a toddler or young child to present with constipation and found by the surgeon to have a previously unrecognized perineal fistula or "anteriorly displaced anus." Although it is easy for an informed observer to discern a perineal fistula, vestibular fistula, and the more severe cloacal anomaly, the other ARM are not readily discernable by physical or radiologic examination. With that said, initial treatment of these patients consisting of a diverting colostomy and an elective contrast-enhanced study of the defunctionalized pouch often give the surgeon a road map of the anatomic defect. ARM are frequently associated with other congenital anomalies. Generally speaking, more complex ARM are more commonly associated with other anomalies. Therefore, the evaluation of a newborn with an ARM should include, at a minimum, cardiac echocardiography, chest x-ray, pelvic x-ray, renal ultrasonography, magnetic resonance imaging of the spine, and chromosomal analysis.

Management The need for a colostomy is in part determined by the defect as well as surgeon experience with definitive repair. **Figs. 4** and **5** outline the management algorithm for boys and girls, respectively. A few principles of colostomy creation warrant specific mention. If a colostomy is required it should be performed as a divided colostomy with the mucous fistula separated from the colostomy to lessen the risk of fecal

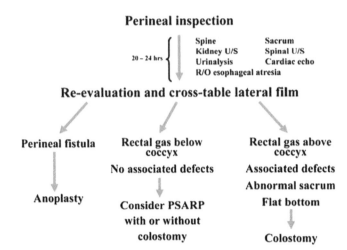

Fig. 4. Treatment algorithm for anorectal malformations in boys. PSAP, posterior sagittal anoplasty; PSARP, posterior sagittal anorectoplasty. (*From* Levitt M, Pena A. Outcomes from the correction of anorectal malformations. Curr Opin Pediatr 2005;17(3):394–401; with permission.)

contamination to the genitourinary system. The colostomy also should performed at the level of the proximal sigmoid colostomy to prevent complications of prolapse, and the surgeon should ensure adequate length of the defunctional pouch is left to allow for a tension-free definitive repair at the subsequent operation. Creation of

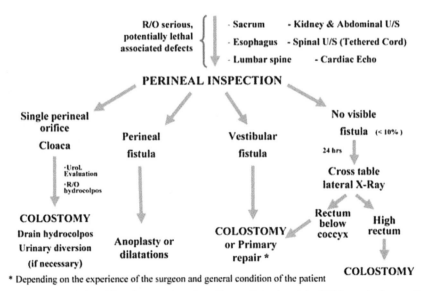

Fig. 5. Treatment algorithm for anorectal malformations in girls. PSAP, posterior sagittal anoplasty; PSARP, posterior sagittal anorectoplasty; PSARVUP, posterior sagittal anorecto-vagino-urethroplasty. (*From* Levitt M, Pena A. Outcomes from the correction of anorectal malformations. Curr Opin Pediatr 2005;17(3):394–401; with permission.)

a mucous fistula at the time of colostomy is helpful to allow a contrast study of the pouch to be performed as a road map before the definitive repair.

The posterior sagittal anorectoplasty (PSARP), described by Alberto Peña, has been the approach adopted by most pediatric surgeons in the United States. A full description of this approach for each type of ARM is beyond the scope of this article, and can be found elsewhere.[14] In general, however, the PSARP allows the surgeon to identify the anatomy of the anal sphincter complex and levator ani musculature allowing the neo-anorectum to be placed in a position to offer the best possible functional outcome. It is well tolerated by newborns postoperatively and creates an incision that is aesthetically invisible. ARM associated with a fistula that communicates high in the genitourinary tract often requires a combined abdominal and perineal approach. Recently, a minimally invasive approach to these ARM has been described with outcomes equal to or better than those of the open approach.[15]

Early complications are infrequent with the PSARP, but include wound infection, injury to the urethra or vagina, and dehiscence and/or retraction of the anoplasty. Treatment of a superficial wound infection includes simple wound care to allow drainage of the infection and healing by secondary intent, provided the fecal stream is diverted proximally. An excellent outcome can still be expected, provided the anoplasty remains intact. Injury to the urethra or vagina is best avoided by anticipation for this potential complication. Even in the most minimal anoplasty, separation of the anterior wall of the rectum from the urethra or vagina is required to prevent tension on the repair. Placement of an indwelling urethral catheter or a Hagar dilatator in the vaginal vault assists in identifying the common wall and helps to prevent or at least identify an injury to either. Dehiscence and retraction of the anoplasty are most often a result of tension on the anoplasty. Tension may arise from inadequate mobilization of the rectum proximally or from either the urethra or vagina anteriorly. If evident in the first few days, successful immediate revision may be feasible. However, if delayed, proximal fecal diversion and local wound care avoid further harm created by attempts to repair the problem with inflamed tissue. Most often, the consequence is formation of a stricture and requires reoperation in a delayed fashion.

Long-term outcomes and complications The majority of adult patients with previously repaired ARM report an excellent quality of life and are highly functional.[16] Several recent reports have demonstrated the functional outcome of adult patients with previously repaired ARM and most at least transiently experience issues of constipation, fecal soiling, and/or fecal incontinence.[16,17] The degree to which these occur depends a variety of factors, including the type of anatomic defect and the presence of associated anomalies (particularly neurologic, and parental involvement.) Despite a well-performed surgery, ARM by definition lacks the presence of the normal anal canal and its sensory innervation involved in maintaining continence. Furthermore, to a varying degree there is an absence of the anal sphincter and levator ani muscles. The more severe the defect, the more likely these structures are incompletely developed (**Table 1**). The presence of spinal cord anomalies or associated developmental delay may lead to inadequate function of these structures as well. Last, strong parental involvement and awareness can overcome most, if not all, of these issues to achieve an acceptable outcome.

Constipation Constipation should be an expected outcome, even in an infant with a favorable defect.[18] Although the cause is not completely understood, hypomotility of the rectosigmoid is common in children with ARM.[14] This may be a consequence

Table 1
Functional outcomes by type of anorectal anomaly

| | Voluntary Bowel Movement | | Bowel Incontinence | | | | | | Constipated | | Urinary Incontinence | |
| | | | Soiling | | Totally Continent | | | | | | | |
	Patients	n (%)	Patients	n (%)	Patients	n (%)			Patients	n (%)	Patients	n (%)
Perineal fistula	39/39	100	3/43	20.9	35/39	89.7			30/53	56.6	0/38	0
Rectal atresia or stenosis	8/8	100	2/8	25	6/8	75			4/8	50	0/8	0
Vestibular fistula	89/97	92	36/100	36	63/89	70.8			61/100	61	—	—
Imperforate anus without fistula	30/35	86	18/37	48.6	18/30	60			22/40	55	1/37	2.7
Bulbar–urethral fistula	68/83	82	48/89	53.9	34/68	50			52/81	64.2	2/85	2.4
Prostatic fistula	52/71	73	67/87	77.1	16/52	30.8			42/93	45.2	7/85	8.2
Cloaca (short common channel)	50/70	71	50/79	63.3	25/50	50			34/85	40	5/18	27.8
Cloaca (long common channel)	18/41	44	34/39	87.2	5/18	27.8			17/45	34.8	37/48	77.1
Vaginal fistula	3/4	75	4/5	80	1/3	33.3			1/5	20	1/5	20
Bladderneck fistula	8/29	28	39/43	90.7	1/8	12.5			7/45	15.6	7/38	18.4

From Levitt M, Pena A. Outcomes from the correction of anorectal malformations. Curr Opin Pediatr 2005;17(3):394–401; with permission.

of incomplete development or acquired in the case of creation of proximal colostomy. It has also been suggested that these children lack the normal sensation of rectal distension that leads to relaxation of the anal sphincter. Untreated constipation leads to an overflow incontinence and eventually nonfunctional mega-sigmoidrectum.[18] It cannot be emphasized enough the surgeon needs to be vigilant in follow-up and in discussing normal and abnormal stooling behaviors in children with ARM. Treatment is centered foremost on prevention. First, the parents and physicians often mistakenly assume that having multiple small stools throughout the day does not represent constipation. Therefore, parents must pay attention to the frequency, volume, and character of the stool. The surgeon should query the parents in follow-up of these details and routinely perform digital rectal examinations to evaluate for the presence of impacted stool and/or a large rectal vault. Plain radiographs can be useful adjuncts. Once constipation is diagnosed, initial management should be medical, including dietary modifications with the addition of fruits and vegetable and natural laxatives in the form of bran or prune juice. Further treatment including stimulants and/or cathartics use should be individualized to the patient's needs. In a large series of patients, Levitt and colleagues[18] reported a high degree of success with minimal morbidity in managing constipation using senna in the long term to provoke daily bowel movements. Enemas should be used if the child fails to have a bowel movement on a daily basis despite these measures and while the medications are adjusted. In children who cannot wean from daily rectal enemas, antegrade enemas via a surgically placed cecostomy can be effective and may be better tolerated than enemas per rectum. Once constipation results in mega-sigmoidrectum, operative resection with immediate anastomosis followed by aggressive medical management is advocated.[18]

   Soiling/fecal incontinence Soiling can be an indication of constipation and overflow incontinence, particularly in children with an isolated favorable ARM. Treatment is directed similar to the management of constipation, as discussed, once the child is disimpacted.[18] Soiling may also represent functional incontinence, particularly in a child with a less favorable ARM or associated anomalies. Treatment options include reoperation, use of a constipating bowel program, or permanent colostomy.[19,20] A proposed algorithm used by Brown and colleagues for the evaluation and treatment for fecal incontinence after repair of ARM is shown in **Fig. 6**. The constipating bowel program involves use of constipating diet and medications, along with the use of daily enemas/colonic irrigations to achieve social continence.

Chronic idiopathic intestinal pseudo-obstruction
Etiology and presentation Chronic idiopathic intestinal pseudo-obstruction presents with the signs and symptoms of obstruction. Although most cases are sporadic and idiopathic, it can be associated with mitochondrial disorders and myopathies. The majority of cases manifest as feeding intolerance in the first few days of life. These must be differentiated from other causes of neonatal obstruction, as discussed. Retrograde contrast enema and small bowel through studies are useful to rule out mechanical obstruction. Rectal biopsy is useful to rule out Hirschsprung disease. Quite often, attempts are made to change enteral formulations, but without success.

Management Management largely is medical and supportive.[21] These infants often require parenteral nutrition; however, all measures to supply at least some enteral nutrition should be exhausted to prevent catheter-related blood stream infections and hepatic failure. This includes jejunal drip feedings via a surgical jejunostomy and proximal decompression by gastrostomy. Not uncommonly, the surgeon is requested to perform full-thickness intestinal biopsies in a newborn not tolerating

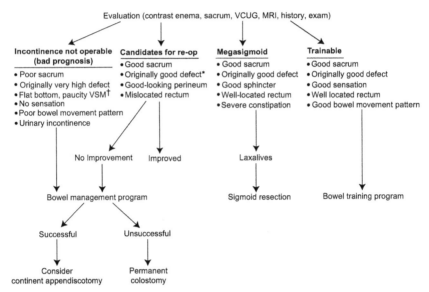

Fig. 6. Algorithm for evaluation and treatment of fecal incontinence after repair of anorectal malformation. MRI, magnetic resonance imaging; VSM, voluntary skeletal muscle; VCUG, voiding cystourethrogram. (*From* Brown RL, Irish MS, Rice HE, et al. Care of the surgical intensive care nursery graduate: the primary care pediatrician's perspective. Pediatr Clin North Am 1998;45(6):1327–52; with permission.)

feeds. These biopsies can be useful in identifying myopathic or neuropathic changes consistent with pseudo-obstruction, but may also be entirely normal. If performed, biopsies should be performed throughout the length of small and large intestine. Pseudo-obstruction is often variable in which portions of intestine are affected and both gastroduodenal and colonic motility studies can be helpful. For those patients with colonic pseudo-obstruction who respond to retrograde enemas, creation of a cecostomy for antegrade enemas often allows easier administration of enemas in older children. In those with colonic pseudo-obstruction who fail medical management, creation of an end ileostomy can be beneficial to restore complete or partial enteral feedings. Colonic resection and creation of ileorectostomy should be delayed until one is confident the small intestine is functional. Intestinal transplantation has been advocated in patients who remain entirely dependent on parenteral nutrition.

Colorectal Disease of Early Childhood

Duplications of the colon and rectum
Etiology and presentation Duplications of the colon and rectum, although far less common than duplications of the small intestine, tend to be remarkably variable in their extent and complexity. Although the etiology of intestinal duplications is unknown, they are most commonly lined with colonic mucosa. As such, in contrast with duplications elsewhere, peptic ulceration is rare. However, the risk of adenocarcinoma in the duplication is much greater than in duplications in other locations. Depending on the extent and location, symptoms of constipation, obstruction, and volvulus are the most common presenting symptoms.

Management Operative resection should be undertaken in all possible cases to treat current symptoms or prevent future complications.[22] Duplications of the colon and rectum can be divided into 3 types helping to define the surgical approach: Midline, tailgut, and bilateral tubular. Midline cysts lie in the mesentery of the colon and/or rectum and have a shared common wall and blood supply. Therefore, one can expect to perform a segmental resection the adjacent bowel. The surgical approach should be individualized based on the location and extent of the cyst. Tailgut cysts are cystic structures between the anus and coccyx. The cysts are separate from the intestinal tract and do not share a common wall or blood supply. On imaging, these cysts seem similar to a sacrococcygeal teratoma and distinction only made after resection and pathologic examination. Resection can often be accomplished through a posterior sagittal approach and should include resection of the coccyx, as one would do with a sacrococcygeal teratoma to prevent recurrence. The last type, bilateral tubular, involves complete duplication of the hindgut and may include a separate anal orifice and extend the entire length of the hindgut. In contrast with midline cysts, these tubular cysts tend not to share a common wall, although they may share a common blood supply. This type of cyst is often associated with genitourinary and spinal anomalies. Given the complexity, surgical management must be individualized. As a result of the shared blood supply and extent of the duplication, resection may not be possible and, therefore, creation of common channel between the duplicated cyst and normal colon may be necessary to achieve drainage and prevent obstructive symptoms. Alternately, complete excision of the duplication and adjacent normal hindgut with a pull-through has been described.[23]

Given the infrequency and heterogeneity of duplications of the colon and rectum, long-term outcomes are highly dependent on the extent and complexity and the duplication as well as the treatment. As stated, development of adenocarcinoma within the duplication can occur and therefore warrants routine evaluation of any residual duplication cyst.

Rectal prolapse

Etiology and presentation Rectal prolapse in young children is relatively common and is a distinct entity from rectal prolapse that occurs in older children and adults. Rectal prolapse in young children most often occurs around the time of toilet training and most commonly includes prolapse of the rectal mucosa only. Although not always provided in the history from the parents, straining and constipation are common. As discussed, rectal prolapse at this age may represent the first manifestation of CF and a sweat chloride test should be performed. In addition, intestinal parasitic infection may be a contributing factor. On rare occasions, severe ileocolonic intussusception, typically presenting with a toxic child and full-thickness prolapse, has been misdiagnosed as rectal prolapse.

Management Most rectal prolapses in young children spontaneously reduce once the child is relaxed, but on occasion require manual reduction. If present, treatment of pancreatic insufficiency related to CF or parasitic infections should be instituted first because this often prevents recurrent prolapse. In absence of these, initial management should include reassurance of the parents as well as treatment for constipation with stool softeners and dietary modifications. Parents should be made aware that early recurrence is common. In cases of recurrent prolapse that only involves the rectal mucosa, submucosal injection of a sclerosing agent has proven efficacious with little to no morbidity.[12,24,25] Older children and those who fail sclerotherapy benefit from a laparoscopic rectopexy.[25,26] Provided successful management of their constipation, these children have an excellent short-term outcome, although there are no studies providing long-term follow-up through adulthood.

Intussusception

Etiology and presentation Intussusception or invagination of 1 segment of intestine into another is a common cause of intestinal obstruction in young children. However, it also occurs in older children and adults, albeit less frequently. For the surgeon, it is important to understand that the likelihood of a pathologic lead point in a child under the age of 5 years is very low, but increases proportionally with advancing age and is as high as 97% in adult patients.[27,28] In children, the most common pathologic lead point is a Meckel's diverticulum, versus adults where more than one half are malignant tumors. Other common lead points include polyps, hamartomas, lymphoma, enteric cysts, submucosal hematomas related to Henoch-Scholein purpura, and inspissated stool from CF. Although intussusception can occur in any region of the intestine, in children it is most often ileocolic. In adults, colocolic intussusception is more common. The classic presentation of intussusception is a child younger than 2 years recently recovering from a viral illness presenting with colicky abdominal pain and "current jelly stools." Between episodes of pain the child seems to be well, or if the illness prolonged, may seem lethargic. Plain films typically lack overly dilated bowel and may, to the untrained, eye seem "nonspecific"; more subtle findings include absence of bowel gas in the right lower quadrant (Dance's sign) and a density in the right upper quadrant. Ultrasound and computed tomography demonstrate a heterogeneous mass with a "bull's eye." These 2 studies can be useful adjuncts if presentation is atypical, and particularly if small intestine intussusception is suspected. Retrograde contrast enema demonstrates the intussusception if it is ileocolic or colocolic, although this is less useful for intussusception located in the small intestine.

Management Reduction of the intussusception is necessary to avoid the progression to ischemia and perforation. These patients should be evaluated and treated as any patient who presents with obstructive symptoms. They should be made nil per os, given resuscitative intravenous fluids, and should be evaluated for signs of peritonitis. If peritonitis is evident, operative exploration should be undertaken.

Infants and toddlers Once resuscitated, and in the absence of peritonitis, either fluoroscopic hydrostatic or pneumatic reduction is reported to be successful in 65% to 75% of patients, with a small but definite risk of perforation. In the absence of recurrence or persistent symptoms, in this age group the risk of pathologic lead point is extremely low and no further evaluation is necessary once reduced. Those who fail radiologic reduction should undergo operative reduction, currently performed in a minimally invasive fashion with simple manual reduction. Necrotic or non-reducible intussusception should undergo resection with re-anastomosis. Although unlikely to be found, a pathologic lead point should always be sought. In young children with intussusception, the mesenteric lymph nodes always seem to be enlarged; yet in the absence of an intestinal mass, biopsy rarely yields positive results. Similarly, the intestine comprising the intussusceptum always feels thick (caused by edema from ischemia) and the surgeon should resist resection, provided it remains viable. If concern remains, a contrast-enhanced study can be obtained a few weeks postoperatively with little morbidity. The appendix is generally removed after reduction of the intussusception. Recurrence in the early postoperative period occurs in fewer than 10% of patients after both radiologic and surgical reduction.[27] These patients can be managed successfully by repeat radiologic reduction and surgery is required only if necessary. Despite the recurrence, the incidence of a pathologic lead point in these patients remains low.[27,29]

Older children Older children are managed similarly to infants and children if no pathologic lead point is identified. However, 3 to 4 weeks after successful operative or radiologic reduction, further diagnostic tests should be performed to rule out a pathologic lead point. Typical test include magnetic resonance imaging enterography or enterocolysis, Meckel's scan, and possible colonoscopy.

Adults Excluding the incidental finding on computed tomography of a transient, asymptomatic small bowel intussusception, intussusception in adults is almost always associated with a pathologic lead point and commonly a malignant neoplasm. Radiologic reduction is rarely successful. Surgical reduction is accomplished by resection, and attempts at reduction should normally be avoided. One should perform the operation with good surgical oncologic technique.

Long-term outcomes and complications In children, long-term outcomes are excellent and complications rare. Recurrence has been described even 3 years after initial presentation. Long-term outcomes older children and adults with pathologic lead point is determined by source of the lead point.

Colorectal Disease of Childhood and Adolescence

Polyps and polyposis syndromes
Juvenile polyps Most polyps found in pediatric patients represent benign hamartomas and are referred to as juvenile polyps. Juvenile polyps are relatively common in pediatric patients and frequently present as either painless rectal bleeding or as a lead point for intussusception in young children. Although it is believed that most juvenile polyps will resolve, there are case reports of malignant degeneration and therefore these should be removed endoscopically when identified.

Juvenile polyposis syndrome Juvenile polyposis syndrome is a rare, autosomal-dominant syndrome defined as 3 our more juvenile polyps in the colon, polyposis involving the entire gastrointestinal tract, or polyps in the setting of a family history for juvenile polyposis syndrome. Classically, patients present in late childhood with painless rectal bleeding from the polyps. With diffuse juvenile polyposis syndrome, polyps number in the 50s to 100s and may present with failure to thrive, anemia, hypoalbuminemia, and abdominal pain during infancy and early childhood. Both upper and lower gastrointestinal tract malignancies occur and screening should begin at age 12 years and repeated every 3 years if negative.[30] Proctocolectomy with ileal pull-through is a reasonable option in both symptomatic patients as well as as a prophylactic procedure to prevent cancer.[31]

Peutz-Jeghers syndrome This rare, autosomal-dominant condition is marked by polyps in association with melanin deposits that may occur anywhere on the body, most commonly in or around the mouth. It often presents with symptoms of intestinal obstruction. These patients are at risk of malignancies both in and outside the gastrointestinal tract and occur in up to 90% of patients.[32,33] Owing to the diffuse nature of these polyps, treatment should be directed at removal of symptomatic lesions and surveillance for malignancy. Given the high lifetime risk of malignancy, screening protocols for various cancers have been developed based on consensus guidelines, and should begin in early adolescence.[33,34]

Familial adenomatous polyposis Familial adenomatous polyposis (FAP) is an autosomal-dominant disease and is the most common genetic polyposis syndrome. In absence of a family history and previous genetic testing, most cases of FAP in pediatric patients present with painless bleeding per rectum. Similar to adults, FAP in children is associated with hundreds of polyps in the colon. Polyps may begin to appear in childhood, but malignant degeneration typically does not occur before the second decade of life. Genetic testing of newborns with a familial history for FAP is reasonable, and if positive for the APC mutation, these children should undergo yearly abdominal ultrasound and serum alpha-fetoprotein screening for hepatoblastoma until age of 10 years, as well as endoscopy at or around age 10 years. Prophylactic proctocolectomy in asymptomatic patients is reasonable beginning at age 10 years given the risk of cancer.

Inflammatory bowel disease

Etiology, presentation, management, and long-term surgical outcomes Pediatric inflammatory bowel disease (IBD) mirrors adult IBD in the etiology, presentation, and management. As such, the reader is referred to other sections of this and other volumes for a discussion of its surgical management. Although IBD is less common in childhood compared with adults, IBD can occur in all pediatric age groups. In a study of the Pediatric IBD Consortium that included 1370 children the mean age at IBD diagnosis was 10.3 years. Of these, 6.1% were diagnosed at younger than 3 years of age, 15.4% at 3 to 6 years, 47.7% at 6 to 12 years, and 36.9% at 13 to 17 years.[35] There are some notable differences in pediatric IBD. Growth retardation and delayed sexual maturity are common findings in pediatric patients with IBD, particularly with Crohn's disease.[36,37] Quite often, these go unnoticed for several months until more classic symptoms of IBD manifest. Therefore, it is not uncommon that pediatric IBD patients present with significant malnutrition. Because this affects both the disease and healing after surgical therapy, this should be considered and addressed early in the management of these patients.

Standardized management of pediatric IBD has been fairly well developed by consensus experts and has allowed for multicenter, prospective studies through the Pediatric IBD Collaborative Research Group.[38–40] This group has demonstrated that corticosteroid dependence in pediatric patients with medically treated Crohn's disease remains high (31%) at 1 year after diagnosis, with an incidence of surgery of 8% over the same time period.[41] Physicians treating patients with IBD must be attentive to the complications of long-term steroid treatment that are generally uncommon in pediatric patients, and particularly those involving thromboembolic events and osteopenia.[40] Additionally, this group has validated the clinical utility of the Pediatric Ulcerative Colitis Activity Index to determine effectiveness of high-dose corticosteroids in the management of severe ulcerative colitis.[42,43] Further studies are currently underway that may link specific genetic abnormalities found in IBD to more successful treatment algorithms.

Surgical treatment of IBD in pediatrics is associated with similar short-term complications to those in adults. Laparoscopic and single-incision laparoscopic procedures for pediatric patients with either Crohn's disease or ulcerative colitis have been well described in the literature and seem to have similar complications and short-term outcomes to adults.[44–46] The recurrence rate after surgical treatment of Crohn's disease in pediatric patients is high (17% at 1 year, 38% at 3 years, and 60% at 5 years.)[47,48] For ulcerative colitis patients who undergo proctocolectomy with ileal pull-through, both straight and pouch procedures are described in the pediatric literature.[49–51] Creation of a J-pouch rather than either a straight or a more complex pouch results in better functional outcomes in the short term.[50,51] Most pediatric patients can expect to achieve 4 to 6 bowel movements a day within the first few months of surgery after creation of a J-pouch. Long-term follow-up suggests that most pediatric patients achieve daytime continence and fewer than 5% report occasional nighttime incontinence.[50,52] The most common long-term complication is pouchitis, and is reported to occur in pediatric patients relatively frequently.[50–52] The approach to the management of pouchitis in children is identical to adult patients. Although overall quality of life seems to be good in pediatric patients who undergo proctocolectomy and ileoanal pull-through, decreased sexual activity and fertility are frequently reported and have a high impact on quality of life.[53]

Unique Aspects of Pediatric Laparoscopy

Most colorectal procedures performed in newborn and pediatric patients are amenable to a minimally invasive approach.[15,54–57] Generally speaking, the techniques in laparoscopy in children are similar to adults, with a few exceptions that warrant mention. Almost all infants and toddlers and many pediatric patients have an open umbilical ring, making this an easy and safe point of initial access. The surgeon must pay close attention to intra-abdominal pressure and flow rates to prevent intra-abdominal hypertension as well as hypothermia.[58] Stab incisions in place of trocars can be used in most infants and young pediatric patients. The thin, pliable abdominal wall allows for a small extension of the umbilical incision through which extracorporeal resection and anastomosis can be performed with relative ease. Until the teenage years, circular stapling devices are often too large to be accommodated for a low rectal anastomosis, and hand-sewn techniques are used.

SUMMARY

Colorectal disease in pediatric patients includes a wide spectrum of diseases, many of which have a significant impact on quality of life and warrant long-term follow-up and treatment into adulthood. Surgeons caring for these patients should have a baseline knowledge of the unique aspects of their care to maximize outcomes.

REFERENCES

1. Langer JC. Hirschprung's disease. In: Colombani PM, Oldham KT, Foglia RP, et al, editors. Principles and practice of pediatric surgery. Philadelphia: Lippincott Williams & Wilkins; 2004.
2. Coe A, Collins MH, Lawal T, et al. Reoperation for Hirschsprung's disease: pathology of the resected problematic distal pull-through. Pediatr Dev Pathol 2012;15(1):30–8.
3. Ieiri S, Nakatsuji T, Akiyoshi J, et al. Long-term outcomes and the quality of life of Hirschsprung disease in adolescents who have reached 18 years or older– a 47-year single-institute experience. J Pediatr Surg 2010;45(12):2398–402.
4. Teitelbaum DH, Coran AG. Enterocolitis. Semin Pediatr Surg 1998;7(3):162–9.
5. Patrus B, Nasr A, Langer JC, et al. Intrasphincteric botulinum toxin decreases the rate of hospitalization for postoperative obstructive symptoms in children with Hirschsprung disease. J Pediatr Surg 2011;46(1):184–7.
6. Beierle EA, Vinocur CD. Gastrointestinal surgery in cystic fibrosis. Curr Opin Pulm Med 1998;4(6):319–25.
7. Dicken BJ, Ziegler MM. Surgical management of pulmonary and gastrointestinal complications in children with cystic fibrosis. Curr Opin Pediatr 2006;18(3):321–9.
8. Fuchs JR, Langer JC. Long-term outcome after neonatal meconium obstruction. Pediatrics 1998;101(4):E7.
9. Escobar MA, Grosfeld JL, Burdick JJ, et al. Surgical considerations in cystic fibrosis: a 32-year evaluation of outcomes. Surgery 2005;138(4):560–71.
10. Angelico M, Gandin C, Canuzzi P, et al. Gallstones in cystic fibrosis: a critical reappraisal. Hepatology 1991;14(5):768–75.

11. Holsclaw DS, Habboushe C. Occult appendiceal abscess complicating cystic fibrosis. J Pediatr Surg 1976;11(2):217–21.
12. Chan WK, Kay SM, Laberge JM, et al. Injection sclerotherapy in the treatment of rectal prolapse in infants and children. J Pediatr Surg 1998;33(2):255–8.
13. Ashcraft KW, Amoury RA, Holder TM. Levator repair and posterior suspension for rectal prolapse. J Pediatr Surg 1977;12(2):241–5.
14. Paidas CN, Levitt MA, Pena A. Rectum and anus. In: Colombani PM, Oldham KT, Foglia RP, et al, editors. Principles and practice of pediatric surgery. Philadelphia: Lippincott Williams & Wilkins; 2004. p. 1395–436.
15. Bischoff A, Levitt MA, Pena A. Laparoscopy and its use in the repair of anorectal malformations. J Pediatr Surg 2011;46(8):1609–17.
16. Hassink EA, Rieu PN, Brugman AT, et al. Quality of life after operatively corrected high anorectal malformation: a long-term follow-up study of patients aged 18 years and older. J Pediatr Surg 1994;29(6):773–6.
17. Rintala RJ, Pakarinen MP. Outcome of anorectal malformations and Hirschsprung's disease beyond childhood. Semin Pediatr Surg 2010;19(2):160–7.
18. Levitt MA, Kant A, Pena A. The morbidity of constipation in patients with anorectal malformations. J Pediatr Surg 2010;45(6):1228–33.
19. Bischoff A, Levitt MA, Bauer C, et al. Treatment of fecal incontinence with a comprehensive bowel management program. J Pediatr Surg 2009;44(6):1278–83.
20. Bischoff A, Levitt MA, Pena A. Bowel management for the treatment of pediatric fecal incontinence. Pediatr Surg Int 2009;25(12):1027–42.
21. Gariepy CE, Mousa H. Clinical management of motility disorders in children. Semin Pediatr Surg 2009;18(4):224–38.
22. Mourra N, Chafai N, Bessoud B, et al. Colorectal duplication in adults: report of seven cases and review of the literature. J Clin Pathol 2010;63(12):1080–3.
23. Craigie RJ, Abbaraju JS, Ba'ath ME, et al. Anorectal malformation with tubular hindgut duplication. J Pediatr Surg 2006;41(6):e31–4.
24. Fahmy MA, Ezzelarab S. Outcome of submucosal injection of different sclerosing materials for rectal prolapse in children. Pediatr Surg Int 2004;20(5):353–6.
25. Shah A, Parikh D, Jawaheer G, et al. Persistent rectal prolapse in children: sclerotherapy and surgical management. Pediatr Surg Int 2005;21(4):270–3.
26. Laituri CA, Garey CL, Fraser JD, et al. 15-Year experience in the treatment of rectal prolapse in children. J Pediatr Surg 2010;45(8):1607–9.
27. Whitehouse JS, Gourlay DM, Winthrop AL, et al. Is it safe to discharge intussusception patients after successful hydrostatic reduction? J Pediatr Surg 2010;45(6):1182–6.
28. Pang LC. Intussusception revisited: clinicopathologic analysis of 261 cases, with emphasis on pathogenesis. South Med J 1989;82(2):215–28.
29. Ein SH. Recurrent intussusception in children. J Pediatr Surg 1975;10(5):751–5.
30. Dunlop MG. Guidance on gastrointestinal surveillance for hereditary nonpolyposis colorectal cancer, familial adenomatous polypolis, juvenile polyposis, and Peutz-Jeghers syndrome. Gut 2002;51(Suppl 5):V21–7.
31. Oncel M, Church JM, Remzi FH, et al. Colonic surgery in patients with juvenile polyposis syndrome: a case series. Dis Colon Rectum 2005;48(1):49–55.
32. Giardiello FM, Brensinger JD, Tersmette AC, et al. Very high risk of cancer in familial Peutz-Jeghers syndrome. Gastroenterology 2000;119(6):1447–53.
33. van Lier MG, Wagner A, Mathus-Vliegen EM, et al. High cancer risk in Peutz-Jeghers syndrome: a systematic review and surveillance recommendations. Am J Gastroenterol 2010;105(6):1258–64.

34. Beggs AD, Latchford AR, Vasen HF, et al. Peutz-Jeghers syndrome: a systematic review and recommendations for management. Gut 2010;59(7):975–86.

35. Heyman MB, Kirschner BS, Gold BD, et al. Children with early-onset inflammatory bowel disease (IBD): analysis of a pediatric IBD consortium registry. J Pediatr 2005;146(1):35–40.

36. Saha MT, Ruuska T, Laippala P, et al. Growth of prepubertal children with inflammatory bowel disease. J Pediatr Gastroenterol Nutr 1998;26(3):310–4.

37. Markowitz J, Daum F. Growth impairment in pediatric inflammatory bowel disease. Am J Gastroenterol 1994;89(3):319–26.

38. Turner D, Griffiths AM. Acute severe ulcerative colitis in children: a systematic review. Inflamm Bowel Dis 2011;17(1):440–9.

39. Turner D, Travis SP, Griffiths AM, et al. Consensus for managing acute severe ulcerative colitis in children: a systematic review and joint statement from ECCO, ESPGHAN, and the Porto IBD Working Group of ESPGHAN. Am J Gastroenterol 2011;106(4):574–88.

40. Rufo PA, Denson LA, Sylvester FA, et al. Health supervision in the management of children and adolescents with inflammatory bowel disease: recommendations of the North American Society for Pediatric Gastroenterology, Hepatology, and Nutrition (NASPGHAN). J Pediatr Gastroenterol Nutr 2012;55(1):93–108.

41. Markowitz J, Hyams J, Mack D, et al. Corticosteroid therapy in the age of infliximab: acute and 1-year outcomes in newly diagnosed children with Crohn's disease. Clin Gastroenterol Hepatol 2006;4(9):1124–9.

42. Turner D, Griffiths AM, Steinhart AH, et al. Mathematical weighting of a clinimetric index (Pediatric Ulcerative Colitis Activity Index) was superior to the judgmental approach. J Clin Epidemiol 2009;62(7):738–44.

43. Turner D, Hyams J, Markowitz J, et al. Appraisal of the pediatric ulcerative colitis activity index (PUCAI). Inflamm Bowel Dis 2009;15(8):1218–23.

44. Potter DD, Tung J, Faubion WA Jr, et al. Single-incision laparoscopic colon and rectal surgery for pediatric inflammatory bowel disease and polyposis syndromes. J Laparoendosc Adv Surg Tech A 2012;22(2):203–7.

45. Laituri CA, Fraser JD, Garey CL, et al. Laparoscopic ileocecectomy in pediatric patients with Crohn's disease. J Laparoendosc Adv Surg Tech A 2011;21(2):193–5.

46. Fraser JD, Garey CL, Laituri CA, et al. Outcomes of laparoscopic and open total colectomy in the pediatric population. J Laparoendosc Adv Surg Tech A 2010; 20(7):659–60.

47. Baldassano RN, Han PD, Jeshion WC, et al. Pediatric Crohn's disease: risk factors for postoperative recurrence. Am J Gastroenterol 2001;96(7):2169–76.

48. Pacilli M, Eaton S, Fell JM, et al. Surgery in children with Crohn disease refractory to medical therapy. J Pediatr Gastroenterol Nutr 2011;52(3):286–90.

49. Coran AG. A personal experience with 100 consecutive total colectomies and straight ileoanal endorectal pull-throughs for benign disease of the colon and rectum in children and adults. Ann Surg 1990;212(3):242–7.

50. Telander RL, Spencer M, Perrault J, et al. Long-term follow-up of the ileoanal anastomosis in children and young adults. Surgery 1990;108(4):717–23.

51. Durno C, Sherman P, Harris K, et al. Outcome after ileoanal anastomosis in pediatric patients with ulcerative colitis. J Pediatr Gastroenterol Nutr 1998;27(5): 501–7.

52. Fonkalsrud EW, Thakur A, Beanes S. Ileoanal pouch procedures in children. J Pediatr Surg 2001;36(11):1689–92.

53. Dalal DH, Patton D, Wojcicki JM, et al. Quality of life in patients post colectomy for pediatric onset ulcerative colitis. J Pediatr Gastroenterol Nutr 2012;55(4):425–8.

54. Diamond IR, Gerstle JT, Kim PC, et al. Outcomes after laparoscopic surgery in children with inflammatory bowel disease. Surg Endosc 2010;24(11):2796–802.

55. Georgeson KE, Robertson DJ. Laparoscopic-assisted approaches for the definitive surgery for Hirschsprung's disease. Semin Pediatr Surg 2004;13(4):256–62.

56. Georgeson KE. Laparoscopic-assisted total colectomy with pouch reconstruction. Semin Pediatr Surg 2002;11(4):233–6.

57. Hebra A, Smith VA, Lesher AP. Robotic Swenson pull-through for Hirschsprung's disease in infants. Am Surg 2011;77(7):937–41.

58. Kalfa N, Allal H, Raux O, et al. Tolerance of laparoscopy and thoracoscopy in neonates. Pediatrics 2005;116(6):e785–91.

Unique Complications of Robotic Colorectal Surgery

Sonia Ramamoorthy, MD[a],*, Vincent Obias, MD[b]

KEYWORDS

- Robotic • Complications • Colorectal

KEY POINTS

- Currently, there are no clear-cut or absolute indications for a robotic approach in colorectal surgery.
- Robotics offer unique advantages that allow for improved visualization and enhanced capabilities that include the use of 4 arms, dual consoles, a single platform for energy, florescence, and single incision surgery.
- Complications or the lack thereof from robotic surgery are yet to be fully realized as this new technology undergoes further scrutiny and use by surgeons.

INTRODUCTION

Few other procedures have been as heavily scrutinized as the minimally invasive approaches used in colorectal surgery. Despite being originally described in 1990 and 1991 for both polyps[1] and cancer,[2,3] a minimally invasive approach for colectomy, especially in malignant cases, has only recently become a more widely accepted and used technique. Early concerns about loss of tactile function, worse outcomes, and malignant port-site implants[4–6] have since been tempered with newer studies showing equivalent oncologic results in malignancy,[7] improved cosmesis,[8] faster return of bowel function,[9] shorter hospital length of stay,[10] and even improved survival with a laparoscopic approach in select studies.[11,12] Although these seemingly straightforward benefits would normally suggest a push toward extensive use, laparoscopic colorectal surgery has yet to gain widespread adoption to this day.[13] This is not without sufficient justification, given that one of the most common indications for laparoscopic colectomy is colorectal cancer. Although concerns of inadequate oncologic resection and tumor aerosolization during laparoscopic colectomy for colon cancer have been largely resolved, other barriers remain to mainstream implementation—even in younger fellowship-trained surgeons.[14]

[a] Rebecca and John Moores' Cancer Center, University of California, San Diego, 3855 Health Sciences Drive, La Jolla, CA 92093, USA; [b] Division of Colon and Rectal Surgery, George Washington University, 2150 Pennsylvania Avenue, Northwest, Washington, DC 20037, USA
* Corresponding author.
E-mail address: sramamoorthy@ucsd.edu

Surg Clin N Am 93 (2013) 273–286
http://dx.doi.org/10.1016/j.suc.2012.09.011
0039-6109/13/$ – see front matter © 2013 Elsevier Inc. All rights reserved.

To some degree, seminal clinical trials, such as the clinical outcomes of surgical therapy (COST) trial in the United States and conventional versus laparoscopic-assisted surgery in colorectal cancer (CLASICC) trial in Europe that show the safety and efficacy of a laparoscopic approach to colorectal cancer have halted the initial moratorium on a minimally invasive approach.[15,16] These trials and others, however, have failed to demonstrate the same efficacy for a minimal invasive approach to rectal cancer.[17] The confines of the bony pelvis, large tumors, and adjacent critical structures are just a few of the underlying reasons for difficulties with a laparoscopic approach to pelvic colorectal disease.[18] At the same time, interest in robotic surgery was growing, particularly in the area of prostate surgery. Over 10 years, robotic surgery had largely replaced all other minimally invasive approaches for prostate resection, and its indications have steadily grown for procedures such as hysterectomy, proctectomy, and colectomy.[19] Although the debate over the application and use for robotics in colorectal surgery remains, the robotic minimally invasive platform continues to gain traction.[20] Here the authors review the potential advantages and disadvantages of robotic approaches, current indications for the use of robotics in colorectal surgery, and future areas of growth and innovation.

CURRENT INDICATIONS

Currently, there are no clear-cut or absolute indications for a robotic approach in colorectal surgery. Successful use of a robotic technique for colonic resection has been described in numerous publications[21,22] as surgeons increasingly use robotics for more common indications such as diverticulitis, colon cancer, and inflammatory bowel disease. The major benefits robotics provide, however, seem to involve its use in the management of rectal cancer and other pelvic disorders (ie, rectal prolapse, proctectomy) where the articulation of the robotic arms and heightened visualization provide an enhanced experience.[23] Early outcome studies from these applications show longer operating times, yet with similar perioperative and postoperative outcomes as laparoscopic techniques (**Table 1**). In the case of segmental resection, traditional multiport laparoscopy and, in certain cases, single incision laparoscopy have been the predominant minimally invasive approaches used.[24] However, with the introduction of new robotic technology such as robotic energy devices, fluorescent dyes to evaluate anastomotic blood flow, and robotic stapling devices, we may see an uptick in the number of cases that are performed using a robotic-assisted approach.

REPORTED ADVANTAGES OF ROBOTIC SURGERY

Robotics is a minimally invasive technique with certain decided advantages over conventional laparoscopic surgery; 3-dimensional visualization, increased degrees of freedom, improved articulation, and the use of 3 instruments at once can help a surgeon perform advanced techniques such as a intracorporeal suturing, operating in a deep pelvis, and aid in identification of important neurovascular structures. This is most apparent when considering rectal procedures because various studies have demonstrated reduced rates of conversion when compared with laparoscopy for rectal cancer (**Table 2**). This is of particular significance when examining overall results, because most prospective randomized trials such as the COST trial have found that those patients who undergo conversion from minimal invasive surgery to open have poorer overall outcomes.[15,25–27] Importantly, the COST trial focused on segmental colectomies for colon cancer and did not address tumors below the peritoneal reflection. Other results have been more mixed, especially in the early reported experiences. Laparoscopy for rectal cancer was assessed in the CLASICC trial and demonstrated

Table 1
Early outcomes from robotic-assisted colorectal surgery

Author	N	Conclusion
Diverticulitis		
Zimmern et al,[53] 2010	16	Safe, Low conversion rate
Abodeely A,[61] 2010	22	Safe, No conversion, no leaks
Raghupathi M,[62] 2011	24	Safe (complicated diverticulitis), No conversions, Low complication rate
Rectal Prolapse		
de Hoog DE,[63] 2009	20	Safe, High recurrence rate
Zimmern et al,[53] 2010	8	Safe
Abodeely A,[61] 2010	10	Safe
Bokhari et al,[38] 2011	5	Safe
Right Hemicolectomy		
De Souza et al,[41] 2010	40 (vs Lap)	Safe, outcomes comparable to lap, higher cost w/robotics, longer op time w/robotics
Luca F,[64] 2011	33 (vs open)	Oncologic outcomes similar, increased EBL w/open, reduced LOS w/robotics, higher cost w/robotics, longer op time w/robotics

Abbreviations: EBL, estimated blood loss; Lap, laparoscopic; LN, lymph node; LOS, length of stay; op, operative.

inferiority of the minimal invasive approach compared with open, mostly because of a significant increase in positive circumferential margins and a high conversion rate of 34%.[16] Subset analyses comparing functional outcomes in the CLASICC trial and the comparison of open versus laparoscopic surgery for mid and low rectal cancer after neoadjuvant chemoradiotherapy (COREAN) trial also found increased sexual and urinary dysfunction in the laparoscopic cohort compared with the open cohort.[28,29] These findings were further supported by a study by Morino and colleagues[30] that also demonstrated an increased rate of sexual and bladder dysfunction after laparoscopic low anterior resections. For these reasons, open rectal cancer surgery remains the gold standard, although clinical trials are underway to assess the safety and efficacy of robotics for rectal cancer surgery. These trials, robotic versus laparoscopic resection for rectal cancer (ROLLAR)[31] and American College of Surgeons Oncology Group (ACOSOG) 6051,[32] specifically examine the quality of the total mesorectal excision (TME) and the status of lymph nodes and circumferential margins. While we await the results of these trials, earlier studies (**Table 3**), such as the one by Choi and

Table 2
Conversion rates for robotic rectal cancer surgery

Author	N	Conversion (%)	Mean BMI (Mean BMI of Converted Cases)
Pigazzi,[65] 2010	143	4.9	26.5 (31.9)
Kim NK,[66] 2010	100	2	23.6
Park YA,[67] 2010	45	2.2	23.56
deSouza,[68] 2010	44	4.5	28.2 (41.5)

Abbreviation: BMI, body mass index.

Table 3
Oncologic outcomes for robotic total mesorectal excision

Author	N	Margin Positivity	Average No. Lymph Nodes
Park YA,[67] 2010	45	1 (2.2%)	13
Kim NK,[66] 2010	100	3 (3%)	14.7
Park et al,[34] 2010	41	2 (4.9%)	17.3
Pigazzi,[65] 2010	143	1 (0.9%)	14.1
deSouza,[68] 2010	44	1 (2.7%)	14
Baik et al,[39] 2009	56	5 (8.9%)	17.5
Choi et al,[33] 2009	50	3 (6%)	20.6

associates,[33] found both decreased conversion to open surgery in laparoscopic versus robotic low anterior resection (LAR) and improved TME in robotic resections. Furthermore, many of these early studies found comparable if not improved oncologic outcomes when compared with standard laparoscopy, despite the prerequisite learning curve associated with the instrumentation.[34,35]

Robotic technology has also been reported to enhance a surgeon's ability to perform difficult cases such as a *low* rectal anastomosis in an obese patient. Before robotics, it was extremely challenging for even the most experienced surgeons to perform an oncologically sound TME with coloanal anastomosis in a deep narrow fatty pelvis. Prasad and colleagues[36] showed a technique whereby after completion of a standard TME, the distal rectum is divided under controlled circumstances, and the specimen is passed through the low rectal (anal) stump. With the aid of the robotic movements, a purse-string suture is placed on the distal rectum stump, allowing a single transanal stapled anastomosis to be performed. Although their experience in these low lesions remains somewhat limited, this group has previously reported their results in 160 patients undergoing a double-purse string technique in mid to upper rectal lesions, finding only one leak (0.6%) requiring diversion, 2.5% having a pelvic abscess, and 96% with no septic complications.[37] With the enhanced visualization and the ability of robotic arms to reach areas that even the human hand cannot access, this has the potential to be the greatest advantage of robotics to colorectal surgery.

DISADVANTAGES OF ROBOTIC SURGERY

Similar to any new technique, there is a learning curve associated with robotic technology. With the loss of tactile sensation and a different overall setup and instrumentation than laparoscopy, robotics offers a unique challenge, but one that is surmountable. Previous investigators have reported that surgeons skilled in laparoscopic colorectal surgery progress through 3 phases when applying robotic techniques. Using cumulative sum (CUSUM) analysis, the authors noted that the initial phase consisted of 15 cases in which the initial learning curve took place. Phase 2 represented a plateau phase in which surgeons primarily were becoming more accustomed to the robotic console and gaining competence. Finally, phase 3 represented the mastery phase after 25 total cases, and consisted of adequate skills needed to perform routine cases skillfully and embark on more challenging cases.[38]

Largely secondary to set up (especially in the early stages), robotics has, on average, longer operating times when compared with laparoscopy.[39,40] As the individual surgeon and the entire team become more accustomed to and facile with the robot, this component remarkably improves. Cost is another consideration, with several studies finding higher costs associated with the use of the robot in colorectal surgery.[40,41] Almost uniformly this metric has gone hand in hand with longer operating times. Yet, it is important to recognize that cost may be defined many ways—those directed to the patient, those directed to the hospital, durable costs, instrumentation costs, and those directed to the health care system or even society. Although certain costs may be consistently higher with robotic surgery, its use in high-volume centers with high-volume surgeons has been found to be cost effective in urologic surgery and is theoretically plausible with colorectal surgery as well, especially after the initial implementation.[42,43] For both the learning curve and the operating time, the importance of having a consistent team familiar with the robot, its setup, potential malfunctions,[44] and operative approaches cannot be emphasized enough to improve overall efficiency and patient outcomes.

Unique Complications Specific to Robotics

Robotics is similar to laparoscopy in that the colon and rectum is accessed through incisions in the abdominal wall, and pneumoperitoneum is maintained while dissection and extraction of the colon is occurring. Complication rates regarding this portion of the operation are similar to those of standard multiport laparoscopy.[31,39] Despite these similarities, surgeons currently using, or who are considering using, this approach should be readily familiar with the unique properties of the robot.

Lack of tactile sensation

Lack of tactile sensation (haptics) is commonly discussed as a possible limitation when doing robotic surgery. Early in the robotic experience, one may quickly learn that lack of tactile sense can lead to organ injury and even perforation. As many robotic surgeons note, however, the improved 3-dimensional view provided by the robot compensates for this by adding a visual haptic sense that allows the surgeon to see how much pressure they are applying to the tissue and respond reflexively. The surgeon has to stay focused on the tissue dissection at hand and cannot rely on pressure to help them discern tension. By carefully observing the robotic instrument's effect on the local tissue (which is easier to do with the high definition 3-dimensional view of the robot and immersion in the operative field), the surgeon can offset the lack of tactile sensation.[45]

External collisions

Although patient positioning and optimal port placement are crucial for all minimally invasive surgery, they are extremely important when performing robotic surgery. The surgeon must keep ports at least 8 cm away from each other to allow for maximal excursion of the robot arms and avoid external collisions (**Fig. 1**). The surgeon also has to adjust the arms externally so that they do not collide with each other. Similar to laparoscopy, triangulation, visualization, and proper traction-countertraction remain keys to adequate ergonomics and technical success using the robot. In laparoscopy, however, the surgeon's main focus is on avoiding instrument collision internally and assistant collisions externally. With robotics, because the surgeon is now at the console, collisions between the surgeon and assistant do not occur. Yet the robotic arms must to positioned ahead of time with proper joint adjustment, making note of the "sweet spot," to minimize external collisions (limiting range of motion) and avoid hitting the instruments internally. In practice this is often more difficult than it sounds.

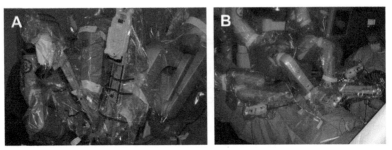

Fig. 1. Positioning of the Robotic arms. (*A*) Poor Robot arm positioning. (*B*) Better arm positioning.

Still, with careful placement of the ports, external collisions can be kept to a minimum as can surgeon frustration and the need to redock.

Proprioceptive and instrument challenges

When performing laparoscopy, it is important that surgeons not lose sight of their instruments to minimize the chances of inadvertent injury to intra-abdominal structures. If this occurs, simply by noting the position of their hands and angle of the instruments surgeons can quickly relocate their instrument and proper position. This is much more difficult in robotics. When training on the robot, the surgeon is heavily educated on how they must look for their instrument and not try and move the instrument into view. Failure to do so may result in bowel wall tears or, more commonly, puncture injuries to mesentery, vessels, or hollow-organs. Although built-in safety mechanisms within the system attempt to minimize any iatrogenic injuries, especially during instrument exchanges, inadvertent injury to the bowel has been reported.[46]

Increased operating times

Although this often is cited by many surgeons as a problem, and is even noted in multiple reports, increased operating times should not be viewed as complications. Recalling the early stages of laparoscopy, the learning curve for surgeons using a minimally invasive approach, gaining familiarity with the equipment, and setup time, all played a role when comparing times with those of open colectomy. Various large, randomized, controlled trials, including a Cochrane review of 25 randomized controlled trials from 1991–2004 comparing laparoscopy with open colectomies, all show an increase in operating time, yet, complications were fewer and outcomes were better.[47] More recent literature has shown similar operating times between the 2 methods.[48] A major factor for this involves the recent overwhelming trend in higher minimally invasive procedures in the operating experience of graduating residents.[49]

It is not surprising, therefore, that similar trends are also being seen in the robotic literature, where operating times were higher in robotics versus laparoscopy.[31,39,40] As more experience is gained using the robot, whether it be purely robotic or a laparoscopic-robotic hybrid procedure, there are scattered reports of similar operating times versus laparoscopy. In a series by D'Annibale and colleagues,[50] there was no difference in total operating times between the laparoscopic and robotic groups, although the operating room and patient preparation times were longer in the robotic cohort. In this case, the time lost in docking the robot was offset by the faster and more accurate dissection the daVinci robot (Intuitive Surgical Inc, Sunnyvale, CA, USA) provides. Furthermore, institutional experience has shown with increasing volume that the gap between robotic and laparoscopy total procedure times is steadily shrinking.[21]

Robotic Training

Most hospitals have a robust protocol for any surgeons wishing to learn robotics. This protocol is unique versus that of laparoscopy and greatly helps the new robotic surge. When a surgeon expresses interest in robotics, several platforms are available to assist in becoming more familiar and facile with the equipment. Initially, the surgeon can gain access to the robot after hours, and the Intuitive (Intuitive Surgical Inc, Sunnyvale, CA) representative can assist the surgeon in identifying the reported advantages of robotics to include the increased articulation of the instruments and 3-dimensional view. The surgeon can practice using the camera, suturing, clutching, and maneuvering objects, all without the need for direct patient contact. Once the surgeon determines they are interested in becoming fully trained, as in laparoscopy, courses are available to develop skills using both cadaveric and pig models. With current robotic training protocols, the surgeon must first observe a case and then be proctored for a set amount of cases before they are deemed sufficiently trained on the robot to proceed independently. This rigorous hands-on training regimen is aimed to help a surgeon overcome their learning curve and improve patient safety. Furthermore, virtual reality simulation has evolved to provide accurate lifelike robotic models that have been shown to allow faster and safer surgeon acquisition of the skills required for incorporation into practice.[51,52]

Conversions

Conversion should be viewed as good judgment and not as a complication. When early in a robotic learning curve, surgeons may feel more comfortable performing certain steps laparoscopically or hand assisted (such as splenic flexure mobilization and major vessel transection), although many robotic surgeons have adapted a hybrid technique as their standard procedure.[53] Another unique aspect in robotics is that the surgeon can convert the procedure to another minimally invasive method (laparoscopy, hand assisted) before converting to open procedure. In general, conversion rates for robotics range from 0%–5% (depending on the operation), with the most common causes listed as adhesions, large tumors, bleeding, and failure to progress.[22,54]

Air leaks

The surgeon may be forced to place extreme stress on the trocars by severe angulation with the robotic arms. Although this is necessary to complete certain steps in the operation, air leaks can occur. This complication causes an obvious impact on the ability to complete the operation. Therefore, it is important to always look for obvious sources of air leakage such as open ports, ports that become pulled out or into the subcutaneous tissue, or those in which the insufflation fell off. When performing a single-incision robotic surgery, anecdotally the authors have found one way to reduce air leakage is by using the Gelpoint device (Applied Medical, Rancho Santa Margarita, CA).

Inability to progress

Failure to progress can be caused by many reasons, such as surgeon comfort when transecting bowel or vessels, large or fixated tumors, or inadequate visualization. Another of the major underlying factors is inadequate patient position. Unlike laparoscopy, once the robot is docked, the patient cannot be repositioned; therefore, it is important to have the patient in ideal position before docking the robot. We have found the hybrid technique to overcome many of these issues. By starting laparoscopically and mobilizing bowel away from the area of dissection, the operative setup is in the best position possible before even docking the robot. In other cases, the patient may be in perfect position for one part of the procedure (ie, the pelvic dissection) but in a poor position for completion of a splenic flexure mobilization. The hybrid procedure also aids in this scenario in which the splenic flexure is initially mobilized laparoscopically and the rest is completed robotically. Other techniques to mobilize the splenic flexure include undocking the robot, using an extra port, and repositioning the patient or flipping one of the robotic arms around so that it can help in splenic flexure mobilization.[55,56]

Lessons Learned

The introduction of new technology

The most successful application of the surgical robot to date has been in urology. Although, the introduction of robotic minimally invasive surgery in urology was rapid, it preceded any evidence-based outcomes to support its widespread use. In a critical review of robotics published in the *New England Journal of Medicine*, Barbash and Glied[57] reported on data from the National Inpatient Sample (NIS) that showed an increase of more than 60% in the number of hospital discharges for prostatectomy (including both robotic and traditional procedures) in the United States between 2005 and 2008. This increase occurred despite a decrease in the underlying incidence of prostate cancer as well as with a conspicuous increase in the number of robot-assisted prostatectomies performed in the United States. The authors suggest that robotic technology may have contributed to the substitution of surgical for nonsurgical treatments for this disease and that the introduction of the robotic technology may have increased both the cost per surgical procedure and the volume of cases treated surgically. This rapid adoption and integration of robotics into urologic practice and training made subsequent attempts at multicenter, randomized trials to confirm its superiority over standard techniques futile. Learning from this experience, 2 multi-center colorectal trials were designed to assess the true benefits of robotic surgery for rectal cancer surgery: ACOSOG 6051[32] (compared with open) and ROLLAR[31] (compared with laparoscopic approaches). The design of these trials is to test for equivalency to standard techniques, which, in the case of robotics, may not be sufficient to justify its use (given outcry over the cost). These pivotal trials, however, are remarkable for more than their clinical outcomes because they represent an important step toward responsible adoption of new technology.

One of the challenges in conducting large retrospective outcomes research has been the appropriate procedure coding, which, in the case of robotics, did not occur until 2008. A study by Anderson and associates[58] examined and compared all robotic procedures with open and laparoscopic procedures when the ICD-9 codes were first available from October 2008–December 2009.[58] This NIS-based study concluded that when compared with procedures performed open, robotic procedures can have decreased odds of death, decreased length of stay, and higher total charges (**Figs. 2** and **3**). When compared with procedures performed laparoscopically, robotic procedures can have decreased odds of death, decreased length of stay in gynecologic procedures, increased prostatectomy and other urologic procedures, and higher overall total cost. Outcomes were most improved in procedures previously performed open, yet its utility is less clear for those procedures that are already successfully performed laparoscopically. This too may be the case for colorectal surgery in which the application of robotics for rectal dissection is found to be advantageous, but its indication for segmental colectomy is debatable.

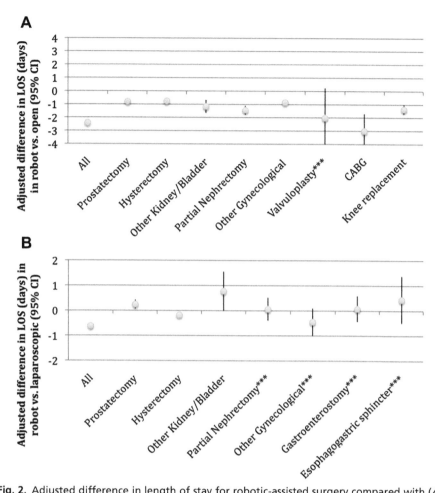

Fig. 2. Adjusted difference in length of stay for robotic-assisted surgery compared with (*A*) open procedures and (*B*) laparoscopic procedures. (*Data from* Barbash GI, Glied SA. New technology and health care costs—the case of robot-assisted surgery. N Engl J Med 2010;363(8):701–4.)

Patient expectations

An important study by Schroek and colleagues[59] described the impact that new technology can have on patients' perceptions of surgical outcomes. The study surveyed more than 1300 patients using a validated prostate cancer–specific quality-of-life questionnaire, which also included questions regarding satisfaction with treatment and regret of treatment choice. Those patients who underwent robotic-assisted prostatectomy were more likely to be regretful and dissatisfied, possibly because of higher expectation of an innovative procedure versus those who underwent radial retropubic prostatectomy. The findings of the study suggest that despite the enthusiasm for new technology and the projected benefits, surgeons must carefully portray the risks and benefits of new procedures during preoperative counseling to minimize regret and maximize satisfaction. Similar reports in robotic rectal surgery show improved quality of life and reduced rates of nerve injury that can result in sexual and urinary

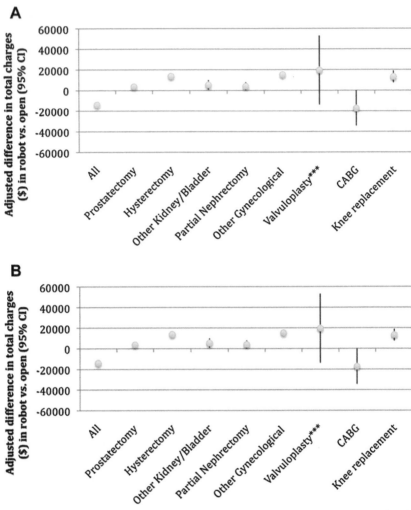

Fig. 3. Adjusted differences in total charges for robotic-assisted surgery compared with (A) nonrobotic laparoscopic procedures and (B) open procedures (***indicates P>.05). (*Data from* Barbash GI, Glied SA. New technology and health care costs—the case of robot-assisted surgery. N Engl J Med 2010;363(8):701–4.)

dysfunction with robotics.[60] These early studies must be verified with multicenter, randomized, control trials before patient-directed advertising and marketing to avoid the same pitfalls of patient misunderstanding and dissatisfaction.

SUMMARY

Robotics offer unique advantages that allow for improved visualization and enhanced capabilities that include the use of 4 arms, dual consoles, a single platform for energy, florescence, and single incision surgery. Robotics may also provide future opportunities for image-guided surgery, simulation, and telementoring. Complications or the lack of complications from robotic surgery are yet to be fully realized as this new technology undergoes further scrutiny and use by surgeons. Early results are encouraging, however, and current recommendations are to perform these procedures under an Institution Review Board (IRB) or within the scope of a clinical trial to allow for proper monitoring of outcomes and to limit unnecessary liability. As new technologies continue to emerge in colorectal cancer, robotics has one of the greatest potentials to change our current practice and create a paradigm shift in surgery as a whole.

REFERENCES

1. Saclariedes TJ, Ko ST, Airan M, et al. Laparoscopic removal of a large colonic lipoma. Dis Colon Rectum 1991;34:1027–9.
2. Schlinkert RT. Laparoscopic-assisted right hemicolectomy. Dis Colon Rectum 1991;34:1030–1.
3. Phillips EH, Franklin M, Carroll BJ, et al. Laparoscopic colectomy. Ann Surg 1992; 216:703–7.
4. Vertruyen M, Cadiere GB, Himpens J, et al. Laparoscopic colectomy for cancer [abstract]. Surg Endosc 1996;10:558.
5. Ramos JM, Gupta S, Anthone GJ, et al. Laparoscopic colon cancer: is the port site at risk. A preliminary report. Arch Surg 1994;127:897–900.
6. Berends FJ, Kazemier G, Bonjer HJ, et al. Subcutaneous metastases after laparoscopic colectomy [letter]. Lancet 1994;344:354–8.
7. Milsom JW, Bohm B, Hammerhofer KA, et al. A prospective, randomized trial comparing laparoscopic versus conventional techniques in colorectal cancer surgery: a preliminary report. J Am Coll Surg 1998;187:46–54.
8. Dunker MS, Bemelman WA, Slors JF, et al. Functional outcome, quality of life, body image, and cosmesis in patients after laparoscopic-assisted and conventional restorative proctocolectomy: a comparative study. Dis Colon Rectum 2001;44:1800–7.
9. Veldkamp R, Kuhry E, Hop WC, et al. Colon cancer Laparoscopic or Open Resection Study Group (COLOR). Lancet Oncol 2005;6:477–84.
10. Bosio RM, Smith BM, Aybar PS, et al. Implementation of laparoscopic colectomy with fast-track care in an academic medical center: benefits of a fully ascended learning curve and specialty expertise. Am J Surg 2007;193:413–5.
11. Lacy AM, Garcia-Valdecasas JC, Delgado S, et al. Laparoscopy-assisted colectomy versus open colectomy for treatment of non-metastatic colon cancer: a randomized trial. Lancet 2002;359:2224–9.
12. Law WL, Lee YM, Choi HK, et al. Impact of laparoscopic resection for colorectal cancer on operative outcomes and survival. Ann Surg 2007;245:1–7.
13. Rea JD, Cone MM, Diggs BS, et al. Utilization of laparoscopic colectomy before and after the clinical outcomes of surgical therapy study group trial. Ann Surg 2011;254:281–8.
14. Steele SR, Stein SL, Bordeianou LG, et al. American Society of Colon and Rectal Surgeons' Young Surgeons Committee. The impact of practice environment on laparoscopic colectomy utilization following colorectal residency: a survey of the ASCRS Young Surgeons. Colorectal Dis 2012;14:374–81.
15. The Clinical Outcomes of Surgical Therapy Study Group. A comparison of laparoscopically assisted and open colectomy for colon cancer. N Engl J Med 2004; 350:2050–9.
16. Guillou PJ, Quirke P, Thorpe H, et al, MRC CLASICC trial group. Short-term endpoints of conventional versus laparoscopic-assisted surgery in patients with colorectal cancer (MRC CLASICC trial): multicentre, randomised controlled trial. Lancet 2005;365:1718–26.

17. Breukink S, Pierie J, Wiggers T. Laparoscopic versus open total mesorectal excision for rectal cancer. Cochrane Database Syst Rev 2006;(4):CD005200.
18. Champagne BJ, Delaney CP. Laparoscopic approaches to rectal cancer. Clin Colon Rectal Surg 2007;20(3):237–48.
19. Wexner SD, Bergamaschi R, Lacy A, et al. The current status of robotic pelvic surgery: results of a multinational interdisciplinary consensus conference. Surg Endosc 2009;23(2):438–43.
20. Jayne DG, Culmer PR, Barrie J, et al. Robotic platforms for general and colorectal surgery. Colorectal Dis 2011;13(Suppl 7):78–82.
21. Deutsch GB, Sathyanarayana SA, Gunabushanam V, et al. Robotic vs. laparoscopic colorectal surgery: an institutional experience. Surg Endosc 2012;26(4): 956–63.
22. Antoniou SA, Antoniou GA, Koch OO, et al. Robot-assisted laparoscopic surgery of the colon and rectum. Surg Endosc 2012;26(1):1–11.
23. Koh DC, Tsang CB, Kim SH. A new application of the four-arm standard da Vinci® surgical system: totally robotic-assisted left-sided colon or rectal resection. Surg Endosc 2011;25(6):1945–52.
24. Li P, Wang DR, Wang LH, et al. Single-incision laparoscopic surgery vs. multiport laparoscopic surgery for colectomy: a meta-analysis of eleven recent studies. Hepatogastroenterology 2012;59(117):1345–9.
25. Lu KC, Cone MM, Diggs BS, et al. Laparoscopic converted to open colectomy: predictors and outcomes from the Nationwide Inpatient Sample. Am J Surg 2011;201(5):634–9.
26. Li JC, Lee JF, Ng SS, et al. Conversion in laparoscopic-assisted colectomy for right colon cancer: risk factors and clinical outcomes. Int J Colorectal Dis 2010;25(8):983–8.
27. Chan AC, Poon JT, Fan JK, et al. Impact of conversion on the long-term outcome in laparoscopic resection of colorectal cancer. Surg Endosc 2008;22(12): 2625–30.
28. Kang SB, Park JW, Jeong SY, et al. Open versus laparoscopic surgery for mid or low rectal cancer after neoadjuvant chemoradiotherapy (COREAN trial): short-term outcomes of an open-label randomised controlled trial. Lancet Oncol 2010;11(7):637–45.
29. Jayne DG, Brown JM, Thorpe H, et al. Bladder and sexual function following resection for rectal cancer in a randomized clinical trial of laparoscopic versus open technique. Br J Surg 2005;92(9):1124–32.
30. Morino M, Parini U, Allaix ME, et al. Male sexual and urinary function after laparoscopic total mesorectal excision. Surg Endosc 2009;23(6):1233–40.
31. Collinson FJ, Jayne DG, Pigazzi A, et al. An international, multicentre, prospective, randomised, controlled, unblinded, parallel-group trial of robotic-assisted versus standard laparoscopic surgery for the curative treatment of rectal cancer. Int J Colorectal Dis 2012;27(2):233–41.
32. Baik SH, Gincherman M, Mutch MG, et al. Laparoscopic vs. open resection for patients with rectal cancer: comparison of perioperative outcomes and long-term survival. Dis Colon Rectum 2011;54(1):6–14.
33. Choi DJ, Kim SH, Lee PJ, et al. Single-stage totally robotic dissection for rectal cancer surgery: technique and short-term outcome in 50 consecutive patients. Dis Colon Rectum 2009;52(11):1824–30.
34. Park JS, Choi GS, Lim KH, et al. Robotic-assisted versus laparoscopic surgery for low rectal cancer: case-matched analysis of short-term outcomes. Ann Surg Oncol 2010;17(12):3195–202.

35. Park JS, Choi GS, Lim KH, et al. Jun SH.S052: a comparison of robot-assisted, laparoscopic, and open surgery in the treatment of rectal cancer. Surg Endosc 2011;25(1):240–8.
36. Prasad LM, deSouza AL, Marecik SJ, et al. Robotic pursestring technique in low anterior resection. Dis Colon Rectum 2010;53(2):230–4.
37. Marecik SJ, Chaudhry V, Pearl R, et al. Single-stapled double-pursestring anastomosis after anterior resection of the rectum. Am J Surg 2007;193(3):395–9.
38. Bokhari MB, Patel CB, Ramos-Valadez DI, et al. Learning curve for robotic-assisted laparoscopic colorectal surgery. Surg Endosc 2011;25(3):855–60.
39. Baik SH, Kwon HY, Kim JS, et al. Robotic versus laparoscopic low anterior resection of rectal cancer: short-term outcome of a prospective comparative study. Ann Surg Oncol 2009;16(6):1480–7.
40. Heemskerk J, de Hoog DE, van Gemert WG, et al. Robot-assisted vs. conventional laparoscopic rectopexy for rectal prolapse: a comparative study on costs and time. Dis Colon Rectum 2007;50(11):1825–30.
41. de Souza AL, Prasad LM, Park JJ, et al. Robotic assistance in right hemicolectomy: is there a role? Dis Colon Rectum 2010;53(7):1000–6.
42. Liberman D, Trinh QD, Jeldres C, et al. Is robotic surgery cost-effective: yes. Curr Opin Urol 2012;22(1):61–5.
43. Lotan Y, Cadeddu JA, Gettman MT. The new economics of radical prostatectomy: cost comparison of open, laparoscopic and robot assisted techniques. J Urol 2004;172(4 Pt 1):1431–5.
44. Agcaoglu O, Aliyev S, Taskin HE, et al. Malfunction and failure of robotic systems during general surgical procedures. Surg Endosc 2012. [Epub ahead of print].
45. Volonté F, Pugin F, Buchs NC, et al. Console-Integrated Stereoscopic OsiriX 3D Volume-Rendered Images for da Vinci Colorectal Robotic Surgery. Surg Innov 2012. [Epub ahead of print].
46. Hung CF, Yang CK, Cheng CL, et al. Bowel complication during robotic-assisted laparoscopic radical prostatectomy. Anticancer Res 2011;31(10):3497–501.
47. Schwenk W, Haase O, Neudecker J, et al. Short term benefits for laparoscopic colorectal resection. Cochrane Database Syst Rev 2005;(3):CD003145.
48. de Campos-Lobato LF, Alves-Ferreira PC, Geisler DP, et al. Benefits of laparoscopy: does the disease condition that indicated colectomy matter? Am Surg 2011;77(5):527–33.
49. Eckert M, Cuadrado D, Steele S, et al. The changing face of the general surgeon: national and local trends in resident operative experience. Am J Surg 2010;199(5):652–6.
50. D'Annibale A, Morpurgo E, Fiscon V, et al. Robotic and laparoscopic surgery for treatment of colorectal diseases. Dis Colon Rectum 2004;47(12):2162–8.
51. Marecik SJ, Prasad LM, Park JJ, et al. A lifelike patient simulator for teaching robotic colorectal surgery: how to acquire skills for robotic rectal dissection. Surg Endosc 2008;22(8):1876–81.
52. Schreuder HW, Wolswijk R, Zweemer RP, et al. Training and learning robotic surgery, time for a more structured approach: a systematic review. BJOG 2012;119(2):137–49.
53. Zimmern A, Prasad L, Desouza A, et al. Robotic colon and rectal surgery: a series of 131 cases. World J Surg 2010;34(8):1954–8.
54. Buchs NC, Pugin F, Bucher P, et al. Totally robotic right colectomy: a preliminary case series and an overview of the literature. Int J Med Robot 2011. [Epub ahead of print]. http://dx.doi.org/10.1002/rcs.404.

55. Peterson CY, McLemore EC, Horgan S, et al. Technical aspects of robotic proctectomy. Surg Laparosc Endosc Percutan Tech 2012;22(3):189–93.
56. Obias V, Sanchez C, Nam A, et al. Totally robotic single-position "flip" arm technique for splenic flexure mobilizations and low anterior resections. Int J Med Robot 2011;7(2):123–6.
57. Barbash GI, Glied SA. New technology and health care costs–the case of robot-assisted surgery. N Engl J Med 2010;363(8):701–4.
58. Anderson JE, Chang DC, Parsons JK, et al. The first national examination of outcomes and trends in robotic surgery in the United States. J Am Coll Surg 2012;215:107–14.
59. Schroeck FR, Krupski TL, Stewart SB, et al. Pretreatment expectations of patients undergoing robotic assisted laparoscopic or open retropubic radical prostatectomy. J Urol 2012;187:894–8.
60. Kim JY, Kim NK, Lee KY, et al. A comparative study of voiding and sexual function after total mesorectal excision with autonomic nerve preservation for rectal cancer: laparoscopic versus robotic surgery. Ann Surg Oncol 2012;19:2485–93.
61. Abodeely A, Lagares-Garcia J, Vrees M, et al. Safety and learning curve in robotic colorectal surgery. Abstract ASCRS 2010. Diseases Colon and Rectum 2010;53(4):514–705.
62. Ragupathi M, Ramos-Valadez DI, Patel CB, et al. Robotic-assisted laparoscopic surgery for recurrent diverticulitis: experience in consecutive cases and a review of the literature. Surg Endosc 2011;25(1):199–206.
63. de Hoog DE, Heemskerk J, Nieman FH, et al. Recurrence and functional results after open versus conventional laparoscopic versus robot-assisted laparoscopic rectopexy for rectal prolapse: a case-control study. Int J Colorectal Dis 2009;24(10):1201–6.
64. Luca F, Ghezzi TL, Valvo M, et al. Surgical and pathological outcomes after right hemicolectomy: case-matched study comparing robotic and open surgery. Int J Med Robot 2011.
65. Pigazzi A, Luca F, Patriti A, et al. Multicentric study on robotic tumor-specific mesorectal excision for the treatment of rectal cancer. Ann Surg Oncol 2010;17(6):1614–20.
66. Kim N-K, Kang J. Optimal total mesorectal excision for rectal cancer: the role of robotic surgery from an expert's view. Journal of the Korean Society of Coloproctology 2010;26(6):377–87.
67. Park YA, Kim JM, Kim SA, et al. Totally robotic surgery for rectal cancer: from splenic flexure to pelvic floor in one setup. Surg Endosc 2010;24(3):715–20.
68. deSouza AL, Prasad LM, Marecik SJ, et al. Total mesorectal excision for rectal cancer: the potential advantage of robotic assistance. Dis Colon Rectum 2010;53(12):1611–7.

Index

Note: Page numbers of article title are in **boldface** type.

A

Abscess(es)
  in Crohn's disease, 168–169
  IPAA and, 110–114
  as unexpected finding in colorectal surgery, 46
Adhesion(s)
  trocars-related
    laparoscopy in colorectal surgery and, 220–221
Adolescent(s)
  colorectal considerations in
    inflammatory bowel disease, 268–269
    polyposis syndromes, 267–268
    polyps, 267–268
American Society of Anesthesiologists' (ASA) Physical Status classification, 3
Anal fissure
  in Crohn's disease, 168
Anastomosis(es)
  colorectal
    complications of, **61–87**. *See also* Colorectal anastomoses, complications of
  complications of
    after surgical management of Crohn's disease, 178–179
  ilial pouch anal, **107–143**. *See also* Ileal pouch anal anastomosis (IPAA)
  pelvic
    low
      anastomotic leak after
        recurrent pelvic surgery for, 204–206
Anastomotic failure
  in colorectal surgery
    mitigating risk for, 75–76
Anastomotic leak
  after low pelvic anastomosis
    recurrent pelvic surgery for, 204–206
Anastomotic stricture
  after colorectal anastomosis, 76–77
Anorectal Crohn's disease, 168–169
Anorectal malformations
  in neonates, 259–263
Anorectal stricture
  in Crohn's disease, 169
Anterior resection syndrome
  treatment of, 99–102

Surg Clin N Am 93 (2013) 287–297
http://dx.doi.org/10.1016/S0039-6109(12)00232-0
0039-6109/13/$ – see front matter © 2013 Elsevier Inc. All rights reserved.

surgical.theclinics.com

Moving?

Make sure your subscription moves with you!

To notify us of your new address, find your **Clinics Account Number** (located on your mailing label above your name), and contact customer service at:

Email: journalscustomerservice-usa@elsevier.com

800-654-2452 (subscribers in the U.S. & Canada)
314-447-8871 (subscribers outside of the U.S. & Canada)

Fax number: 314-447-8029

Elsevier Health Sciences Division
Subscription Customer Service
3251 Riverport Lane
Maryland Heights, MO 63043

*To ensure uninterrupted delivery of your subscription, please notify us at least 4 weeks in advance of move.

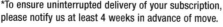
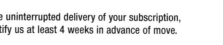